D1490273

MANUAL OF RADIOLOGY: ACUTE PROBLEMS AND ESSENTIAL PROCEDURES

Second Edition

MANUAL OF RADIOLOGY: ACUTE PROBLEMS AND ESSENTIAL PROCEDURES

Second Edition

Edited by

Clifford R. Weiss, MD

Fellow, Vascular and Interventional Radiology
The Russell H. Morgan Department of Radiology and Radiological Science
The Johns Hopkins University School of Medicine
Baltimore, Maryland

Oleg M. Teytelboym, MD

Resident/Fellow, Nuclear Medicine
The Russell H. Morgan Department of Radiology and Radiological Science
The Johns Hopkins University School of Medicine
Baltimore, Maryland

Nafi Aygun, MD

Assistant Professor of Radiology
The Russell H. Morgan Department of Radiology and Radiological Science
The Johns Hopkins Medical Institution
Baltimore, Maryland

John Eng, MD

Associate Professor of Radiology
Joint Appointment in Health Sciences Informatics
The Russell H. Morgan Department of Radiology and Radiological Science
The Johns Hopkins University School of Medicine
Baltimore, Maryland

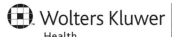 Wolters Kluwer | Lippincott Williams & Wilkins
Health
Philadelphia · Baltimore · New York · London
Buenos Aires · Hong Kong · Sydney · Tokyo

Acquisitions Editor: Lisa McAllister
Managing Editor: Kerry Barrett
Project Manager: Jennifer Harper
Marketing Manager: Angela Panetta
Senior Manufacturing Manager: Benjamin Rivera
Art Director: Risa Clow
Production Services: Laserwords Private Limited, Chennai, India

© 2008 by LIPPINCOTT WILLIAMS & WILKINS, a Wolters Kluwer business

530 Walnut Street
Philadelphia, PA 19106 USA
LWW.com

First edition, © 1997 by Lippincott-Raven Publishers

Printed in the USA

Library of Congress Cataloging-in-Publication Data
Manual of radiology / Clifford R. Weiss ... [et al.].—2nd. ed.
    p. ; cm.
Includes bibliographical references and index.
ISBN 978-0-7817-9964-5
1. Radiology, Medical—Handbooks, manuals, etc. I. Weiss, Clifford R.
[DNLM: 1. Radiography—methods—Handbooks. WN 39 M295 2008]
RC78.M242 2008
616.07'57—dc22

                                                    2007041348

Care has been taken to confirm the accuracy of the information presented and to describe generally accepted practices. However, the authors, editors, and publisher are not responsible for errors or omissions or for any consequences from application of the information in this book and make no warranty, expressed or implied, with respect to the currency, completeness, or accuracy of the contents of the publication. Application of this information in a particular situation remains the professional responsibility of the practitioner.

The authors, editors, and publisher have exerted every effort to ensure that drug selection and dosage set forth in this text are in accordance with current recommendations and practice at the time of publication. However, in view of ongoing research, changes in government regulations, and the constant flow of information relating to drug therapy and drug reactions, the reader is urged to check the package insert for each drug for any change in indications and dosage and for added warnings and precautions. This is particularly important when the recommended agent is a new or infrequently employed drug.

Some drugs and medical devices presented in this publication have Food and Drug Administration (FDA) clearance for limited use in restricted research settings. It is the responsibility of the health care provider to ascertain the FDA status of each drug or device planned for use in their clinical practice.

To purchase additional copies of this book, call our customer service department at (800) 638-3030 or fax orders to (301) 223-2320. International customers should call (301) 223-2300.

Visit Lippincott Williams & Wilkins on the Internet: at LWW.com. Lippincott Williams & Wilkins customer service representatives are available from 8:30 am to 6 pm, EST.

                                        10 9 8 7 6 5 4 3 2 1

Laura Amodei, MD
Director of MRI
Charleston Breast Center
Charleston, South Carolina

Nafi Aygun, MD
Assistant Professor of Radiology
The Russell H. Morgan Department
of Radiology and Radiological
Science
The Johns Hopkins University School of
Medicine
Baltimore, Maryland

Brad P. Barnett
Medical Student
The Johns Hopkins University School of
Medicine
Baltimore, Maryland

Visveshwar Baskaran, MD
Chief Resident, Diagnostic Radiology
The Russell H. Morgan Department
of Radiology and Radiological
Science
Johns Hopkins University School of
Medicine
Baltimore, Maryland

Norman J. Beauchamp, Jr., MD, MHS
Professor and Chair
Department of Radiology
University of Washington
Seattle, Washington

Simon Bekker, MD
Resident, Diagnostic Radiology
The Russell H. Morgan Department
of Radiology and Radiological
Science
Johns Hopkins University School of
Medicine
Baltimore, Maryland

Ari M. Blitz, MD
Assistant Professor of Radiology
The Russell H. Morgan Department of
Radiology and Radiological Science
Johns Hopkins University School of
Medicine
Baltimore, Maryland

Paul D. Campbell, Jr.
Resident, Diagnostic Radiology
The Russell H. Morgan Department of
Radiology and Radiological Science
Johns Hopkins University School of
Medicine
Baltimore, Maryland

Claire S. Cooney, MD
Fellow, Body Imaging
The Russell H. Morgan Department of
Radiology and Radiological Science
Johns Hopkins University School of
Medicine
Baltimore, Maryland

Azar P. Dagher, MD
Annapolis Radiology Associates
Anne Arundel Medical Center
Annapolis, Maryland

Mandeep Dagli, MD
Fellow, Vascular and Interventional
Radiology
The Russell H. Morgan Department of
Radiology and Radiological Science
Johns Hopkins University School of
Medicine
Baltimore, Maryland

Michael W. D'Angelo, MD, MS
Fellow, Muskuloskeletal Imaging
The Russell H. Morgan Department of
Radiology and Radiological Science
Johns Hopkins University School of
Medicine
Baltimore, Maryland

v

Joseph P. DiPietro, MD
Resident, Diagnostic Radiology
The Russell H. Morgan Department of
Radiology and Radiological Science
Johns Hopkins University School of
Medicine
Baltimore, Maryland

W. Dee Dockery, MD
Partner, American Radiology Associates,
P. A.
Dallas, Texas

Daniel J. Durand, MD
Resident, Diagnostic Radiology
The Russell H. Morgan Department of
Radiology and Radiological Science
Johns Hopkins University School of
Medicine
Baltimore, Maryland

Timothy S. Eckel, MS, MD
Director, Diagnostic and Interventional
Neuroradiology
Annapolis Radiology Associates
Anne Arundel Medical Center
Annapolis, Maryland

John Eng, MD
Associate Professor of Radiology
Joint Appointment in Health Sciences
Informatics
The Russell H. Morgan Department of
Radiology and Radiological Science
Johns Hopkins University School of
Medicine
Baltimore, Maryland

Bradley R. Foerster, MD
Fellow, Neuroradiology
The Russell H. Morgan Department of
Radiology and Radiological Science
Johns Hopkins University School of
Medicine
Baltimore, Maryland

David J. Grelotti, MD
Clinical Fellow
Department of Psychiatry
Harvard Medical School;
Resident in Psychiatry
Department of Psychiatry
Massachusetts General Hospital and
McLean Hospital
Boston, Massachusetts

Edward H. Herskovits, MD, PhD
Associate Professor
Department of Radiology
University of Pennsylvania
Philadelphia, Pennsylvania

Andrew L. Holz, MD, MBA
Resident Fellow, Nuclear Medicine
The Russell H. Morgan Department
of Radiology and Radiological
Science
Johns Hopkins University School of
Medicine
Baltimore, Maryland

Karen M. Horton, MD
Associate Professor of Radiology
The Russell H. Morgan Department
of Radiology and Radiological
Science
Johns Hopkins University School of
Medicine
Baltimore, Maryland

Krishna Juluru, MD
Assistant Professor
Department of Radiology
Weill Medical College of Cornell University
New York, New York

Satomi Kawamoto, MD
Assistant Professor of Radiology
The Russell H. Morgan Department
of Radiology and Radiological
Science
Johns Hopkins University School of
Medicine
Baltimore, Maryland

Alexander M. Kowal, MD
Resident, Diagnostic Radiology
The Russell H. Morgan Department
of Radiology and Radiological
Science
Johns Hopkins University School of
Medicine
Baltimore, Maryland

George P. Kuo, MD
Resident, Diagnostic Radiology
The Russell H. Morgan Department of
Radiology and Radiological Science
Johns Hopkins University School of
Medicine
Baltimore, Maryland

Loralie D. Ma, MD
Clinical Asst. Professor of Radiology
Department of Radiology
The Johns Hopkins Hospital;
Medical Director
Department of Radiology
Greater Baltimore Medical Center
Baltimore, Maryland

Aimee Lynn Maceda, MD
Fellow, Body Imaging
The Russell H. Morgan Department of
    Radiology and Radiological Science
Johns Hopkins University School of
    Medicine
Baltimore, Maryland

Cathleen F. Magill, MD
Chief Resident
Department of Internal Medicine
The Johns Hopkins University
Chief Resident
Department of Internal Medicine
The Johns Hopkins Bayview Medical
    Center
Baltimore, Maryland

Sarah Mezban, MD
Resident, Diagnostic Radiology
The Russell H. Morgan Department of
    Radiology and Radiological Science
Johns Hopkins University School of
    Medicine
Baltimore, Maryland

Jason Oaks, MD, MA
Resident, Diagnostic Radiology
The Russell H. Morgan Department of
    Radiology and Radiological Science
Johns Hopkins University School of
    Medicine
Baltimore, Maryland

Rick W. Obray, MD
Resident Physician
Department of Radiology
The Johns Hopkins University
Baltimore, Maryland

Marcus W. Parker, MD
Resident, Diagnostic Radiology
The Russell H. Morgan Department of
    Radiology and Radiological Science
Johns Hopkins University School of
    Medicine
Baltimore, Maryland

Myria Petrou, MD
Fellow, Neuroradiology
The Russell H. Morgan Department of
    Radiology and Radiological Science
The Johns Hopkins University School of
    Medicine
Baltimore, Maryland

Valerie A. Pomper, MD
Staff Radiologist
Department of Radiology
Washington Adventist Hospital
Takoma Park, Maryland

Douglas E. Ramsey, MD
Radiology Resident
Russell H. Morgan Department of
    Radiology and Radiological Sciences
The Johns Hopkins University School of
    Medicine
Baltimore, Maryland

Hari Charan P. Reddy, MD
Fellow, Neuroradiology
The Russell H. Morgan Department of
    Radiology and Radiological Science
Johns Hopkins University School of
    Medicine
Baltimore, Maryland

Christopher L. Smith, MD
Assistant Professor of Radiology
The Russell H. Morgan Department of
    Radiology and Radiological Science
Johns Hopkins University School of
    Medicine
Baltimore, Maryland

Kevin A. Smith, MD
Chief Resident, Diagnostic Radiology
The Russell H. Morgan Department of
    Radiology and Radiological Science
Johns Hopkins University School of
    Medicine
Baltimore, Maryland

Joshua Smith, MD
Fellow, Neuroradiology
The Russell H. Morgan Department of
    Radiology and Radiological Science
Johns Hopkins University School of
    Medicine
Baltimore, Maryland

Jennifer E. Swart, MD
Resident, Diagnostic Radiology
The Russell H. Morgan Department of
  Radiology and Radiological Science
Johns Hopkins University School of
  Medicine
Baltimore, Maryland

Oleg M. Teytelboym, MD
Resident/Fellow, Nuclear Medicine
The Russell H. Morgan Department of
  Radiology and Radiological Science
Johns Hopkins University School of
  Medicine
Baltimore, Maryland

Benjamin Tubb, MD
Fellow in Magnetic Resonance Imaging
Department of Radiology
The University of Pennsylvania
Pennsylvania, Philadelphia

D. Darrell Vaughn, MD
Jefferson Regional Medical Center
Pittsburgh, Philadelphia

Jens Vogel-Claussen, MD
Assistant Professor of Radiology
The Russell H. Morgan Department of
  Radiology and Radiological Science
Johns Hopkins University School of
  Medicine
Baltimore, Maryland

Kenneth C. Wang, MD, PhD
Resident, Diagnostic Radiology
The Russell H. Morgan Department of
  Radiology and Radiological Science
Johns Hopkins University School of
  Medicine
Baltimore, Maryland

Monica D. Watkins
Fellow, Neuroradiology
The Russell H. Morgan Department of
  Radiology and Radiological Science
Johns Hopkins University School of
  Medicine
Baltimore, Maryland

David A. Weiland, MD
Advanced Medical Imaging
Denver, Colarado

Clifford R. Weiss, MD
Fellow, Vascular and Interventional
  Radiology
The Russell H. Morgan Department of
  Radiology and Radiological Science
Johns Hopkins University School of
  Medicine
Baltimore, Maryland

$\mathcal{T}$he Manual of Radiology has been created by The Johns Hopkins radiology residents and faculty to help radiology residents during night call. Radiology is a massive field, encompassing all organ systems, age groups and patient populations. For any given problem or suspected disease process, there are many diagnostic pathways to choose from. Any on-call radiologist needs to be able to manage all of these challenges efficiently and effectively. The same is true of the on-call medical or surgical residents, who are requesting the radiological tests.

This manual focuses on the imaging essentials of the disease processes most commonly encountered by the on-call resident. Using a direct and simple format, each chapter includes a brief description of pathophysiology and clinical presentation, followed by key imaging findings. The manual emphasizes selecting the best imaging modality, choosing the appropriate protocol, and identifying the key findings needed to establish the diagnosis, detect life-threatening complications, and avoid common pitfalls. As in the first edition, we have included a collection of essential procedures and practical references, which we have found useful in our daily practice as radiology residents.

The manual has been extensively updated since the first edition and now includes multiple figures and images which illustrate key disease presentations, complications, and imaging pitfalls. Multiple new topics have been added, including chapters on cardiac imaging and CNS infections. Imaging protocols have been extensively updated to reflect current, state-of-art imaging.

This manual is targeted for radiology residents who are starting night call, for medical and surgical residents who are requesting imaging studies, and for medical students beginning their clinical rotations.

We would like to thank senior faculty of the Johns Hopkins radiology department and particularly Dr. Stanley Siegelman for his mentoring and long-standing commitment to resident education.

 INVITATION FOR COMMENTS

I sincerely invite any suggestions, corrections, criticisms, or other comments about this book and would greatly value any such feedback. Please address comments to me through the publisher or send them by electronic mail to cweiss@jhmi.edu. All electronic mail will be answered.

Clifford R. Weiss, MD
Oleg M. Teytelboym, MD
Nafi Aygun, MD
John Eng, MD

*T*his manual was written primarily for radiologists in training, especially junior residents who are beginning to learn how to perform common radiological procedures or who may be facing the first months of on-call responsibilities. These are times which provoke a certain amount of anxiety, even though few would admit to this by the time they have become senior residents. This manual may also help to jog the memories of many radiology subspecialty fellows who, upon finishing their fellowships, are about to perform their first barium study outside of academia.

The radiology trainee's anxiety stems from the unknown, of course. What kinds of clinical problems will I face when I am on call? How will I know what to do? How do I decide if an imaging exam is appropriate? This manual attempts to encapsulate the core information needed to answer such questions in practical terms, a necessary step in becoming an effective consultant. It is impossible to answer all possible questions in one volume, but I hope to provide a basic framework of knowledge to which the reader can more easily add new knowledge and practices gained from experience and further reading. I hope that this will make preparation for the on-call experience much less nebulous and more enlightening.

Many of the protocols in the Procedures section have not been published in as explicit a format as in this manual. This format should not imply dogma—the protocols are intended to be detailed suggestions to which each reader should add personal variations gained from experience. However, I feel that it is very important for a trainee to start with *someone's* way of doing a procedure rather than *no one's* way.

ORGANIZATION OF THE MANUAL

In rough anatomical order, the first five sections of this book cover the acute clinical problems for which radiologic consultation is commonly requested. The sixth section, "Procedures," contains protocols for common procedures in diagnostic radiology. The seventh and final section, "Reference," is a collection of diagrams and tables which may come in handy at the reading board.

INVITATION FOR COMMENTS

I sincerely invite any suggestions, corrections, criticisms, or other comments about this book and would greatly value any such feedback. Please address comments to me through the publisher or send them by electronic mail to jeng@rad.jhu.edu. All electronic mail will be answered.

John Eng, MD

CONTENTS

Contributor List v
Preface ix
Preface to the First Edition xi

I: HEAD AND SPINE

Trauma

1 **Traumatic Brain Injury** 1
  Ari M. Blitz

2 **Skull Fractures** 7
  Norman J. Beauchamp, Jr. and Andrew L. Holz

3 **Traumatic Facial Injury** 10
  Aimee Lynn Maceda and Monica D. Watkins

4 **Orbital Fractures** 13
  George P. Kuo and David J. Grelotti

5 **Cervical Spine Trauma** 17
  Simon Bekker and Oleg M. Teytelboym

6 **Thoracolumbar Spine Trauma** 26
  David A. Weiland

7 **Soft Tissues Injury of the Neck** 32
  Oleg M. Teytelboym and Kevin A. Smith

Infection

8 **Intracranial Infections** 36
  Bradley R. Foerster and Myria Petrou

9 **Orbital and Periorbital Infections** 46
  David J. Grelotti and Nafi Aygun

10 **Head and Neck Infections** 51
  Hari Charan P. Reddy and Oleg M. Teytelboym

Cerebrovascular

11 **Stroke** 56
  Nafi Aygun

12 Subarachnoid Hemorrhage **66**
Bradley R. Foerster and Myria Petrou

13 Intracranial Venous Thrombosis **71**
Bradley R. Foerster and Myris Petrou

Miscellaneous Topics

14 Hydrocephalus and Shunt **76**
Monica D. Watkins

15 Brain Herniation **80**
Joshua Smith

16 Spinal Cord Compression **86**
Azar P. Dagher and Andrew L. Holz

17 Headache **91**
Timothy S. Eckel

II: CHEST

18 Stridor and Wheezing **93**
David A. Weiland

19 Foreign Body Aspiration **97**
Alexander M. Kowal

20 Pulmonary Embolism **102**
Krishna Juluru

21 Thoracic Aortic Aneurysm and Dissection **110**
Paul D. Campbell, Jr. and Edward H. Herskovits

22 Thoracic Aortic Injury **117**
Jens Vogel-Claussen and Edward H. Herskovits

23 Myocardial Ischemia and Infarction **121**
Jens Vogel-Claussen and Oleg M. Teytelboym

III: ABDOMEN

24 Abdominal Abscess **131**
Marcus W. Parker and D. Darrell Vaughn

25 Abdominal Aortic Aneurysm and Dissection **136**
Valerie A. Pomper and Paul D. Campbell, Jr.

26 Abdominal Trauma **142**
Marcus W. Parker

27 Appendicitis **147**
Oleg M. Teytelboym

28 Cholecystitis **153**
Oleg M. Teytelboym

29 Diverticulitis **159**
Michael W. D'Angelo

30 Gastrointestinal Hemorrhage **162**
Mandeep Dagli and W. Dee Dockery

31 Intestinal Obstruction **167**
Simon Bekker and D. Darrell Vaughn

32 Intussusception **176**
Alexander M. Kowal

33 Liver Transplantation **181**
Christopher L. Smith

34 Nephrolithiasis **187**
Daniel J. Durand and Karen M. Horton

35 Renal Failure **194**
Brad P. Barnett and Satomi Kawamoto

36 Renal Transplantation **200**
Benjamin Tubb

37 Retroperitoneal Hemorrhage **208**
Mandeep Dagli

38 Necrotizing Enterocolitis **212**
Douglas F. Ramsey

39 Malrotation and Midgut Volvulus **215**
Sarah Mezban

40 Hypertrophic Pyloric Stenosis **220**
Jennifer E. Swart

41 Urinary Tract Infections **223**
Daniel J. Durand and Karen M. Horton

IV: PELVIS

42 Bladder and Ureteral Injury **231**
Visveshwar Baskaran

43 Ectopic Pregnancy **236**
Claire S. Cooney and Loralie D. Ma

44 Ovarian Torsion **240**
Claire S. Cooney

45 Pelvic Fractures **244**
Visveshwar Baskaran

46 Testicular Torsion **249**
Karen M. Horton and George P. Kuo

47 Tubo-Ovarian Abscess **255**
Aimee Lynn Maceda and Satomi Kawamoto

48 Retained Products of Conception **261**
Laura Amodei

V: EXTREMITIES

49 Deep Venous Thrombosis **264**
Christopher L. Smith

50 Osteomyelitis **270**
Rick W. Obray, Cathleen F. Magill, and Oleg M. Teytelboym

51 Peripheral Vascular Injury **276**
Christopher L. Smith

52 Septic Arthritis **281**
Rick W. Obray and Cathleen F. Magill

VI: PROCEDURES

53 Arteriography Primer **285**
Kevin A. Smith

54 Arthrogram, Hip **288**

55 Arthrogram, Shoulder **291**

56 Barium Studies **295**

57 Intussusception Reduction **306**
Alexander M. Kowal

58 Nephrostomy **309**

59 Spinal Puncture and Myelography **313**

60 Retrograde Urethrogram **316**

61 Voiding Cystourethrogram **317**

62 Saline Infusion Sonohysterography **319**
Laura Amodei

VII: REFERENCES

63 Bones 324

64 Contrast 336
Kenneth C. Wang

65 Dermatomes 342

66 Disk Nomenclature 344

67 Dosimetry 345
Joseph P. DiPietro

68 Radionuclides 348

69 Thorax 351

70 Ultrasound 354

71 Vascular Anatomy 359

72 Vesicoureteral Reflux Grading 375

Index 377

MANUAL OF RADIOLOGY: ACUTE PROBLEMS AND ESSENTIAL PROCEDURES

Second Edition

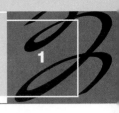

TRAUMATIC BRAIN INJURY
Ari M. Blitz

CLINICAL INFORMATION

Traumatic brain injury (TBI) presenting in isolation or as a component of polyorgan trauma accounts for much of trauma-related morbidity and mortality. Urgent diagnosis and treatment is critical and is most often guided by computed tomography (CT) findings. CT findings which correlate most strongly with poor outcome are subfalcine herniation (also known as midline shift), effacement of basal cisterns (due to edema or herniation), and subarachnoid hemorrhage.

This chapter discusses various forms of traumatic intracranial hemorrhage, as well as other acute injuries such as diffuse axonal injury (DAI), and cerebral contusion. Acute TBI is categorized into extracerebral hemorrhages and intraparenchymal injuries for ease of discussion, although these two forms of injury often coexist. Skull fractures are discussed in Chapter 2, "Skull Fractures", and patterns of herniation are discussed in Chapter 15, "Herniation".

IMAGING WITH COMPUTED TOMOGRAPHY AND MAGNETIC RESONANCE

Indications.   Because of its speed, availability, and high sensitivity for acute hemorrhage, CT is the primary imaging modality for the assessment of TBI. Magnetic resonance imaging (MRI) is most often used in the subacute stage, and is particularly sensitive to DAI and nonhemorrhagic contusions.

Computed Tomographic Protocol.   Noncontrast head CT reconstructed with both soft tissue and bone algorithms is the imaging standard. Computed tomographic angiography (CTA) may be performed in select patients to look for vascular injuries such as dissection/occlusion and caroticocavernous fistula (CCF).

Magnetic Resonance Imaging Protocol.   Noncontrast MRI evaluation typically includes: sagittal T1, axial T2, fluid attenuated inversion recovery (FLAIR) axial, and diffusion weighted axial with calculated apparent diffusion coefficient (ADC) map. Gradient echo or susceptibility weighted sequences are critical, as they have a high sensitivity for acute and chronic hemorrhage.

EXTRACEREBRAL (EXTRA-AXIAL) HEMORRHAGE

Extracerebral hemorrhage may be confined to the epidural space, subdural space, or subarachnoid space. A working knowledge of the anatomy of the meninges and cranial sutures is therefore necessary to appropriately discuss and diagnose intracranial and extra-axial hemorrhage and will often significantly impact upon clinical decision making. Hemorrhage can be superficial to the dura (epidural hemorrhage), subjacent to the dura but superficial to the arachnoid (subdural hemorrhage), and between the arachnoid and the pia mater (subarachnoid hemorrhage).

Epidural Hematoma

Epidural hematoma (Fig. 1-1) typically occurs in association with a linear fracture of the temporal bone that causes laceration of the middle meningeal artery or one of its branches,

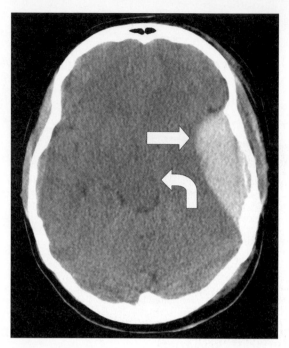

Figure 1-1. Noncontrast head computed tomography (CT) showing lens-shaped left temporal epidural hematoma (*straight arrow*) causing uncal herniation (*curved arrow*).

resulting in extravasated arterial blood under high pressure dissecting between the inner table of the skull and the closely applied outer layer of the dura mater. Because epidural hematoma has an arterial source 80% of the time there can be very rapid accumulation of blood, increased intracranial pressure, and subsequent brain herniation. Posterior fossa epidural hematomas are associated with occipital bone fractures and disruption of the transverse sinus. The classic clinical scenario is blunt trauma to the temporal region, loss of consciousness followed by a lucid interval of minutes to a few hours, with subsequent rapid deterioration into coma and even death as the mass effect grows. Epidural hematoma is a neurosurgical emergency.

- The dura and bone are essentially fused at sutures, so epidural hematomas do not cross sutures, and therefore take on a characteristic biconvex shape. Epidural hematomas can cross midline.
- Thirty percent of conservatively managed epidural hematomas will enlarge in the first 24 hours. Alternating regions of lower attenuation creating a "swirl" appearance can be seen in acute epidural hematomas and may be associated with ongoing hemorrhage, but enlarging epidural hematomas do not consistently show this sign.
- The transverse sinuses are often asymmetric in size and a prominent sinus can mimic an extra-axial hematoma. Look for an associated skull fracture and scalp hematoma and use coronal/sagittal reconstructions for clarification.

Subdural Hematoma

Subdural hematoma (Fig. 1-2) is usually secondary to disruption of bridging veins between the cerebral cortex and dural sinuses allowing blood to collect in the potential space between the inner layer of the dura mater and the pia arachnid. While majority are traumatic, spontaneous subdural hematoma can occur in elderly and coagulopathic individuals.

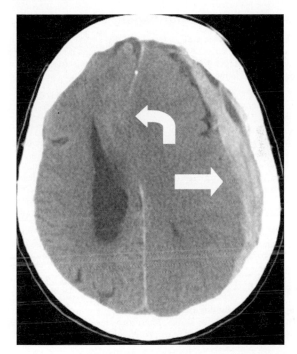

Figure 1-2. Noncontrast head computed tomography (CT) demonstrating left sided subdural hematoma (*straight arrow*) causing midline shift (*curved arrow*).

- Acutely, CT will show a crescentic high-attenuation rim of blood between the skull and gray matter, often with apparent disproportionately large mass effect on the ipsilateral ventricular system, probably reflecting additional brain injury.
- Subdural hematoma can spread along the ipsilateral cerebral convexity, freely crossing sutures, appearing thin on any axial section, but representing a large volume of blood.
- Because it is confined by major dural structures, hemispheric subdural hematoma docs not cross the midline but can be bilateral.

Chronic Subdural Hematoma

Chronic subdural hematoma is difficult to diagnose clinically because of an insidious onset of decline in cognition, typically in patients who already have significant brain atrophy. The typical scenario is an elderly patient with a history of minor head trauma who shows progressive cognitive decline, sometimes with focal neurologic symptoms and headache. This occurs because of gradual enlargement of the subdural hematoma due to repeated hemorrhages.

- The transverse sinuses are often asymmetric in size and a prominent sinus can mimic an extra-axial hematoma. Look for an associated skull fracture and scalp hematoma and use coronal/sagittal reconstructions for clarification.
- Bilateral isodense subdural hematoma on CT usually demonstrates no asymmetric mass effect on the ventricles, given the equally increased pressures on both sides of the falx cerebri. However, the gray–white matter junction, which should normally be less than 1 cm from the inner table of the skull, may be displaced medially by chronic subdural hematoma.
- Bilateral subdural hematoma can manifest as bilateral uncal herniation and basal cistern effacement or diffuse effacement of the cortical sulci.

Traumatic Subarachnoid Hemorrhage

The subarachnoid space contains CSF, surrounds the entire brain and spinal cord, and communicates with the ventricular system through the paired lateral foramina of Luschka, the midline foramen of Magendie which allow CSF to exit from the fourth ventricle. Therefore, subarachnoid hemorrhage is sometimes seen with intraventricular hemorrhage.

- Usually seen in the cortical sulci near the site of blunt impact or along the path of a penetrating wound.
- Usually associated with parenchymal brain injury.
- Intracranial hemorrhage, such as diffuse subarachnoid hemorrhage due to aneurysmal rupture may also precede and precipitate traumatic injury. Although a driver of a vehicle, for instance, may present with subarachnoid hemorrhage due to trauma alone, consider the possibility of an underlying etiology such as antecedent aneurysmal rupture in the appropriate circumstances.

Intraventricular Hemorrhage

Intraventricular hemorrhage without blood in other intracranial compartments is unusual. Intraventricular hemorrhage typically occurs as an extension from intraparenchymal or subarachnoid hemorrhage. Intraventricular hemorrhage is a common cause of hydrocephalus.

Scalp Hematoma

- Scalp hematomas are rarely clinically significant by themselves, but may point to the site of traumatic impact to the skull. Therefore, look for skull fractures and brain injuries just beneath (coup) and on the opposite side (contra-coup) from the scalp hematoma.
- Posttraumatic subgaleal hematomas occur deep to the galea aponeurotica, in the loose connective tissue layer just outside the periosteum of the skull bones.
- Soft tissue hematomas occur superficial to the galea aponeurotica.
- In neonates, posttraumatic cephalhematomas occur beneath the periosteum, separating it from the outer table to which it is relatively loosely applied. These are almost always related to birth trauma and have a predilection for the parietal region.

 INTRAPARENCHYMAL (INTRA-AXIAL) HEMORRHAGE

Cerebral contusions (Fig. 1-3) are the most common type of TBI and occur at the cortical surfaces and underlying white matter. Typical locations are the inferior/anterior surfaces of the frontal and temporal lobes as a result of translational movements of the brain on bony surfaces of the anterior and middle cranial fossa. Occasionally, traumatic forces are transmitted on a relatively straight line accounting for "coup-contrecoup" type injuries. Contusions are serious injuries often resulting in long term neurologic sequela including intellectual decline, focal deficits, and epilepsy.

- Contusions can be hemorrhagic or nonhemorrhagic. Only about one half of contusions show hemorrhage on CT.
- There is always associated edema which may take several hours to emerge, leading to the typical CT appearance of mottled high-attenuation blood surrounded by low-attenuation edema. Nonhemorrhagic contusions appear as focal or regional low attenuation and brain swelling and may be difficult to identify on initial CT.
- Both hemorrhagic and nonhemorrhagic contusions become more conspicuous with time due to increasing edema and mass effect. Occasionally, delayed hemorrhage into nonhemorrhagic contusions occurs.
- MRI is more sensitive to contusions, particularly the nonhemorrhagic ones, than CT at all stages of injury. Diffusion weighted and susceptibility weighted images emerge as the most sensitive pulse sequences.

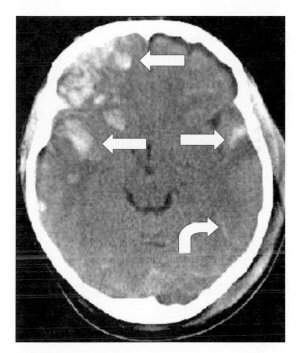

Figure 1-3. Noncontrast head computed tomography (CT) showing bilateral frontal and temporal lobe contusion (*straight arrows*) and associated subarachnoid hemorrhage (*curved arrow*).

 AXONAL SHEARING INJURY

Axonal shearing injury is a potentially devastating result of blunt trauma or rapid acceleration/deceleration of the head in which axons and small vessels are severed due to rotational forces which cause shearing at regions of changes in tissue density. These injuries can be focal and are associated with relatively mild deficits, but are often generalized, a condition called *diffuse axonal injury*. DAI is seen in severe, closed head trauma with immediate loss of consciousness followed by a persistent vegetative state.

■ The most common locations of damage are the cerebral gray–white matter junction, the inferior aspect of the corpus callosum, the dorsolateral midbrain, and the junction of the internal capsule and basal ganglia.
■ CT is often completely normal other than diffuse cerebral edema, but small punctate "tissue tear" hemorrhages (secondary to small vessel disruption) at the above sites, can be seen. Conversely, the presence of tissue tear hemorrhages does not always indicate axonal injury. MRI, diffusion weighted images in particular, is much more sensitive for DAI.
■ In the brainstem, axonal shearing injuries are life threatening, and the detection of tissue tear hemorrhages at these locations indicates a poor prognosis. Susceptibility weighted sequences are the most sensitive to small hemorrhages.

 DEEP GRAY MATTER INJURY

Injury to the thalamus, caudate nucleus, putamen, and globus pallidus accounts for approximately 5% of TBI. These can be hemorrhagic and nonhemorrhagic and are associated with poor outcomes.

INTRACRANIAL TRAUMA IN CHILDREN

Subdural hematomas are the most common intracranial consequence of child abuse. Cerebral contusion may also occur. In addition to the considerations above, a careful search for subdural blood adjacent to the falx cerebri should be undertaken in children.

Chronic subdural hematomas, skull fractures of varying ages, or ischemic injury in particular should prompt consideration of the possibility of nonaccidental trauma. Infarction has been found to be six times more likely in head trauma in abused children, when compared with nonabused children.

Further Readings

Barkovitch AJ. *Pediatric neuroimaging.* Philadelphia: Lippincott Williams & Wilkins, 2005.

Eisenberg HM, Gary HE, Aldrich EF, et al. Initial CT findings in 753 patients with severe head injury: a report from the NIH traumatic coma data bank. *J Neurosurg* 1990;73: 688–698.

Grossman RI, Yousem DM. *Neuroradiology—the requisites,* 2nd ed. Philadelphia: Mosby, Elsevier Inc., 2003.

Ransom GH, Mann FA, Vavilala MS, et al. Cerebral infarct in head injury: relationship to child abuse. *Child Abuse Negl* 2003;27(4):381–392.

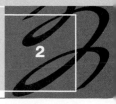

SKULL FRACTURES
Norman J. Beauchamp, Jr. and Andrew L. Holz

 CLINICAL SIGNIFICANCE

Skull fractures can be seen with blunt or penetrating trauma. The skull is, in most circumstances, a structure requiring significant force to fracture. One might expect that this indicates a direct correlation with intracranial injury, however the presence of a skull fracture is not predictive of intracranial injury as detected by computed tomography (CT). Forces applied to the skull are often insufficient to fracture the bone but more than sufficient to injure the meningeal structures and brain parenchyma. Therefore, the absence of a fracture does NOT exclude intracranial injury.

 COMPLICATIONS

Infection. Skull fractures are considered "open fractures" if there is extension into the paranasal sinuses, middle ear cavities, or mastoid air cells, or when there is an overlying superficial soft tissue laceration. Basilar skull fractures, which often enter the paranasal sinuses, middle ear cavities, or mastoid air cells, can be detected clinically if rhinorrhea or otorrhea is present and are suggested by periorbital or postauricular ecchymosis. Both the nonbasilar open fractures and basilar skull fractures put the patient at risk of infection.

Meningeal or Parenchymal Injury. Skull fractures in general, but especially those depressed more than 5 mm deep to the inner table, may lacerate the dura or cause brain parenchymal injury. Significantly depressed skull fractures, greater than 5 mm deep to the inner table, are associated with seizures and should be elevated urgently.

Vascular Injury. Fractures in the temporal and occipital bones are associated with epidural hematomas due to involvement of the middle meningeal artery and transverse sinus, respectively. Skull base fractures that involve the carotid canal may be associated with carotid occlusion and brain infarct. Caroticocavernous fistula may result from sphenoid fractures.

Indication of Alternative Etiology of Injury. Fractures in the pediatric population are also of concern in that they may alert the clinician to nonaccidental trauma/child abuse.

Potential Leptomeningeal Cyst Formation. A rare complication of skull fracture is a leptomeningeal cyst. This occurs in children and is associated with a diastatic fracture through which cerebrospinal fluid (CSF) pulsations prevent closure of the fracture. This is seen as a "growing fracture" sign.

 IMAGING WITH RADIOGRAPHS

Indications. Radiographs have been supplanted by CT for evaluation of skull fractures and only routinely obtained in children to screen for nonaccidental trauma.

Possible Findings

■ Acute fractures appear as a linear lucency that is sharply demarcated and do not have a sclerotic margin. These are to be differentiated from vascular grooves and sutures, which have a serpentine course and a sclerotic border. Knowledge of sutural anatomy is important as the fracture may run nearly parallel to the suture.

■ Fracture may extend into a suture and result in sutural separation, that is, a diastatic fracture. This may be best visualized by comparing sutural widths bilaterally.

■ Depressed fractures appear as a step-off on a tangential view.

■ Basilar skull fractures can be subtle, and are far better assessed on CT, but pneumo-cephalus is a detectable secondary sign.

 ## IMAGING WITH COMPUTERIZED TOMOGRAPHY

Protocol.   Thin slices are preferred for evaluation of head trauma. Slices measuring 0.5 to 1 mm with multiplanar reconstructions should be performed if temporal bone fracture is suspected.

Possible Findings (Figs. 2-1 and 2-2)

■ Disruption of calvarium is sharply defined and without sclerotic borders. Symmetry is helpful, and the consideration of fracture is important in the presence of an abnormality which resembles a suture.

■ Fluid in the sphenoid and frontal sinuses, mastoid air cells, or middle ear cavity represents fracture until proven otherwise.

■ Pneumocephalus suggests basilar skull fracture. Look for frontal sinus posterior wall, sphenoid sinus, and temporal bone fractures.

■ Depression of bone. Discrete sharply defined calvarial disruption may not be visible in rare cases of depressed fractures. CT enables accurate measurement of the degree of fragment depression.

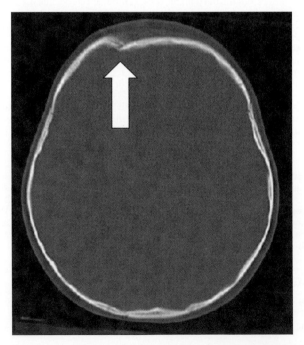

Figure 2-1. Noncontrast head computed tomographic (CT) findings showing depressed fracture of right frontal bone (*straight arrow*).

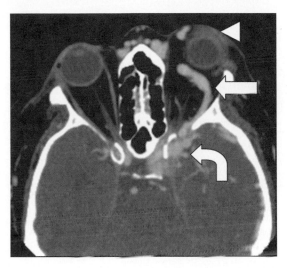

Figure 2-2. Contrast-enhanced head computed tomography (CT) demonstrating cavernous carotid fistula in a patient with sphenoid fracture with exophthalmus (*arrowhead*), engorgement of left superior opthalmic vein (*straight arrow*), and prominence of left cavernous sinus (*curved arrow*).

■ Associated lesions. Contusion, shearing injury, extracerebral hematoma, shaken baby syndrome findings in other imaged body parts.

 IMAGING TIPS

■ Always look for skull fractures on cervical spine series. Fractures that the clinicians were not suspecting will be found.
■ Always look on the CT scout topograms for skull fractures. When reviewed without the reference lines, the topogram is similar to the lateral skull radiograph and will enable detection of the in-plane axial fractures that would otherwise only be seen with three-dimensional (3D) processing.
■ Children younger than 2 years have a complex pattern of cranial sutures, particularly at and caudal to the level of pterion. Be cautious not to overcall fractures in these areas.

 ISSUES AFTER IMAGING

■ Neurosurgery should be notified immediately for depressed (>5 mm) skull fractures.
■ All fractures occurring in the pediatric population should be brought to the immediate attention of the requesting physician.
■ Skull base fractures are associated with CSF leak and increased risk of meningitis.
■ Temporal bone fractures are associated with hearing loss and facial paralysis.
■ Sphenoid bone and carotid canal fractures are associated with carotid artery injury.

Further Readings

Davis KR, Taveras JM, Roberson GH, et al. Computed tomography in head trauma. *Semin Roentgenol* 1977;12:53–62.
Grossman RI, Yousem DM. *Neuroradiology—the requisites*, 2nd ed. Philadelphia: Mosby, Elsevier Science, 2003.
Harwood-Nash CE, Hendrick EB, Hudson AR. The significance of skull fractures in children: a study of 1,187 patients. *Radiology* 1971;101:151–156.

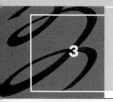

TRAUMATIC FACIAL INJURY
Aimee Lynn Maceda and Monica D. Watkins

$\mathcal{R}$adiologic consultation for facial trauma is common in the emergency room setting. Most facial fractures occur secondary to direct blow to the face with the remainder mainly due to automobile accidents. Nasal fractures are the most common, followed by mandibular and zygomatic fractures. High speed automobile accidents commonly result in zygomaticomaxillary and LeFort midfacial fractures.

Adequate evaluation of facial fractures requires thin slice computed tomography (CT) with multiplanar reconstructions. The probability of facial fracture is extremely low if there is no nasal bone fracture and fluid in the paranasal sinuses.

 MIDFACIAL FRACTURES

- Unilateral facial fractures most commonly represent zygomaticomaxillary complex (ZMC) fracture. Orbital fracture account for most other unilateral fractures (discussed in Chap. 4, "Orbital Fractures").
- Nearly all bilateral facial fractures represent Le-Fort fractures.
- All LeFort fractures involve pterygoid processes.
- Each LeFort fracture has a unique component.

LeFort I: "Floating Palate" (Fig. 3-1)

- Frequency: 20–30% of LeFort fractures.
- Examination: maxillary teeth moveable on physical examination.
- Mechanism: directed horizontal impact to the premaxilla.
- Unique component: inferior orbital rim.
- All components: horizontal fracture through inferior nasal septum, floor of the maxillary sinuses (anterior, medial, lateral, and posterior walls), and bilateral pterygoid plates.

LeFort II: "Floating Maxilla, Pyramidal Fracture" (Fig. 3-1)

- Frequency: 35–55% of LeFort-type maxillary fractures; the most common type.
- Examination: the midportion of the face is detached resulting in movement of the maxillary teeth and nose relative to the remainder of the skull.
- Mechanism: horizontal blow to the midportion of the face.
- Unique component: inferior orbital rim.
- All components: pyramidal-shaped fracture with the nasofrontal suture at the apex and the teeth as the base. Fracture passes through the nasal ala across the frontal process of the maxilla and medial orbital wall. The fracture then extends through the infraorbital rim and then involves the posterior and lateral wall of the maxillary sinus. The fracture line then crosses the pterygomaxillary fossa and through the pterygoid plates.
- Association with ZMC fracture on the side of impact.

Le-Fort III: "Craniofacial Disjunction" (Fig. 3-1)

- Frequency: 5–15% of LeFort fractures.
- Examination: the maxillary teeth, nose, and zygomata move in relation to the skull.
- Mechanism: occurs with massive facial trauma and is commonly associated with intracranial injuries.
- Unique component: zygomatic arch.

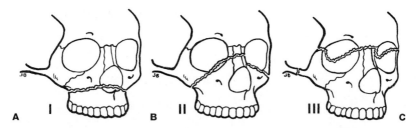

Figure 3-1. Midfacial fractures according to LeFort Classification. **A:** Le Fort I. **B:** LeFort II. **C:** LeFort III craniofacial disjunction. (Modified from Ralston EL. Handbook of fractures. St. Louis: Mosby, 1967. Reprinted with permission from Harris JH Jr, Harris WH. The radiology of emergency medicine, 4th ed. Philadelphia: Lippincott Williams & Wilkins, 2000:437–581.)

■ All components: arises high on the nasal side of the frontonasal suture line, resulting in nasal bone fractures and then crosses the frontal processes of the maxilla and lacrimal bones and through the lamina papyracea and ethmoid sinuses. The fracture line passes posterior to the inferior orbital fissure with one fracture line extending across the lateral orbital wall to the sphenozygomatic junction continuing to separate the zygomatic arch. A second fracture line extends across the posterior maxilla to involve the pterygoid plates.

■ Frequently results in airway compromise due to hematoma caused by pharyngeal artery injury.

Le-Fort Variations

■ Incomplete: fracture does not follow the entire course of the expected fracture line.
■ Hemi-LeFort: fracture involves the pterygoid plates and maxillary on one side only.
■ Mixed: fracture on both sides of the face is of different LeFort types.
■ Combination: more than one type of LeFort fracture on the same side of the face.

ZMC Fracture

(sometimes called *tripod, trimaleolar,* or *quadropod fracture*) (Fig. 3-2):

■ Examination: flattening of malar eminence, cheek and eyelid bruise, trismus, diplopia (up to 30%).
■ Mechanism: direct blow to the zygoma (malar eminence).
■ Fractures: lateral wall maxillary sinus, orbital rim close to the infraorbital foramen, floor of orbit, zygomatic arch (or zygomaticofrontal suture). May result in pterygoid plate fracture.
■ Association with greater wing of sphenoid fracture which can result in middle meningeal artery injury and epidural hematoma.

 ## NASOETHMOIDAL-ORBITAL FRACTURES

■ Examination: enophthalmus, diplopia excessive bleeding.
■ Mechanism: direct blow to the dorsum of nose.
■ Fractures: comminuted fractures of the nasal bones with involvement of at least one of the following; the frontal bone and sinus, ethmoid air cells, lamina papyracea (medial orbital wall), orbital roof, and cribriform plate.
■ Associated brain injury, dural tear, cerebrospinal fluid (CSF) leak, ocular injury, and injury to the lacrimal apparatus. Surgical intervention is virtually always necessary.

 ## MANDIBULAR FRACTURES

■ Examination: trismus and malocclusion.
■ Mechanism: direct blow to the zygoma (malar eminence).

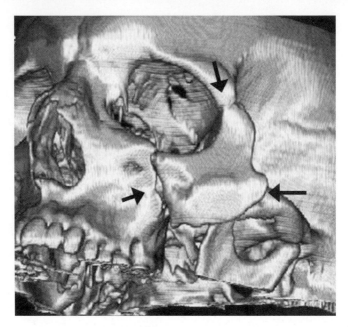

Figure 3-2. Three-dimensional volume rendered noncontrast head computed tomography (CT) showing left zygomaticomaxillary complex fracture (*arrows*).

- Fractures
  - Fifty percent single fracture (typically direct blow), 40% two fractures, and 10% three fractures (automobile accidents).
  - Areas of weakness: body at the mental foramen, angle, and condylar neck.
  - Fracture line entering a root of a tooth is considered an open fracture.

 NASAL FRACTURES

- Mechanism: direct blow.
- Fractures: usually transverse with displacement or depression. Fifteen percent have other facial fractures.

 ISSUES AFTER IMAGING

- Facial fractures are usually repaired surgically to restore stability. However, these patients frequently have other traumatic injuries requiring more immediate surgical intervention.

Further Readings

Harris HJ Jr, Harris WH. *The radiology of emergency medicine*, 4th ed. Philadelphia: Lippincot Williams & Wilkins, 2000:437–581.

Rhea JT, Novelline Robert. How to simplify the ct diagnosis of Le Fort fractures. *Am J Roentgenol* 2005;184:1700–1705.

Rhea JT, Rao PM, Novelline RA. Helical CT and three dimensional CT of facial and orbital injury. *Radiol Clin North Am* 1999;37:489–451.

Sun Julie, LeMay Daniel. Imaging of facial trauma. *Neuroimaging Clin N Am* 2002;12: 295–309.

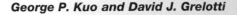

ORBITAL FRACTURES

George P. Kuo and David J. Grelotti

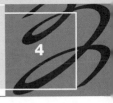

4

Orbital fractures are a common result of direct blunt trauma to the eye, such as being struck with a fist or baseball. The orbital floor and/or medial wall are most commonly involved. Superior rim and orbital roof fractures occasionally occur, particularly if the adjacent frontal sinus is well developed. Orbital floor fractures result from sudden increased intraorbital pressure caused by the eyeball's transmission of the force of a blow. The orbit is also involved in a number of other facial fractures including LeFort II and III fractures, nasoethmoidal complex fractures, and zygoma fractures.

Mechanism. The type of orbital fracture is thought to relate to the nature of the injury. Orbital rim fractures generally result from a direct blow to the bony orbit. Orbital wall fractures, on the other hand, are believed to be the result from a sudden increase in intraorbital pressure caused by a blow to the orbit and subsequent transmission of the force to the orbital wall. Fracture fragments are typically directed away from the orbit causing a "blow-out" fracture. However, it is also possible to sustain an orbital wall injury as a result of blunt trauma to the frontal bone or maxilla with subsequent transmission of the force to the orbital roof or floor. With this mechanism, it is not uncommon to find fracture fragments within the orbital space or a "blow-in" fracture.

 CLINICAL INFORMATION

Vision-threatening injuries can co-occur with orbital fracture. Prompt attention should be paid to individuals experiencing monocular diplopia, loss of vision, severe eye pain, evidence of corneal laceration or hyphema, or a triad of eye pain, proptosis, and central retinal artery pulsations (suggesting orbital hemorrhage). These are ophthalmologic emergencies and require urgent evaluation and possible surgical intervention by an ophthalmologist.

Symptoms and Signs. With an appropriate history of trauma, an orbital floor fracture is suspected if one or more of the following are present:

- Diplopia, the most common symptom, is caused by entrapment or contusion of extraocular muscle(s) near the fracture.
- Decreased ocular motility, especially on vertical gaze (classically, a loss of upward gaze).
- Enophthalmos occurs especially if the fracture is large, but may be masked if intraorbital edema and/or hemorrhage is present, which can even cause initial proptosis (exophthalmos).
- Hypoesthesia (hypesthesia) of the ipsilateral cheek is a particularly reliable sign and is caused by concomitant injury to the infraorbital nerve, which travels in a groove and canal in the orbital floor.

Differential Diagnosis primarily includes orbital edema and/or hematoma without a fracture. These can cause any of the first three clinical findings listed in the preceding text.

Entrapment is a clinical diagnosis in which there is severe restriction of eye movement, often causing diplopia, due to "catching" of the orbital contents by edges of the fracture. Certain computed tomographic (CT) findings support the diagnosis of entrapment, but CT cannot rule in or out the entrapment (see subsequent text).

Inferior rectus muscle entrapment, a rare but severe form of entrapment, can result in ischemic strangulation of the muscle and is the only indication for emergency surgery.

IMAGING WITH COMPUTED TOMOGRAPHY

Indications.   CT is the preferred modality for the detection of orbital fractures. Emergency CT is necessary if soft tissue swelling prevents adequate physical examination of the eye (e.g., to look for a ruptured globe) or if inferior rectus entrapment is clinically suspected. A nonemergent CT is customarily performed in all cases of suspected orbital fracture, in order to:

- Establish the presence of a fracture.
- Document fracture's size, extent, and amount of depression.
- Look for other associated fractures.
- Look for involvement of orbital soft tissues.

Protocol.   Noncontrast contiguous 1-mm axial slices with coronal (essential) and sagittal reconstructions. Bone and soft tissue windows.

Possible Findings (Figs. 4-1 and 4-2)

- Step-off of orbital floor, fracture fragment usually displaced inferiorly (maxillary blow-out).
- Inferior prolapse of orbital contents (i.e., fat and/or muscle) into the maxillary sinus, a common finding; prolapse through a very narrow or nonvisualized fracture opening may correlate with the clinical finding of entrapment, but entrapment cannot be ruled in or out by CT.

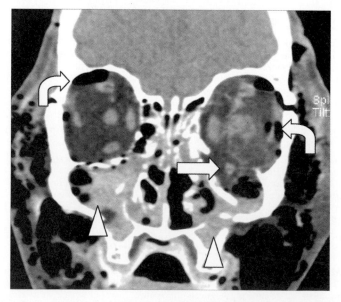

Figure 4-1. Noncontrast coronal facial computed tomography (CT) demonstrating multiple bilateral facial fractures with hemorrhage in the sinuses (*arrowheads*), herniation of left inferior rectus through orbital floor (*straight arrow*), and extensive orbital (*curved arrows*) and soft tissue air.

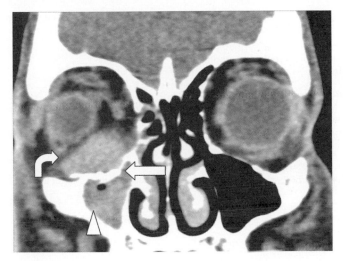

Figure 4-2. Noncontrast coronal facial computed tomography (CT) demonstrating right orbital floor fracture (*straight arrow*), orbital hematoma (*curved arrow*), and right maxillary sinus hemorrhage (*arrowhead*).

- Inferior rectus entrapment—the inferior rectus muscle appears caught in a very narrow or nonvisualized fracture opening, causing a "trapdoor" mechanism.
- Medial wall (lamina papyracea) fracture (ethmoid blow-out) may be isolated or present in 20–30% cases of orbital floor fracture, not usually seen on radiographs, may be a more important determinant of enophthalmos.
- Associated rim involvement.
- Orbital air or hematoma.
- Enophthalmos or proptosis.
- Swelling and/or hematoma of eyelid and surrounding soft tissue.

Routine Checks

- Measure the transverse dimensions of the fracture defect and amount of depression (used for prognosis).
- Check for globe rupture—any thickening or loss of roundness may require emergency surgery—not usually associated with floor fracture.
- Check for swelling of the optic nerve, retrobulbar stranding of fat and hematoma.
- Check for intracranial air and hematoma adjacent to roof fractures.
- Check for associated nasal bone fractures.

 IMAGING TIPS

- **Groove and canal of the infraorbital nerve** can cause the appearance of a fracture on both radiograph and CT; use symmetry.
- **Fluid and/or blood** in the ipsilateral sinuses: if none is present on CT scan, a fracture is extremely unlikely or old if present.

 ISSUES AFTER IMAGING

Except for cases of inferior rectus entrapment, the decision for surgical repair of an orbital floor fracture is made after waiting 7–10 days for the orbital swelling to subside.

The timing of surgery is somewhat controversial. Indications for subsequent surgery are:

- Persistent diplopia, that is, continued functional entrapment.
- Cosmetically unacceptable enophthalmos.
- Large fractures equal to or greater than half the area of the floor.

Further Readings

Albert DM, Jakobiec FA, eds. *Principles and practice of ophthalmology*, 2nd ed. Philadelphia: WB Saunders, 1999.

Chang EL, Bernardino CR. Update on orbital trauma. *Curr Opin Ophthalmol* 2004;5: 411–415.

Cruz AA, Eichenberger GC. Epidemiology and management of orbital fractures. *Curr Opin Ophthalmol* 2004;5:416–421.

Lee HJ, Jilani M, Frohman L, et al. CT of orbital trauma. *Emerg Radiol* 2004;4:168–172.

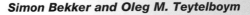

CERVICAL SPINE TRAUMA

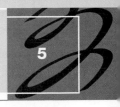

Simon Bekker and Oleg M. Teytelboym

5

Epidemiology. The cervical spine is the most common site of spinal injury in blunt trauma or automobile accidents. C1-2 are the most commonly involved levels, followed by C5-7. Approximately 20% of patients with cervical spine fracture will have more than one fractures. Majority of cervical cord injuries occur at the time of the fracture, however up to 15% may develop later due to fracture instability.

Symptoms and Signs. Cervical spine fractures are always symptomatic. However, patients may be unconscious, intoxicated, or have distracting injury rendering the history and examination inaccurate. Patients usually present with posterior neck pain which is accentuated on palpation. Cervical cord injury can manifest with weakness, paresthesias, areflexia, flaccidity, and loss of sphincter tone.

Mechanism. Knowing the mechanism of injury is essential for understanding its radiographic features. C-spine injuries can be classified according to the causative mechanism and its sequelae, but most cases are likely the result of multiple simultaneous forces with one predominant force (see Table 5-1 for major fracture types).

- Hyperflexion.
- Hyperflexion and rotation.
- Hyperextension.
- Hyperextension and rotation.
- Vertical compression.
- Lateral flexion.
- Other mechanism.

Stability. Cervical spine can be separated into three columns—anterior, middle, and posterior. Injuries to one column are considered stable. If two columns are disrupted the injury is unstable, increasing the probability of delayed spinal cord injury.

- **Anterior.** Anterior longitudinal ligament, anterior two thirds of the vertebral body and intervertebral disk.
- **Middle.** Posterior longitudinal ligament, posterior one third of the vertebral body and intervertebral disk.
- **Posterior.** Posterior bony elements (pedicles, transverse processes, articular facets, laminae, and spinous processes).

 IMAGING WITH RADIOGRAPHS

Indications. C-spine radiographs are indicated in all trauma patients presenting with localized neck pain, deformity, altered mental status, distracting injury, neurologic deficits, or head injury. If the radiograph findings are negative in a trauma patient who has neck pain, neurologic deficits, or other reason for high clinical suspicion, a computed tomography (CT) should be performed subsequently.

Protocol. A cross-table lateral radiograph is usually performed first to avoid moving the patient in case a C-spine fracture is present. If this appears normal, routine views are then

TABLE 5-1   **Cervical Spine Fractures. Listed are the Major Types, Organized by Predominant Mechanism of Injury**

Mechanism	Fracture type	Stability	Description
Hyperflexion	Anterior subluxation	Stable	Disruption of the posterior ligament complex only (supraspinous, infraspinous, interfacetal joint capsule, and posterior longitudinal ligaments); the anulus fibrosus may be partially disrupted. The anterior longitudinal ligament is intact
	Bilateral interfacetal dislocation	Unstable	Complete disruption of the posterior ligament complex PLUS the anulus fibrosus and possibly the anterior longitudinal ligament
			Results in bilateral jumped facets; neurologic injury common
	Simple wedge fracture	Stable	Anterior compression fracture of vertebral body; the posterior ligament complex is stretched but intact; the anulus fibrosus and anterior longitudinal ligament are intact
	Clay Shoveler's fracture	Stable	Avulsion fracture of spinous process of C7, C6, or T1 (in order of frequency).
	Flexion tear-drop fracture	Unstable	Complete disruption of all ligament groups (posterior complex, anulus fibrosus, and anterior longitudinal) nteriorly displaced triangular fracture fragment from the anterior-inferior corner of the vertebral body
			Angulation and displacement of vertebral body causes spinal canal narrowing; often associated with anterior cervical cord syndrome; the most serious C-spine injury
Rotation-flexion	Unilateral interfacetal dislocation	Stable	Complete unilateral disruption of facet joint capsule and posterior longitudinal ligament; partial disruption of the anulus fibrosus and the opposite facet joint capsule
			Results in unilateral locked facet; fracture of involved facet is common; commonly associated with vertebral artery injury
Rotation-extension	Pillar fracture	Stable	Vertical fracture of one of the lateral masses, usually in a lower cervical vertebra

Compression	Jefferson's fracture C1	Unstable	Fractures of anterior and posterior arches of C1 with disruption of the transverse ligament of C1 and lateral displacement of the articular masses of C1
			Atlantodental interval greater than 3 mm. Can be difficult to see — watch for prevertebral soft tissue swelling
	Burst fracture (lower C-spine)	Stable	Comminuted vertical fracture of vertebral body, usually a lower cervical vertebra, caused by forcing of nucleus pulposus through inferior endplate
			Posterior fracture fragment commonly displaced posteriorly into spinal canal
Extension	Extension Tear-drop fracture	Unstable	Avulsion fracture involving the anterior-inferior corner of the vertebral body, disrupting the attachment of the anterior longitudinal ligament
			Commonly associated with preexisting degenerative joint disease (DJD)
	Posterior neural arch fracture C1	Stable	Fracture only of the posterior arch of C1
			Caused by compression of the arch between the occiput and the arch of C2
	Hangman's fracture	Unstable	Bilateral fracture of C2 pedicles
			Usually results in anterior dislocation of C2 on C3; usually caused by rapid deceleration (head against windshield) followed by rebound flexion, causing the dislocation
	Hyperextension fracture-dislocation	Unstable	Comminuted fracture of lateral masses and posterior elements caused by compressive extension; anterior and posterior longitudinal ligaments may or may not be disrupted
			The involved vertebral body usually displaced ANTERIORLY, although injury was due to extension
	Hyperextension dislocation	Unstable	Complete disruption of anterior longitudinal ligament; the upper vertebral body momentarily slides posteriorly into spinal canal, causing cord injury; the intervertebral disc is separated from the inferior endplate and the posterior longitudinal ligament is torn away from the posterior surface of the lower vertebral body
			The radiographs may appear NORMAL

(continued)

TABLE 5-1 *(Continued)*

Mechanism	Fracture type	Stability	Description
Complex	Type I odontoid	Stable unless there is severe ligamentous injury	Avulsion fracture of the tip of the odontoid; uncommon. May be associated with severe ligamentous disruption of the craniovertebral junction
	Type II odontoid	Variable, delayed instability common	Usually a transverse fracture at the base of the odontoid process; two thirds of all odontoid fractures; nonunion is common
	Type III odontoid	Unstable	Fracture through the base of the odontoid that extends to the body of C2 and often to the articular surface
Complex, distraction	Atlantooccipital dissociation	Unstable	Ligamentous disruption without fracture unless associated with other fractures; the distance between the tip of the clivus and tip of the odontoid process is greater than 12 mm; severe neurologic injury
Complex, distraction	Atlantoaxial dissociation	Unstable	Ligamentous disruption without fracture unless associated with other fractures; increased distance between the lateral masses of C1 and C2; severe neurologic injury

performed, including anteroposterior (AP) and open-mouth odontoid views. The routine C-spine examination can also include angled 45 degree oblique and flexion-extension views. One should be able to see the seven cervical segments and the cervicothoracic junction for a cervical spine series to be complete. Flexion-extension views are particularly useful for detection of ligamentous disruption when the routine views (and sometimes even CT) are normal. The patient must perform the flexion and extension voluntarily without any assistance. Any external force can cause severe injury if a fracture or dislocation is present. Flexion-extension views are contraindicated if the patient is disoriented, uncooperative, or intoxicated.

Possible Findings (Figs. 5-1 and 5-2)

- **Count the vertebral bodies.** All seven cervical vertebral bodies along with the superior aspect of T1 should be visualized. If the lower C-spine is obscured by the shoulders and the upper C-spine is normal (especially looking for atlanto-occipital and atlantoaxial abnormalities), repeat the film with downward traction on both arms or with one arm extended above the head ("swimmer's view"). If these maneuvers fail and the clinical suspicion remains high, proceed with CT to visualize the C7-T1 region.
- **Overall curvature.** A gradual, smooth lordotic curve is characteristic of the normal C-spine. A cervical collar and/or muscle spasm may alter the degree of the curve.
- **Prevertebral soft tissues.** The soft tissue line should be smooth in contour, with a sharp and distinct interface between air and soft tissue. An abnormality in this line may be the only, or the most obvious, radiographic sign of cervical injury, possibly reflecting underlying edema and/or hemorrhage. Anterior to the body of C3, the width of the prevertebral soft tissue should be 3–4 mm. Anterior to C2, the soft tissue should be no thicker than the AP diameter of the adjacent odontoid process. At C4 and lower, the prevertebral soft tissue can be as thick as the width of the adjacent vertebral body. In

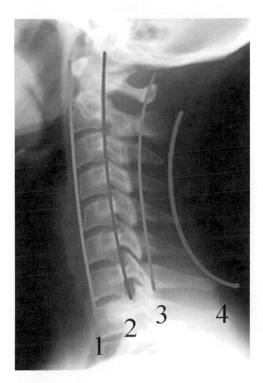

Figure 5-1. Lateral radiograph of cervical spine illustrating spinal lines: *1*-anterior vertebral, *2*-posterior vertebral, *3*-spinolaminar, *4*-posterior spinous line.

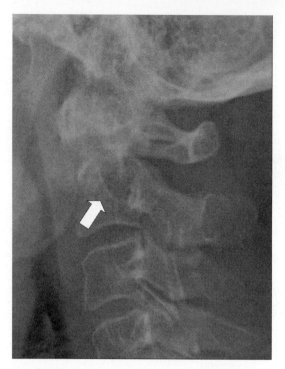

Figure 5-2. Lateral radiograph of cervical spine demonstrating odontoid fracture with disruption of Harris, ring (*arrow*) and disruption of spinal lines due to anterior displacement of C1.

children, the prevertebral soft tissue can appear thickened or otherwise abnormal if the child is crying, swallowing, or if the head is flexed.

- **Line 1. Anterior vertebral body line.** This line should be smooth, uninterrupted, and generally parallel to the other lines. Anterior osteophytes should be ignored in drawing this line.
- **Line 2. Posterior vertebral body line.** This line should be smooth, uninterrupted, and generally parallel to the other lines.
- **Line 3. Spinolaminar line.** This line represents the posterior "wall" of the spinal canal and should be smooth, uninterrupted, and generally parallel to the other lines. Because the spinal cord lies between lines 3 and 4, a stepoff of these lines may represent existing or impending spinal cord injury. The distances between two adjacent laminae should be roughly equal.
- **Line 4. Posterior spinous line.** The spinous processes should be approximately evenly spaced. The C7 spinous process is often the largest. A spinous process fracture is not serious if isolated, but it can sometimes involve the lamina and be associated with spinal instability.
- **C1-2 relationship.** The distance between the anterior arch of C1 and the odontoid process should not be greater than 2.5 mm (Fig. 5-1), except in children where up to 5 mm can be normal. If this distance is greater, then disruption of the transverse ligament between C1 and C2 should be suspected.
- **Odontoid view** odontoid process should be centered between the lateral masses of C1, which in turn should be aligned with the lateral masses of C2. The teeth or occipital bone can occasionally cause false fracture lines, which on closer inspection are seen to extend beyond the odontoid. Incorrect positioning such as head rotation can cause apparent asymmetry; repeat the view as necessary.

- **Harris ring.** On lateral radiographs the junction of the central and lateral portions of the C2 body forms two rings that should overlap and be complete except in its inferoposterior border. Disruption of the ring shadow indicates type III odontoid fracture.
- **Disc spaces.** Should not be widened or narrowed. Before attributing disc space narrowing to degenerative arthritis (the most common cause), be sure that associated osteophytes and/or sclerosis are present.
- **Articular processes.** Should overlap on a lateral radiograph. A small nonoverlap seen at multiple adjacent levels can occur in rotated spines. Nonoverlap isolated to one level is suspicious for posterior element fracture.
- **Vertebral body volume and shape.** Should be evaluated to exclude compression. The superior and inferior endplates of each vertebral body should be approximately parallel. The cortical margins should be sharp and unbroken.
- **Anteroposterior view.** The spinous processes should form a straight line at the midline and be approximately evenly spaced. The spinous processes may have a bifid appearance, which is a normal variant. The interpediculate distances should be uniform and unwidened, the uncovertebral joints aligned, and the lateral cortical margins intact. The trachea should be seen as a midline air column; displacement or narrowing of this column may indicate hematoma or edema from injury.
- **Flexion-extension views.** A change in alignment when comparing the flexion view to the one in extension is evidence for ligamentous instability.
- **Oblique views.** The size of the neuroforamina, alignment of all facet joints, and integrity of the pedicles should be evaluated.
- **Pseudosubluxation.** Laxity of the longitudinal ligaments is normally present in children, which causes the body of C2 to appear slightly anteriorly subluxed on C3. Traumatic subluxation can be excluded if the posterior neural arches of C1, C2, and C3 are aligned.

 IMAGING WITH COMPUTED TOMOGRAPHY

Indications. CT should be performed if there is any acute, trauma-related abnormality on the radiographs. As discussed earlier, CT should also be performed if the radiograph findings are negative when there is a high clinical suspicion due to the patient's symptoms or signs and when radiographs are inadequate due to obesity or technical factors. Typically, more fractures will be seen on CT than on the radiographs; reported sensitivities of cervical radiographs in detecting cervical spine pathology range between 74 and 86%, while CT has been shown to detect up to 97–100% of cervical spine fractures.

Protocol. Thin section images with multiplanar reconstructions are required for adequate evaluation of cervical spine. Bone windows (specific bone kernel reconstruction) for osseous injury and soft tissue windows should be reconstructed.

Possible Findings (Fig. 5-3)

- Discontinuity of the neural arch at any of the C-spine levels. This requires following the portions of each neural arch through multiple slices. Be careful not to confuse normal facet joints with fractures and vice versa.
- Discontinuity of the articular facets which could indicate jumped, perched, or locked facets, and commonly associated fractures of the articular masses and laminae.
- Bony fragments in the spinal canal, which can impinge upon the spinal cord.
- Fractures parallel to the axial plane: examination of sagittal and coronal reconstructions can help identify type II odontoid fractures or vertebral body burst fractures.
- Soft tissue hematomas or other abnormalities.
- Skull fractures, specifically the occipital condyles.

 IMAGING WITH MAGNETIC RESONANCE

Indications. Magnetic resonance imaging (MRI) is the test of choice for evaluation of ligamentous injury, cord injury, epidural hematoma, and intervertebral disc herniation.

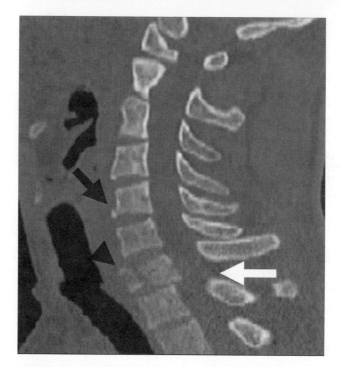

Figure 5-3. Saggital reconstruction of cervical spine computed tomography (CT) demonstrating multiple fractures with disruption of all three columns. There is a burst fracture of C7 (*arrowhead*) with widening of interspinous distance indicating ligamentous rupture (*white arrow*). There is a flexion tear drop fracture of C5 (*black arrow*).

MRI is indicated in evaluating patients with complete, incomplete, or progressive neurologic deficit after cervical spine injury, if feasible given the patient's clinical predicament.

Protocol.   Standard sequences include sagittal and axial T1-weighted spin echo for evaluation of bony anatomy, sagittal T2-weighted spin echo and short inversion time inversion recovery (STIR) to evaluate ligamentous structures and pathologic processes, axial gradient echo sequences to optimize detection of hemorrhage and distinguish osteophytes from disc material.

Possible Findings (Fig. 5-4)

- Ligamentous injuries are associated with soft tissue edema that is best seen on STIR.
- Bone marrow edema has high T2 signal and implies underlying fracture.
- Fracture line can appear as T1 dark line.
- Cortical discontinuity and/or facet subluxation or dislocation.
- Cord edema has high T2 signal.
- Acute cord hemorrhage usually has low T2 signal.

 ISSUES AFTER IMAGING

Emergency treatment of spinal fractures is determined primarily by whether the injury is stable or unstable. Unstable injuries usually require surgical management, especially if there is evidence of spinal cord compression.

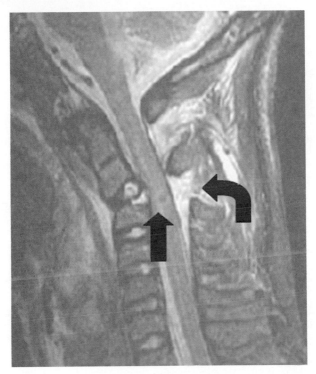

Figure 5-4. Saggital, short inversion time inversion recovery–magnetic resonance imaging (STIR–MRI) image demonstrates cord injury (*straight arrow*) and epidural hematoma (*curved arrow*) in setting of angulated Hangman's fracture. There is also disruption of posterior longitudinal ligament, C2-3 disc, and posterior ligamentous injury with adjacent soft tissue edema.

Further Readings

Berlin L. CT versus radiography for initial evaluation of cervical spine trauma: What is the standard of care? *Am J Roentgenol* 2005;180:911–915.

Blackmore CC. Clinical prediction rules in trauma imaging: Who, how, and why? *Radiology* 2005;235:371–374.

Daffner RH. Helical CT of the cervical spine for trauma patients. *Am J Roentgenol* 2001;177:677–679.

Ferrucci JT. *Radiology: diagnosis, imaging, and intervention.* Philadelphia: Lippincott Williams & Wilkins, 2003. revised ed.

Harris HJ, Harris WH. *The radiology of emergency medicine.* 4th ed. Philadelphia. Lippincott Williams & Wilkins, 2000:437–581.

Helms CA. Trauma. In: Brant WF, Helms CA, eds. *Fundamentals of diagnostic radiology*, 2nd ed. Baltimore: Lippincott Williams & Wilkins, 1999:997–1023.

Li AE, Fishman EK. Cervical spine trauma: Evaluation by multidetector CT and three-dimensional volume rendering. *Emergency Radiology* 2003;10:34–39.

Stuart EM, Kathirkamanthan S. *Imaging in trauma and critical care*, 2nd ed. Philadelphia: Elsevier Science, 2003.

Van Goethem JW, Maes M, Ozsarlak O, et al. Imaging in spinal trauma. *Euro Radiol* 2005;15:582–590.

Watura R, Cobby M, Taylor J. Multislice CT imaging of trauma of the spine, pelvic, and complex foot injuries. *Br J Radiol* 2004;77:46–63.

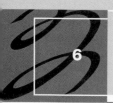

6

THORACOLUMBAR SPINE TRAUMA
David A. Weiland

Epidemiology.   Most thoracolumbar spine injuries occur as a result of motor vehicle accidents, although in the inner-city emergency room gunshot wounds are also very common. With the aging of the adult population, the frequency of compression fractures related even to minor trauma is also increasing.

Location.   Spinal fractures occur most frequently at C1-2, C5-7, and T12-L2. In the thoracolumbar spine, 60% of fractures occur between T12 and L2, with 90% between T11 and L4. The increased susceptibility of the thoracolumbar junction to trauma is thought to result from (1) loss of stabilization from the ribs and thoracic musculature, (2) change of thoracic kyphosis to lumbar lordosis, and (3) change in orientation of the facet joints from coronal to sagittal. In the pediatric population, there is a higher incidence of fractures in the midthoracic and upper lumbar spine.

Classification.   Flexion, compression, and shearing forces predominate in the thoracolumbar spine. The three-column classification system of Denis divides the spine into an anterior column consisting of the anterior longitudinal ligament and the anterior two thirds of the vertebral body and disc, a middle column comprising the posterior one third of the vertebral body and disc and the posterior longitudinal ligament, and a posterior column that includes the remaining posterior elements. Injuries involving more then one column are considered unstable.

A newer classification system has been proposed by Magerl to address some of the shortcomings of the Denis system. In this classification scheme, there are three types (A, B, and C) with subcategories within each group. Type A injuries include compression fractures of the vertebral body. Type B is a distracting injury resulting in disruption of two columns from either a hyperflexion or hyperextension type mechanism. Type C injuries involve a superimposed rotational component on a type B.

Mechanism.   The mechanism of injury is occasionally useful in predicting the type of spine injury. For example, a patient with a lap belt injury should be carefully evaluated for a possible Chance fracture; a patient with calcaneal fractures who jumped from a height should be examined for vertebral body compression fractures in the lower thoracic and lumbar spine. Upper thoracic spine trauma requires considerable force because of its inherent stability, and 17% of these injuries are associated with other noncontiguous spinal fractures. When injury does occur in this region, there is a very high incidence of associated spinal cord injury, which is probably related to the narrow spinal canal in the upper thoracic spine.

Complications.   Neurologic injury occurs in two thirds of burst fractures and three fourths of fracture-dislocations. Magnetic resonance imaging (MRI) is the best method for evaluation of cord injury, ideally performed within 24–48 hours of injury. Cord edema has a relatively good prognosis and demonstrates normal T1 signal and increased T2 signal. Cord hemorrhage has a poor prognosis and demonstrates abnormal signal of both T1 and T2 weighted images. Kummell's disease is delayed posttraumatic vertebral body collapse. It can follow minimal trauma without overt fracture and is thought to be a form of avascular necrosis.

Differential Diagnosis. Upper thoracic spine fractures can demonstrate mediastinal widening, an apical pleural cap, pleural effusion, paraparesis, or paraplegia—all of which are also seen with aortic transection.

 IMAGING WITH RADIOGRAPHS

Indications. Radiographs are still the first line in the diagnosis of thoracolumbar trauma at most institutions. Obtaining good quality images can be a problem in an acutely injured patient, and the lateral spine views are notoriously difficult to obtain with the upper thoracic vertebrae almost always being obscured. Therefore, it is not unusual that the diagnosis is made on the basis of the anteroposterior (AP) films alone.

Possible Findings

- Paraspinal soft tissue swelling.
- Pleural effusion.
- Abnormal kyphosis.
- Posterior rib fractures.
- Widening of the interpedicular distance.
- Disruption or bulging of the posterior vertebral body line.
- Anterior vertebral body wedging.
- Indistinct endplates.
- Loss of height of vertebral bodies and discs.
- Increased or decreased distance between adjacent spinous processes.
- Fractures through the pedicles on the AP view (Chance fracture).

 IMAGING WITH COMPUTED TOMOGRAPHY

Indications. Computed tomography (CT) should be performed if there is any acute, trauma-related abnormality on the radiographs. CT should also be performed if the radiographs are negative when there is a high clinical suspicion due to the patient's symptoms or signs. The sensitivity of CT in detecting unstable fractures varies between 97 and 100% whereas the sensitivity of plain radiographs is 33–57%.

Protocol. Thin section images with multiplanar reconstructions are required for adequate evaluation of thoracolumbar spine. Bone windows (specific bone kernel reconstruction) for osseous injury and soft tissue windows should be reconstructed.

Possible Findings (Figs. 6-1 and 6-2)

- Discontinuity of the neural arch.
- Discontinuity of the articular facets.
- Bony fragments in the spinal canal, which can impinge upon the spinal cord.
- Posterior rib fractures.
- Soft tissue hematomas or other abnormalities.

 IMAGING WITH MAGNETIC RESONANCE

Indications. MRI is the test of choice for evaluation of ligamentous injury, cord injury, epidural hematoma, and intervertebral disc herniation. MRI is indicated in evaluating patients with complete, incomplete, or progressive neurologic deficit after spine injury, if feasible given the patient's clinical predicament.

Protocol. Standard sequences include sagittal and axial T1-weighted spin echo for evaluation of bony anatomy, sagittal and axial T2-weighted spin echo, and short inversion time inversion recovery (STIR) to evaluate ligamentous structures and pathologic processes.

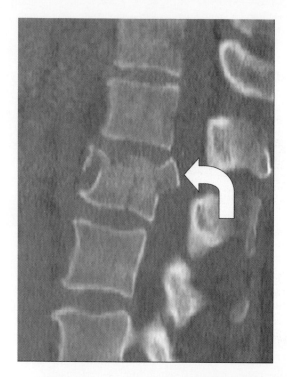

Figure 6-1. Sagittal reconstruction of lumbar spine computed tomographic (CT) scan demonstrating L1 burst fracture with fragment retropulsion into the central canal (*curved arrow*).

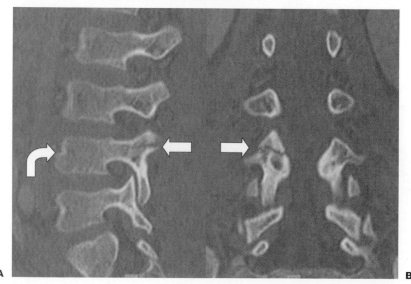

A   B

Figure 6-2. **A:** Sagittal and **(B)** coronal reconstruction of lumbar spine computed tomographic (CT) scan demonstrating chance fracture of L4 involving vertebral body (*curved arrow*) and posterior elements (*straight arrows*).

Possible Findings

- Ligamentous tears demonstrate high T2 signal, best seen on sagittal STIR.
- Bone marrow edema has high T2 signal and implies underlying fracture.
- Fracture line can appear as T1 dark line.
- Cortical discontinuity and or facet subluxation or dislocation.
- Cord edema has high T2 signal.
- Cord hemorrhage can have high T1 signal.

 COMMON FRACTURE TYPES

Wedge Compression Fractures

Frequency. Most common injury, representing 50% of thoracolumbar spine fractures.

Mechanism. Forward flexion about the axis of the middle column with an element of axial compression.

Possible Findings

- Anterior wedging or depression of superior or inferior endplate
- Normal height of the posterior vertebral cortex is maintained.
- In osteoporotic spines this fracture may be more comminuted.

Stability. Stable because the middle and posterior columns are intact.

Differential Diagnosis

- Old osteoporotic compression fracture. Look for soft tissue swelling and cortical disruption in acute wedge fractures.
- Compression fracture due to vertebral body metastasis. MRI can be helpful in distinguishing these possibilities.
  - Complete marrow replacement which is best seen as low signal on T1-weighted MRI images involving the entire vertebral body. Contrast-enhanced images can confuse diagnosis because enhancing metastasis can appear similar to normal fatty marrow.
  - Convex posterior border, unlike osteoporosis or trauma-related compression fractures which tend to have sharp angles.

Burst Fractures

Frequency. Fourteen percent of spinal fractures, two thirds will have associated neurologic deficit.

Mechanism. Axial compression with some element of flexion.

Possible Findings

- Comminuted fracture involving superior, inferior, or both endplates and extending backward to the posterior vertebral margin which is often associated with retropulsion of bone fragments into the spinal canal.
- Radiographs can show (1) anterior wedging, (2) sagittal fracture line through the vertebral body on the AP view, (3) widening of interpedicular distance, and (4) loss of continuity or malalignment of the posterior vertebral body line on the lateral view.
- Always obtain CT to locate fragments. There is relatively poor correlation between CT findings and extent of neurologic deficits, probably because CT only demonstrates the final position of the fragment and not the maximum displacement at the time of injury.

Stability. Always unstable because these fractures always involve the anterior and middle columns, sometimes the posterior column.

Chance Fractures

Frequency.   Five percent of spinal fractures, frequently associated with lap belts, often have associated abdominal injuries.

Mechanism.   Hyperflexion about an axis located anteriorly, related to the lap belt. The entire spine is subject to tension stress, with distraction of posterior elements predominating.

Possible Findings

■ Classic fracture consists of a horizontal component through the posterior arch and pedicles extending into the posterior vertebral body; however, more than one level can be involved, or the injury can be entirely ligamentous. Mild anterior compression may also be seen.
■ Radiographs can show (1) well-defined fracture through posterior elements on lateral view, (2) minimal vertebral body compression, (3) "empty" vertebral body on AP view because of disruption and angulation of posterior elements, (4) pedicle or spinous process fracture on AP view, and (5) increased or decreased distance between adjacent spinous processes on AP view.
■ Always obtain CT to definitively access extent of fracture, presence of spinal canal compromise, and soft tissue injury.

Stability.   Unstable because of disruption of the posterior and middle columns.

Fracture-Dislocation

Frequency.   Sixteen percent of spinal fractures, neurologic deficit in 75%.

Mechanism.   Flexion, axial compression, and shear stress.

Possible Findings

■ Anterior displacement of spine above level of injury with variable degree of anterior wedging below. Posterior column injuries include tears of interspinous ligaments, disruption of facet joints, fractures of laminae and facets, and perched or locked facets.
■ CT is essential to evaluate position of articular facets and extent of spinal canal compromise.

Stability.   Unstable because of failure of all three columns.

Gunshot Wound

Mechanism.   Disruption of bone by projectile.

Possible Findings

If radiographs or clinical examination suggests spinal injury, CT is indicated to look for fractures and to locate bullet fragments.

Stability.   Although fractures are frequently seen in gunshot injuries, the fractures are usually a minor component of the total injury and the spine is seldom unstable.

 ISSUES AFTER IMAGING

Emergency treatment of spinal fractures is determined primarily by whether the injury is stable or unstable. Unstable injuries usually require surgical management, especially if there is evidence of spinal cord compression. Gunshot injuries to the spine are treated as open wounds of the spinal cord or dura.

Further Readings

Brandser EA, El-Khoury GY. Thoracic and lumbar spine trauma. *Radiol Clin North Am* 1997;35(3):533–557.

Denis F. The three column spine and its significance in the classification of acute throcacolumbar spinal injuries. *Spine* 1983;8:817–831.

Gray L, Vandermark R, Hays M. Thoracic and lumbar spine trauma. *SeminUltrasound CT MR* 2001;22(2):125–134.

Herzog C, Ahle H, Mack MG, et al. Traumatic injuries of the pelvis and thoracic and lumbar spine: Does thin-slice multidetector-row CT increase diagnostic accuracy? *Eur Radiol* 2004;14:1751–1760.

Magerl F, Aebi M, Gertzbein SD, et al. A comprehensive classification of thoracic and lumbar spine injuries. *Eur Spine J* 1994;3:184–201.

Oner FC, van Gils AP, Dhert WJ, et al. MRI findings of thoracolumbar spine fractures: A categorization based on MRI examinations of 100 fractures. *Skeletal Radiol* 1999;28(8):433–443.

Oner FC, Ramos LMP, Simmermacher RKJ, et al. Classification of thoracic and lumbar spine fractures: Problems of reproducibility. A study of 53 patients using CT and MRI. *Eur Spine J* 2002;11:235–245.

Roos JE, Hilfiker P, Platz A, et al. MDCT in emergency radiology: Is a standardized chest or abdominal protocol sufficient for evaluation of thoracic and lumbar spine trauma? *Am J Roentgenol* 2004;183(4):959–968.

Sledge JB, Allred D, Heyman J. Use of magnetic resonance imaging in evaluating injuries to the pediatric thoracolumbar spine. *J Pediatr Orthop* 2001;21(3):288–293.

Wintermark M, Mouhsine E, Theumann N, et al. Thoracolumbar spine fractures in patients who have sustained severe trauma: Depiction with multi-detector row CT. *Radiology* 2003;227:681–689.

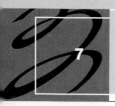

SOFT TISSUES INJURY OF THE NECK
Oleg M. Teytelboym and Kevin A. Smith

Penetrating and blunt (nonpenetrating) neck trauma can cause injury to any of the vital structures (in order of frequency): (1) great vessels, (2) larynx and trachea, (3) pharynx and esophagus, (4) spinal cord and brachial plexus, and (5) thoracic duct. If physical examination reveals clear signs of injury to one of these structures, immediate surgical exploration and repair is usually indicated. Patients who are asymptomatic can often be evaluated with noninvasive tests.

 ANATOMY

- Lateral neck is divided by the sternocleidomastoid muscle into an anterior and posterior triangle.
- Anterior triangle is the most common site of penetrating injury of the neck. Penetrating wounds into the anterior triangle can injure the internal and external carotid arteries, the jugular vein, and the vagus nerve.
- Wounds in the posterior triangle are often less associated with serious visceral and vascular injuries, unless they are located inferiorly, where injuries can involve the internal jugular vein, phrenic nerve, brachial plexus, and subclavian arteries and veins.
- Anterior neck describes injuries near the anterior midline, where the trachea and esophagus are most susceptible.
- The neck can be divided into three zones on the basis of the site of injury. Zone of injury has significant implications for patient management.
- **Zone I.** Below the sternal notch can be fatal due to injury of great vessels and esophagus. These injuries may be clinically silent requiring thorough evaluation of every patient regardless of symptoms.
- **Zone II.** Above the sternal notch and below the angle of the mandible. Zone II is the most frequent site of injury. Older surgical literature suggested surgical evaluation of any injury that penetrated the platysma. Modern protocols increasingly rely on noninvasive testing to avoid surgery in asymptomatic patients.
- **Zone III.** Above the angle of the mandible. Penetrating injuries can result in injury of major blood vessels and cranial nerves. Up to 25% of patients with significant arterial trauma are asymptomatic at presentation. Routine surgical exploration is not feasible due to the complex anatomy in this zone.

 CLINICAL INFORMATION

Symptoms and Signs. Most laryngotracheal injuries cause acute symptoms and physical findings, whereas vascular and pharyngoesophageal injuries are more often occult on initial presentation. Penetrating projectiles are associated with a higher incidence of severe injury than stab wounds.

- Vascular injury, pulsatile arterial bleeding, hematoma, diminished distal arterial pulsation, bruit, unexplained shock, and neurologic changes are indicative of an ischemic or embolic event. Brain infarction and hemorrhage are major sequelae and may occur acutely or remotely after the injury.

■ Aerodigestive injury, stridor, dysphonia, aphonia, hemoptysis, and subcutaneous emphysema are among the most common findings in airway (laryngotracheal) injury. Hematemesis, dysphagia, odynophagia (pain on swallowing), subcutaneous emphysema, hydropneumothorax, and widened mediastinum suggest an injury to the esophagus or pharynx.

Penetrating Injury Management Protocol

■ Twenty-five percent of patients with penetrating injury to the neck will have arterial injury.
■ Hypotensive shock requires immediate surgery.
■ Symptoms of vascular or aerodigestive injury require surgical explorations. However, patients with zone I and III injuries should undergo conventional or computed tomographic angiography (CTA) before surgery.
■ Asymptomatic patients are usually evaluated with CTA and clinical observation. Patients with zone I injuries require esophageal evaluation with endoscopy and or contrast esophagram.

Nonpenetrating Trauma

■ Results in arterial injury in less than 1% of cases.
■ Arterial dissection or pseudoaneurysm can result from blunt trauma or hyperextension/rotational injuries.
■ Basilar skull fractures may disrupt the intrapetrous portion of the carotid artery.
■ Injury to cavernous carotid artery can result in carotid cavernous fistula.
■ Cervical spine fractures with disruption of foramen transversarium should be evaluated for vertebral artery injury.

 ARTERIAL INJURY

Most Common Location

■ **Carotid:** cervical internal carotid artery (ICA) just below skull base. The dissection usually does not extend intracranially because petrous carotid is anchored to periosteum.
■ **Vertebral:** above C2.

Possible Findings (Figs. 7-1 and 7-2)

■ **Digital subtraction angiography (DSA).** Gold standard for evaluation of vascular injury. Can detect injuries missed out with CTA.
  • Tapered irregular luminal stenosis extending to skull base.
  • Pseudoaneurysm.
  • Arteriovenous fistula (carotid cavernous sinus fistula > vertebral artery fistula > external carotid fistula).
■ **CTA:** Usually the test of choice given the high accuracy and ready availability.
  • Intimal flap/dissection.
  • Pseudoaneurysm.
  • Irregular vessel contour.
  • Intramural hematoma.
  • Three-dimensional (3D) reconstructions are often useful in establishing the diagnosis and explaining imaging findings to the referring clinicians in a comprehensive manner.
■ **Ultrasonography:** rarely performed because superior portion of internal carotid cannot be evaluated.
  • Echogenic intimal flap.
  • Doppler evaluation may show velocity elevation due to narrowing of vessel lumen by dissection. High resistance waveform can be present with near occlusion.
■ **Magnetic resonance imaging (MRI):** not practical for acute trauma due to logistic constraints, such as the need for rapid availability and the presence of patient monitoring equipment.

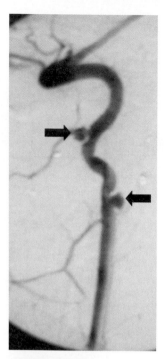

Figure 7-1. Digital subtraction angiogram showing multiple pseudoaneurysms (*arrows*) of a vertebral artery in a patient after gunshot wounds to the neck.

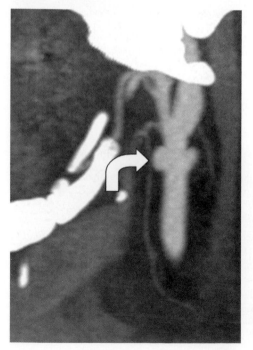

Figure 7-2. Carotid computed tomographic angiography (CTA) demonstrates pseudoaneurysms of common carotid artery (*arrow*) after stab wound to the neck.

- Intimal flap: flowing blood (in the true and false lumens) will manifest signal void on spin- echo sequences, and as high signal on black-blood sequences. It may be difficult to distinguish thrombus from slowly flowing blood in the false lumen.
- Intramural hematoma has high T1 signal and absence of normal flow void on T2-weighted imaging (T2-WI) sequence.
- Lumen narrowing on magnetic resonance angiography (MRA). Postgadolinium MRA is preferred to time of flight techniques because of decreased motion artifact.

Pitfalls

■ CTA may be limited because of dental artifacts, bullet fragments, and technical factors such as poor contrast opacification and venous contamination. Have a low threshold for recommending DSA when CTA is suspicious or limited.

 ## LARYNGOTRACHEAL INJURY

■ Can result from automobile accidents, assault, attempted strangulation, gunshot, and stab wounds.
■ Flexible endoscopy is usually the study of choice.
■ Computed tomography (CT) can be helpful in evaluating the location and extent of injury where endoscopy is not feasible.

 ## PHARYNGOESOPHAGEAL INJURY

■ Pharyngoesophageal injuries should always be suspected when there are injuries to nearby structures. Early identification of esophageal injuries is especially important to reduce subsequent mortality.
■ Contrast esophagram (should performed with water soluble contrast) is both sensitive and specific for detecting esophageal perforation and is the study of choice if the patient can tolerate the study. Endoscopy is equally accurate and is the study of choice in intubated patients.

Further Readings

Dahnert Wolfgang. *Radiology review manual*, 5th ed. Philadelphia: Lippincott Williams & Wilkins, 2003.
Grossman RI, Yousem DM. *Neuroradiology: the requisites*, 2nd ed. Philadelphia: Mosby, 2003.
Mirvis S, Shanmuganathan K. *Imaging in trauma and critical care*, 2nd ed. Philadelphia: WB Saunders, 2003.

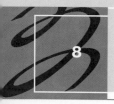

8

INTRACRANIAL INFECTIONS
Bradley R. Foerster and Myria Petrou

 ## MENINGITIS

Etiology and presentation. Leptomeningeal inflammation most often occurs after hematogenous spread of bacteria. In the early phase, the pia and arachnoid matter become congested and hyperemic. Later, the leptomeninges becomes thickened and an exudate can cover the brain particularly in the dependent regions such as the basal cisterns. Inflammatory changes can interfere with cerebrospinal fluid (CSF) drainage, potentially causing hydrocephalus. Infants can have a varied clinical picture including mental status changes, fever, irritability, and vomiting. Adults have a more typical presentation with symptoms including fever, headache, meningismus, and photophobia. Bacterial meningitis is a clinical diagnosis based on history and physical examination and confirmed by CSF laboratory testing. Imaging is important to exclude a mass lesion, other potential diagnoses, and to look for potential complications of meningitis.

Differential diagnosis includes migraine, subarachnoid hemorrhage, brain abscess, subdural empyema, and viral encephalitis.

Complications

- Hydrocephalus is the most common complication and results from disruption of CSF resorption or obstruction.
- Spread of infection may cause brain abscess and subdural empyema (see subsequent text).
- Infarction from vasculitis, arterial ischemia, or venous thrombosis.
- Ventriculitis is a possible complication of meningitis. Ventricles are enlarged with surrounding high T2 signal and subependymal enhancement.
- Permanent neurologic deficits and death (in 10 to 30% of patients with bacterial meningitis).

Cerebrospinal Fluid Evaluation

Noncontrast head computed tomography (CT) is usually performed before lumbar puncture (LP) to exclude a mass lesion despite lack of evidence to support the routine use of this practice. Obtaining the head CT should not delay the LP and initiation of antibiotic therapy. CSF is sent for protein and glucose concentrations, cell count, Gram stain, and culture.
    CSF findings in different types of infection are given in Table 8-1.

Possible Findings (Fig. 8-1)

- Normal imaging is the most common finding in early meningitis.
- Enhancement of the leptomeninges is better seen on magnetic resonance (MR) than on CT.
- Enlargement of CSF spaces, particularly in the basal cisterns and interhemispheric fissure.
- High intensity of subarachnoid fluid on fluid attenuation inversion recovery (FLAIR) imaging.
- Communicating hydrocephalus with enlargement of temporal horns and effacement of basal cisterns.

	Bacterial	Viral	Tuberculosis	Fungal
TABLE 8-1		**Cerebrospinal Fluid Findings in Infections**		
Cell type	PMNs	Lymphocytes	Lymphocytes	Mixed
Protein	High	Normal to mildly high	Normal to high	Normal to high
Glucose	Low	Normal to mildly low	Normal to mildly low	Normal to mildly low
PMN, polymorphonuclear.				

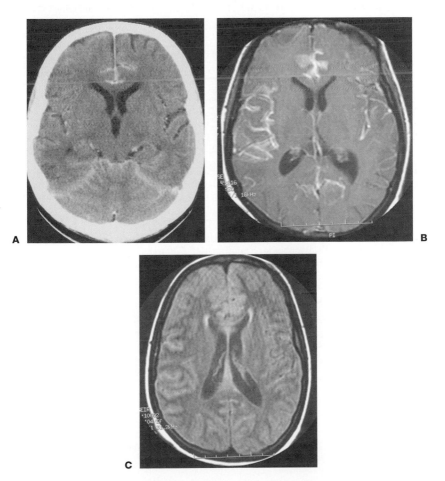

Figure 8-1. Meningitis on computed tomography (CT) and magnetic resonance imaging (MRI). **A:** Contrast-enhanced axial CT and **(B)** postcontrast axial MRI images demonstrate diffuse leptomeningeal enhancement. **C:** Axial fluid attenuation inversion recovery (FLAIR) image on MRI demonstrates bright cerebrospinal fluid (CSF) signal in the subarachnoid spaces.

- Brain infarct.
- Cerebral edema/inflammation (cerebritis).

Pitfalls

- Diffuse pachymeningeal enhancement can occur with intracranial hypotension following LP.

 BRAIN PARENCHYMAL ABSCESS

Etiology and presentation.   Cerebral abscesses are most commonly caused by hematogenous dissemination. Brain abscesses can be divided into four stages: (1) early cerebritis (1 to 3 days), (2) late cerebritis (4 to 9 days), (3) early capsule formation (10 to 13 days), and (4) late capsule formation (>13 days). Magnetic resonance imaging (MRI) is the study of choice for diagnosis of brain abscesses.

Possible Findings

- **Noncontrast CT**
  - Low-density abnormalities with mass effect and surrounding edema.
- **Contrast-enhanced CT**
  - Uniform ring enhancement is virtually always present in later phases.
- **MRI**
  - Early phase can have patchy enhancement, low T1 signal, and high T2 signal.
  - Later phase is characterized by development of ring enhancement.
  - The abscess typically has low T1 and high T2 signal with surrounding edema, which has high T2 signal.
  - Restricted diffusion (bright signal on diffusion weighted imaging [DWI] and low signal on apparent diffusion coefficient [ADC] map) helps differentiate abscesses from necrotic neoplasms (usually not restricted), however not all abscesses follow this rule.

Pitfalls

- Ring enhancement is nonspecific. Differential diagnosis includes neoplasm, tumefactive multiple sclerosis, lymphoma, hematoma, and infarct. Thickness, irregularity, and nodularity of the enhancing ring suggest tumor (majority of cases) or fungus.

 HERPES SIMPLEX

Etiology and presentation.   Herpes simplex virus (HSV) is the most common cause of fatal endemic encephalitis. Both type 1 and type 2 viruses produce encephalitis. Type 1 affects children and adults, and presents with viral prodrome, seizures, fever, headache, and mental status changes. Type 2 infection occurs during the neonatal period. Mortality due to HSV encephalitis is reduced from approximately 75% to 25% with early diagnosis and prompt acyclovir therapy.

Possible Findings (Fig. 8-2)

- Type 1 (children and adults)
  - **CT**
    - Findings are subtle with lower density areas in the swollen temporal lobe and insular cortex.
    - Hemorrhage is uncommon.
  - **MRI**
    - High signal on T2-weighted imaging with predilection for limbic system (temporal lobes, cingulate gyri, inferior frontal lobes).
    - Restricted diffusion (bright signal on DWI and low signal on ADC map).
    - Enhancement is usually gyriform.

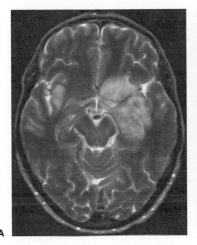
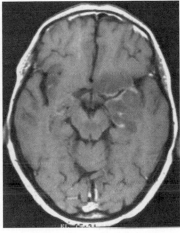

A   B

Figure 8-2. Herpes encephalitis on magnetic resonance imaging (MRI). **A:** Axial T2-weighted MRI demonstrates increased signal in bilateral temporal lobes. **B:** Axial postcontrast T1-weighted MRI demonstrates enhancement in bilateral temporal lobes.

■ Type 2 (neonates)
  • Subtle regions of low density on CT in various regions of the brain with subsequent enlargement, and meningeal and gyriform enhancement.
  • Calcification can be seen several weeks after disease onset.
  • Thalamic hemorrhage is possible.

Pitfalls

■ MR findings in type 2 HSV can have limited sensitivity. Normal neonatal findings of low T1 signal of white matter and high T2 signal limit sensitivity. Loss of gray-white matter differentiation which can be an early finding of this disease can be incorrectly interpreted as poor quality images.

 TUBERCULOSIS

Etiology and presentation. Tuberculosis has made a comeback in recent years with the advent of acquired immunodeficiency syndrome (AIDS) and drug-resistant strains. Patients can present with tuberculous meningitis, intracranial tuberculoma, or both (10% of patients). The initial focus of infection is usually pulmonary with secondary hematogenous spread. Tuberculomas have varied clinical course ranging from complete resolution to rupture with meningoencephalitis. Patients present with confusion, fevers, headache, lethargy, and meningismus. Symptoms can progress to stupor, coma, decerebrate rigidity, cranial nerve palsy, and stroke. There is no evidence of extracranial active disease in 19% of patients.

Possible Findings

■ **CT**
  • Basal and sylvian cisterns poorly visualized without contrast because of dense exudates, which can subsequently enhance with contrast.
  • Tuberculomas appear as low to high density nodules on CT.
■ **MRI**
  • High FLAIR signal in basal cisterns secondary to proteinaceous exudate.
  • Cisterns can demonstrate enhancement extending over cortical surfaces.

- Noncaseating tuberculomas often have high signal on T2-weighted imaging with nodular enhancement.
- Caseating tuberculomas have isosignal or low signal on T2-weighted imaging and ring enhancement.
- Hydrocephalus and infarction secondary to arteritis are sequelae of central nervous system (CNS) tuberculosis.

 CYSTICERCOSIS

Etiology and presentation.   Cysticercosis is the most common CNS infection worldwide and the most common cause of epilepsy. This parasite is endemic in Mexico, South America, Asia, Africa, and Eastern Europe and is acquired by ingestion of undercooked pork. The larvae develop into tapeworm in the gastrointestinal tract and then enter the blood stream to spread to other regions including the CNS. Patients are typically asymptomatic until the larvae die inciting an acute inflammatory reaction. The most common neurologic symptom is seizure. The larvae progress through different stages with varying degrees of edema and enhancement.

Possible Findings

■ **CT**
- Characteristic calcifications in the brain parenchyma which are slightly off-center spherical in shape.

■ **MRI**
- Multiple cysts with changing signal characteristics as the larvae progress through different stages.
- Hydrocephalus can occur with meningeal involvement.

 COCCIDIOIDOMYCOSIS

Etiology and presentation.   Coccidioidomycosis is an endemic fungus present in southwestern United States and Mexico. The spore is inhaled causing a primary pulmonary infection which can then be hematogenously spread. Thick basilar meningitis with meningeal and parenchymal granulomas can then ensue.

Possible Findings

■ Poor visualization of basal and sylvian cisterns on noncontrast CT secondary to dense exudate, which may show increased density.
■ Hydrocephalus and enhancing nodules are occasionally seen.

 EPIDURAL ABSCESS AND SUBDURAL EMPYEMA

Extra-axial infectious collections of the brain are more common in children than adults and are usually secondary to spread of infection from the paranasal sinuses and mastoids.

Possible Findings (Fig. 8-3)

■ Opacification of the sinuses and mastoids with or without bone defect.
■ Slightly hypoattenuating, partially enhancing subdural or epidural collection. Restricted diffusion on DWI.
■ Brain edema.
■ Dural sinus thrombosis.

 SPINAL EPIDURAL ABSCESS

Etiology and presentation.   Spinal epidural abscesses result from either hematogenous spread or direct extension from adjacent vertebral osteomyelitis, with *Staphylococcus*

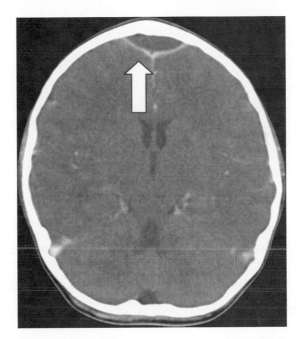

Figure 8-3. Epidural abscess on axial contrast-enhanced computed tomography (CT) demonstrates with extra-axial rim enhancing collection crossing midline in a patient with orbital cellulitis.

being the most common pathogen (45%). Patients present with fever, elevated white cell counts, back pain, spine tenderness, and progressive neurologic deficits. Risk factors include immunosuppression, intravenous drug abuse, concurrent infection, and prior hematoma due to blunt trauma. The thoracic spine is most commonly involved. MRI is the study of choice.

Possible Findings

■ **MRI**
- Epidural mass with low T1 signal compared to the spinal cord and high T2 signal.
- The mass can have diffuse enhancement, representing early phlegmon, peripheral enhancement representing frank abscess formation or have a combined pattern.
- Changes in the adjacent disk spaces and vertebrae (low T1, high T2 and enhancement) indicate coexisting discitis/osteomyelitis.

 HUMAN IMMUNODEFICIENCY VIRUS AND THE IMMUNOCOMPROMISED PATIENT

Etiology and presentation. HIV is a retrovirus infecting the brain in 30 to 80% of all patients with AIDS. This disease has become much less common with antiretroviral therapy. The virus causes subacute encephalitis and a syndrome of progressive dementia with cognitive, motor, and behavioral abnormalities. Pathology shows microglial nodules and multinucleated cells in the white matter.

Possible Findings

■ **CT**
- Frequently unremarkable.
- Progressive brain atrophy.

■ **MRI**
- Bilateral patchy and confluent high T2 signal changes in the white matter predominately affecting frontal and parietal lobes.
- No contrast enhancement.
- Progressive brain atrophy.

Complications

■ Progressive multifocal leukoencephalopathy (PML) which is caused by the JC papovirus. High T2 signal in the bilateral white matter typically affecting occipital and parietal lobes. No mass effect and no contrast enhancement.

■ Meningitis including cryptococcosis, toxoplasmosis, tuberculosis, and cytomegalovirus (CMV) infections.

■ Infarction which can be caused by vasculitis, medications, infection, and endocarditis. Can produce high T1 signal in basal ganglia.

■ Mass lesions including lymphoma and toxoplasmosis.

 HERPES ZOSTER

Etiology and presentation.   Herpes varicella zoster virus affects the elderly and immunocompromised patients. It is caused by reactivation of latent varicella zoster virus that has remained dormant in cranial nerve and dorsal root ganglia. It can occur without a rash and presents with headache, altered mental status, neurologic deficit, and CSF pleocytosis.

Possible Findings

■ **CT**
- Low-density regions with mass effect.
■ **MRI**
- High signal regions on T2-weighted imaging.
- Gyriform enhancement in the segmental distribution of vasculitis.

 ASPERGILLOSIS

Etiology and presentation.   Aspergillus primarily infects immunocompromised hosts and gains entry either from direct extension of the sinuses or hematogenously. Aspergillosis produces meningitis and meningoencephalitis with subsequent hemorrhagic infarction. Patients present with confusion, fever, headache, lethargy, and meningismus. Symptoms can progress to stupor, coma, decerebrate rigidity, cranial nerve palsy, and stroke. Aspergillus is angioinvasive with mortality exceeding 85%.

Possible Findings

■ Predilection for basal ganglia and corpus callosum.
■ **CT**
- Abnormalities are usually subtle with varying densities and minimal mass effect.
- Poor contrast enhancement and no ring formation.
■ **MRI**
- High signal lesions on T2-weighted imaging and at times on T1-weighted imaging.
- Enhancement depends on immune status.

 TOXOPLASMOSIS

Etiology and presentation.   Toxoplasmosis is a commonly found protozoan parasite and typically affects immunocompromised patients as they experience reactivation of latent infection. Toxoplasmosis is the most common mass lesion in AIDS patients, affecting up to 10% of this population. Toxoplasmosis can cause vascular thrombosis resulting in infarction or abscess formation.

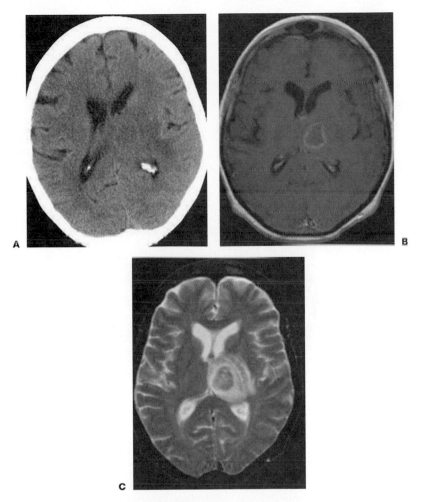

Figure 8-4. Toxoplasmosis on computed tomography (CT) and magnetic resonance imaging (MRI). **A:** Noncontrast-enhanced axial CT demonstrates low-density lesion in the left thalamus with mass effect and surrounding edema. **B:** Postcontrast axial MRI demonstrates ring enhancement of the lesion. **C:** Axial T2-weighted image on MRI demonstrates surrounding edema.

Possible Findings (Fig. 8-4)

- Multiple abscess formation with propensity for basal ganglia, corticomedullary junction, white matter, or periventricular region.
- CT
  - Areas of low density with little/no enhancement or isodense nodules that enhance.
- MRI
  - Multiple high T2-weighted signal lesions with vasogenic edema.
  - Ring or nodular enhancement.

Pitfalls

- Appearance overlaps with lymphoma. High density masses on noncontrast CT and periventricular lesions with subependymal spread suggest lymphoma. Thallium-201 single photon emission computed tomography (SPECT) and fluorodeoxyglucose positron emission tomography (FDG-PET) have been shown to have increased uptake in lymphoma but not toxoplasmosis. MR spectroscopy shows markedly elevated lactate and lipid concentration in toxoplasmosis; lymphoma has moderately increased lactate and lipid levels and markedly increased choline (Cho).

CRYPTOCOCCOSIS

Etiology and presentation.   Cryptococcus is a yeast with a polysaccharide capsule that stains with Indian ink. Eleven percent of patients with AIDS develop cryptococcosis which ranks third behind HIV and toxoplasmosis as the cause of infection in those patients. Pathologic findings include meningitis, meningoencephalitis, or granuloma formation.

Possible Findings

- MRI findings can be normal.
- Dilated Virchow-Robin spaces in young immunocompromised patients represent gelatinous cysts which may or may not enhance.
- Multiple enhancing parenchymal and leptomeningeal nodules with involvement of the choroid plexus and spinal cord. In contrast, Tb and bacterial meningitis have diffuse confluent leptomeningeal enhancement.
- Basal ganglia lesions: differential includes toxoplasmosis and lymphoma.

MUCORMYCOSIS

Etiology and presentation.   Mucor is an inhaled fungus and affects patients with altered cellular immunity. Diabetic patients are particularly susceptible to this infection as are AIDS patients. Mucor usually spreads from the paranasal sinuses into the skull base or cribriform plate affecting orbits, frontal lobes, and basal ganglia. Clinical symptoms include facial pain, bloody nasal discharge, chemosis, exophthalmos, cranial nerve palsy progressing rapidly to stroke, encephalitis, and death.

Possible Findings

- CT
  - Rim of soft tissue thickness along walls of paranasal sinuses.
- MRI
  - Low intensity of the sinuses may be present on T1-weighted and T2-weighted imaging.
  - Orbital extension from the ethmoid sinuses produces proptosis, chemosis, superior ophthalmic vein thrombosis, extension through orbital apex, and subsequent thrombosis of cavernous sinus.
  - Proliferates along vascular structures producing arteritis, pseudoaneurysm, abscess formation, and infarction.

CANDIDIASIS

Candida has a propensity for neutropenic patients receiving steroids. Imaging findings include hydrocephalus, enhancing nodules (granulomas) with edema, infarction, and abscess formation.

NORCARDIOSIS

Nocardia is associated with a compromised immune system. Brain abscess occurs due to hematogenous spread typically from pulmonary focus. An enhancing capsule is common. Meningitis is rare.

Further Readings

Bradley GW, Daroff RD, Renichel GM, eds. *Neurology in clinical practice*, 3rd ed. Woburn: Butterworth-Heinemann, 2000.

Castillo M. *Neuroradiology*, 1st ed. Philadephia: Lippincott Williams & Wilkins, 2002.

Grossman RI, Yousem DM. *Neuroradiology: the requisites*, 2nd ed. Philadephia: Mosby, 2003.

Levy AD, Koeller KK, Chung EM, eds. *Radiologic pathology*, 4th ed. Washington, DC: Armed Forces Institute of Pathology, 2005.

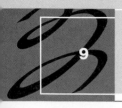

ORBITAL AND PERIORBITAL INFECTION

David J. Grelotti and Nafi Aygun

Anatomy. The orbits are conical in shape and contain the globes, cranial and autonomic nerves, extraocular muscles, vessels, lacrimal gland and tear ducts, and fat and connective tissue. Seven bones make up the orbit and the periosteum of these bones borders the orbit. An extension of the periosteum, the orbital septum, covers the anterior margin of the orbit and attaches over the front of the tarsal plates. The periosteum and orbital septum together form a relative barrier against the spread of infection into the orbit. An inflammatory process is described as either periorbital or preseptal if it is localized to the skin and subcutaneous areas of the eyelid (i.e., anterior to the septum). An inflammatory process within the orbit is described as either orbital or postseptal (i.e., posterior to the septum).

Pathophysiology. Despite the barrier formed by the periosteum and septum, infection still reaches the intraorbital space. The most common origin is from the paranasal sinuses, with extension occurring through numerous tiny foramina in the lamina papyracea that separate the orbits from the ethmoid sinuses. Additionally, an extensive venous system surrounds the orbit and consists of valveless veins that can serve as conduits for infection into the orbit from the paranasal sinuses as well as from the soft tissues of the face. In a similar manner, infection can be transmitted from the orbit into the intracranial compartment, which is often catastrophic. Less commonly, orbital and periorbital infections can occur secondary to trauma, foreign bodies, or bacteremia. Detecting extension into the subperiosteal or postseptal space is important in that surgical intervention may be required, whereas preseptal cellulitis typically responds to antibiotics.

 CLINICAL INFORMATION

Clinical Presentation. Infections involving the region of the orbit occur most commonly in children. Periorbital cellulitis is more common than orbital cellulitis (90% versus 10%) and is unilateral 90% of the time.

- Periorbital cellulitis occurs at any age group without gender preference but is more common in children with a mean age of 21 months. It is caused by infection with *Staphylococcus aureus* or group A *Streptococcus* secondary to trauma (e.g., insect bites) or caused by infection with *Streptococcus pneumoniae* secondary to bacteremia. It is characterized by soft tissue swelling, often involving the eyelid, with associated erythema, warmth, and tenderness. There is no proptosis, chemosis, or decreased ocular motility.
- Orbital cellulitis occurs in older children and adults. It can occasionally be the result of infection after penetrating trauma, but it most often occurs in the setting of sinusitis. *S. pneumoniae, Haemophilus influenzae, Moraxella catarrhalis*, group A *Streptococcus, S. aureus*, and/or anaerobes are the likely causative agents. In the early stages of orbital cellulitis, the infection is limited by the periosteum and presents as subperiosteal phlegmon or abscess. Later, infection infiltrates the periorbital and retrobulbar fat and causes thrombosis of the ophthalmic vein and cavernous sinus. The clinical presentation is characterized by diffuse inflammatory edema, proptosis, chemosis, decreased ocular motility, decreased visual acuity, swelling and erythema involving the periorbital regions, fever, and/or leukocytosis. With intracranial involvement, neurologic symptoms appear.

IMAGING WITH COMPUTED TOMOGRAPHY

Indications.   If orbital cellulitis is suspected, a computed tomography (CT) should be performed.

Protocol.   Intravenous contrast may obscure foreign matter, but it is useful in locating and characterizing the extent of the underlying inflammatory process. To provide the best visualization of an abscess in the inferior and superior orbit, scans should be studied in both axial and coronal planes.

Possible Findings (Figs. 9-1 and 9-2)

- Paranasal sinuses infection.
- Air fluid levels in the frontal, maxillary, and sphenoid sinuses or fluid opacification of ethmoid sinuses indicate acute sinusitis.
- Areas of increased attenuation in the sinuses should raise the possibility of fungal disease.
- Bone erosion or osteomyelitis.
- Preseptal cellulitis.
- Soft tissue swelling and stranding of structures anterior to the orbital septum.
- No extension of the inflammation into the postseptal region. Use the contralateral orbit as an internal reference. Careful evaluation for extension of the inflammation into the postseptal region is imperative.
- Orbital infection.
- Abnormalities and irregularities of the intraorbital and extraconal fat (outside the intraocular muscle cone). Subtle areas of increased attenuation relative to fat subperiosteal phlegmon.

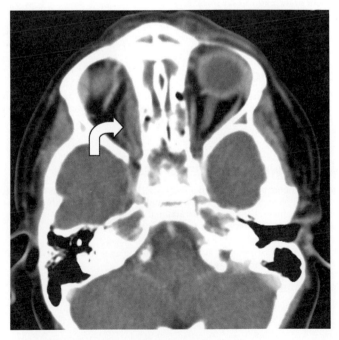

Figure 9-1. Subperiosteal phlegmon. Axial computed tomography (CT) scan shows obliteration of fat planes adjacent to the right medial rectus muscle (*curved arrow*).

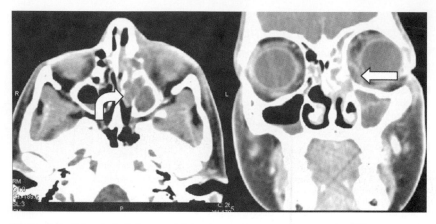

Figure 9-2. Subperiosteal abscess. Axial and coronal computed tomography (CT) scan showing sinusitis (*curved arrow*) and a rim enhancing collection adjacent to the medial wall of the left orbit (*straight arrow*).

- Focal fluid collection between the periorbita and the involved sinus displacing the periosteum indicates subperiosteal abscess.
- Diffuse infiltration of the intraconal and extraconal fat or abscess formation within the orbital fat suggest an orbital abscess (orbital abscess is rare).
- Proptosis.
- Displacement of the extraocular muscles.
- Edema of the medial rectus muscle.
- Foreign matter or other potential source of infection, especially when the paranasal sinuses are clear.

 COMPLICATIONS

- Superior ophthalmic vein (SOV) or cavernous sinus thrombosis presenting with marked asymmetric prominence of SOV or heterogeneous enhancement of cavernous sinus.
- Intracranial extension of infection which can cause meningitis, epidural abscess, subdural empyema, cerebritis, or brain abscess.

 IMAGING WITH MAGNETIC RESONANCE

Indications. Magnetic resonance imaging (MRI) is not routinely performed for evaluation of orbital infections because CT is faster and more readily available. However, MRI is the test of choice for evaluation of intracranial complications such as cavernous sinus thrombosis or intracranial extension of the infection.

Protocol. Axial and coronal T1- and T2-weighted images of the orbits. Postgadolinium axial and coronal T1-weighted images of the orbits.

Possible Findings (Figs. 9-3–9-5)

MRI findings are similar to CT.

Pitfalls

Clinical setting is very important in distinguishing the etiology for similar radiographic appearances. Trauma to the eye can present with fluid in the sinus (fracture), proptosis,

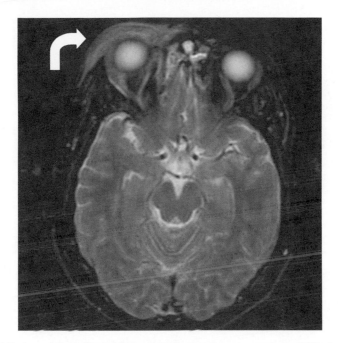

Figure 9-3. Preseptal cellulitis. Axial T2-weighted magnetic resonance image (MRI) shows eyelid and facial edema (*curved arrow*).

swelling, and increased attenuation in the soft tissues. A carotid cavernous fistula can also present with proptosis, chemosis, pain, and increased attenuation in the soft tissues. In the latter case, the SOV will typically be prominent. Although the SOV can be prominent due to postinfectious thrombosis, further clinical history and physical examination for a supraorbital bruit from a fistula should be recommended when this finding is present. A thrombosed SOV will not enhance on postcontrast images as opposed to carotid cavernous fistula. The differential diagnosis also includes pseudotumor (idiopathic inflammatory

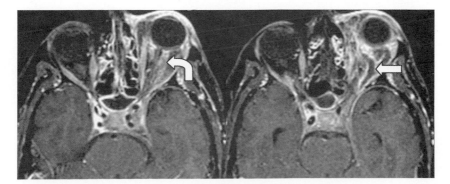

Figure 9-4. Orbital cellulitis. Axial T1-weighted images after contrast showing an abnormal enhancement of the retroseptal tissues (*curved arrow*). Lack of enhancement of the left superior ophthalmic vein signifies thrombosis (*straight arrow*).

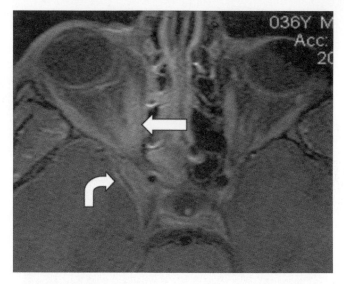

Figure 9-5. Intracranial extension of orbital cellulitis. Axial postgadolinium T1-weighted magnetic resonance image (MRI) shows right orbital (*straight arrow*) and right middle cranial fossa extra-axial (*curved arrow*) enhancement.

syndromes of the orbit). This should be considered in a patient with normal paranasal sinuses and no demonstrable infectious source.

 ISSUES AFTER IMAGING

Most orbital infections are treated medically, but surgery is indicated with CT evidence of abscess formation, initial presentation with severe orbital complaints (e.g., decreased visual acuity or blindness, diminished papillary reflex, gaze restriction), rapid progression of orbital signs despite treatment, or no improvement within 48 hours despite treatment. Neurologic deterioration suggests intracranial extension, thrombophlebitis of a major dural sinus, or meningitis.

Further Readings

Eustis HS, Mafee MF, Walton C, et al.. MR imaging and CT of orbital infections and complications in acute rhinosinusitis. *Radiol Clin North Am* 1998;36(6):1165–1183,xi.

Givner LB. Periorbital versus orbital cellulitis. *Pediatr Infect Dis J* 2002;21(12):1157–1158.

Hawkins DD, Clark RW. Orbital involvement in acute sinusitis. *Clin Pediatr (Phila)* 1977;16:464–471.

Mafee MF, Dobben GD, Valvassori GE. The orbit proper. In: Som PM, Bergeron RT, eds. *Head and neck imaging.* St. Louis: Mosby-Year Book, 1991:747–813.

Teele DW. Management of the child with a red and swollen eye. *Pediatr Infect Dis J* 1983;2:258–262.

Younis RT, Anand VK, Davidson B. The role of computed tomography and magnetic resonance imaging in patients with sinusitis with complications. *Laryngoscope* 2002;112(2):224–229.

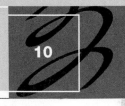

TONSILLAR/PERITONSILLAR ABSCESS

Etiology and Presentation. Tonsillar abscess most commonly occurs in adolescents or young adults, typically beginning as acute tonsillitis. Clinical presentation usually includes sore throat, dysphasia, fever, and cervical adenopathy. Progression of symptoms despite antibiotic therapy suggests development of an abscess. Acute tonsillitis can be treated with antibiotics; however an abscess should be treated with needle aspiration and or surgical drainage.

Complications. Tonsillar infection is typically confined to the pharyngeal mucosal space by the middle layer of the deep cervical fascia; however the infection can spread to adjacent parapharyngeal or masticator spaces causing parapharyngeal abscess. Bilateral tonsillar abscesses can cause airway obstruction.

Possible Findings (Fig. 10-1)

- Contrast-enhanced computed tomography (CT)
  - Enlarged tonsil with low density in the tonsil or peritonsillar regions with peripheral enhancement.
  - Edema and stranding of adjacent fat.
  - Enlarged cervical lymph nodes.
- Magnetic resonance imaging (MRI)
  - Enlarged tonsil with peripheral enhancement.
  - High T2 and low T1 central signal.

Pitfalls

- Important to differentiate from tonsillitis or phlegmon which present with tonsillar enlargement and edema without well-defined central fluid collection.

RETROPHARYNGEAL ABSCESS

Etiology and Presentation. True retropharyngeal abscess is rare. Most of the retropharyngeal space infections represent adenitis, suppurative adenitis, or phlegmon which can however progress to true abscess. There is usually an infection (i.e., pharyngitis, tonsillitis, adenitis, sinusitis, otitis) that spreads to the retropharyngeal nodes. Common organisms include *Staphylococcus, Streptococcus*, anaerobes, and tuberculosis. Infection can also spread directly from an adjacent space such as the parapharyngeal, submandibular, or prevertebral spaces or from direct inoculation through instrumentation or penetrating trauma/foreign body. Symptoms are variable depending on the age of the patient. Infants show neck swelling (97%), fever (85%), poor oral intake (55%), rhinorrhea, lethargy, and cough. Children older than 1 year can present with sore throat (84%), fever, neck stiffness, odynophagia, and cough. Adults demonstrate sore throat, fever, odynophagia, dysphagia, neck pain, and dyspnea. Inspection of the pharynx will show redness and edema. Treatment of retropharyngeal abscess usually requires surgical drainage.

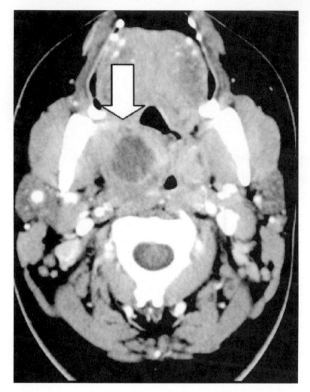

Figure 10-1. Peritonsillar abscess on contrast-enhanced computed tomography (CT) (*arrow*) manifesting as fluid collection with rim enhancement.

Complications.   Retropharyngeal infection can directly spread to mediastinum causing mediastinitis with up to 50% mortality. Soft tissue swelling can result in airway compromise. Infection can also spread to adjacent neck spaces causing internal jugular vein thrombosis.

Possible Findings (Fig. 10-2)

- **Radiographs**
  - Prevertebral soft tissue swelling (>6 mm at C2 regardless of age; >22 mm at C6 in adults and >14 mm at C6 in children younger than 15 years).
  - Foreign body may be noted.
- **Contrast-enhanced CT**
  - Fluid collection with rim enhancement in retropharyngeal space.
  - Prevertebral soft tissue swelling and edema.
- **MRI**
  - Fluid collection (central high T2 and low T1 signal) with rim enhancement in retropharyngeal space.

Pitfalls

- Important to differentiate from **adenitis and phlegmon** which do not have well-defined central fluid collection.
- Prevertebral soft tissues in children can be significantly accentuated by neck flexion.

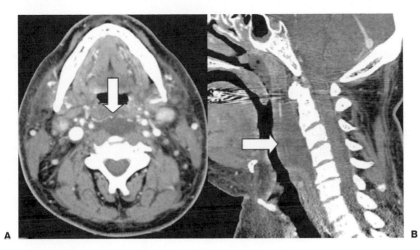

Figure 10-2. **A:** Axial and **(D)** sagittal contrast-enhanced computed tomography (CT) demonstrating retropharyngeal phlegmon (*arrows*) in a patient with neutropenia.

 DENTAL ABSCESS

Etiology and Presentation. The great majority of infectious lesions in the face are of dental origin. Facial swelling, cellulitis, and pain are common presenting signs and symptoms. Abscesses in masticator space are usually caused by molar tooth infection. Most patients are older and have a history of poor dentition. Trismus is a sign that indicates involvement of muscles of mastication. Other symptoms and signs can include cheek swelling, tenderness, fever, and leukocytosis. Treatment usually includes intravenous antibiotics and may require surgical drainage. Mandibular osteomyelitis requires long-term intravenous antibiotics.

Possible Findings

■ **Contrast-enhanced CT**
- Lucency around the root of the tooth (periapical or radicular cyst) suggests underlying infection. Best seen on bone windows.
- Small periodontal abscess near the periapical lucency and stranding of subcutaneous fat, best seen on soft tissue windows.
- Cortical erosion and periosteal reaction or subperiosteal abscess due to mandibular osteomyelitis.
- Loss of fat planes and fluid collection with rim enhancement in masticator space.
■ **MRI**
- Mandibular osteomyelitis with low T1 and high T2 marrow signal.
- Subperiosteal fluid collection/abscess with high T2 signal.
- Fluid collection (central high T2 and low T1 signal) with rim enhancement in masticator space.

Pitfalls

■ Differential diagnosis of lucency around the root of the tooth on CT includes periapical or radicular cyst (due to infection), dentigerous cyst (cyst from unerupted tooth), odontogenic keratocyst (developmental cyst with aggressive features and high recurrence rate), ameloblastoma (enhancing soft tissue component), and basal cell nevus syndrome (congenital syndrome with multiple odontogenic keratocysts).

LUDWIG'S ANGINA

Etiology and Presentation.   Ludwig's angina is a cellulitis of the floor of the mouth that develops secondary to dental infection or penetrating injury. Pain, neck swelling, fever, and difficulty breathing are the presenting symptoms. Rapid swelling may cause life-threatening airway compromise.

Possible Findings (Fig. 10-3)

■ **Contrast-enhanced CT**
  • Loss of fat planes in the floor of the mouth and abscess formation in advanced cases.
  • Lucency about the dental roots.
  • Airway compromise.

 PAROTITIS AND SUBMANDIBULAR SIALOADENITIS

Infections of the salivary glands usually present with pain and tenderness and are usually self-limited. Imaging is rarely indicated for bacterial or viral parotitis. Sialithiasis should be suspected as an underlying factor. Infected first branchial apparatus fistulas may be associated with parotitis.

Possible Findings

■ **Contrast-enhanced CT**
  • Mild swelling of the parotid with stranding of the surrounding fat.

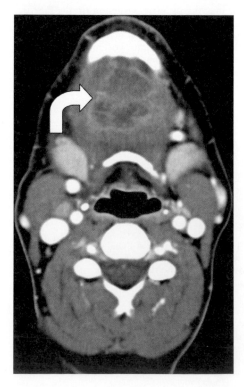

Figure 10-3. Ludwig's angina on contrast-enhanced computed tomography (CT) demonstrating abscess in the floor of the mouth (*curved arrow*).

- Calcifications (stones) of varying sizes within the glands and salivary ducts.
- Dilatation of the intra- and extraglandular salivary ducts.
- Tubular enhancing fistula that opens to the skin.

Further Readings

Grossman RI, Yousem DM. *Neuroradiology: the requisites*, 2nd ed. Philadelphia: Mosby, 2003.

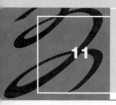

STROKE
Nafi Aygun

$\mathcal{S}$troke is a sudden loss of neuronal function that can be ischemic or hemorrhagic. Ischemic stroke can be thrombotic, embolic, and due to diffuse hypoperfusion whereas hemorrhagic stroke can be intraparenchymal and subarachnoid. By convention, an ischemic event is classified as a transient ischemic attack (TIA) when the neurologic symptoms have resolved within 24 hours (although most neurologic symptoms lasting >20 minutes have positive findings on magnetic resonance imaging [MRI] suggesting permanent tissue damage); if the symptoms persist for more than 24 hours, the attack is termed an *ischemic stroke*.

 ## ISCHEMIC STROKE
Mechanisms of Ischemic Stroke

- **Thrombotic.** Stenosis/occlusion of a large extracranial or intracranial vessel typically due to atherosclerosis leading to regional hypoperfusion. Nonatheromatous causes of arterial stenosis/occlusion include dissection and vasculitis.
- **Embolic.** Approximately 20% of brain infarcts are due to emboli originating from the heart. Emboli may also arise from atheromatous plaques in the cerebral vessels (artery-to-artery embolism).
- **Watershed infarcts** develop after episodes of global hypoperfusion, such as seen in cardiorespiratory arrest and prolonged hypotension.
- **Lacunar infarcts** are small round infarcts in the internal capsules, thalami, and basal ganglia due to stenosis/occlusion of small penetrating vessels typically seen in the setting of chronic hypertension and diabetes.

Clinical Information

Symptoms and Signs. It is important to determine precisely the temporal course and physical distribution of all neurologic symptoms. The symptoms of ischemic stroke have an all at once onset but may be either transient or permanent. TIAs due to stenosis are characteristically short in duration and highly stereotyped, often occurring in clusters. Artery-to-artery embolic TIAs may also be stereotypical and are usually more long lasting. Cardioembolic TIAs tend to be quite long lasting (from 1 to several hours), do not recur frequently, and may present with symptoms from different vascular territories in separate attacks. Vascular dissections may be neurologically asymptomatic, and may become symptomatic days to weeks after.

Carotid distribution TIA or stroke, suggestive symptoms:

- Contralateral paralysis, weakness, or clumsiness.
- Contralateral sensory loss: paresthesia and numbness.
- Dysarthria (disturbance in articulation), not in isolation.
- Ipsilateral amaurosis fugax (transient monocular blindness).
- Rarely, homonymous hemianopsia.
- Dysphasia (words not arranged in understandable way).

Vertebrobasilar distribution TIA or stroke, suggestive symptoms:

- Weakness, bilateral or shifting.
- Sensory loss, bilateral or shifting.

- Homonymous hemianopsia.
- Vertigo, diplopia, dysphagia, dysarthria, ataxia (two or more together).
- "Top of the basilar artery" related symptoms including cardiorespiratory compromise, coma, "locked-in syndrome"—considered life threatening.

Symptoms, not evidence of TIA or stroke include syncope, dizziness, confusion, incontinence, and generalized weakness.

Diagnostic Hints. The combination of amaurosis fugax and ipsilateral focal neurologic signs, as those listed in the preceding text, is highly suggestive of carotid disease. Alternating neurologic symptoms, such as left then right hemiparesis, suggest vertebrobasilar disease, cardiac embolism, or diffuse vascular disease.

Clinical Differential Diagnosis. A number of entities can resemble TIA or stroke clinically. Migraine presents with a march of neurologic symptoms that last 5–20 minutes. Seizures present with a rapid sequence of neurologic signs that last for less than a minute. Occasionally, primary and metastatic brain tumors produce transient focal neurologic findings. Supratentorial meningioma and arteriovenous malformations (AVMs) can also mimic TIAs. Less common etiologies of strokelike symptoms include subacute subdural hematoma, especially in elderly patients, and amyloid angiopathy (AA), which usually causes lobar hemorrhages but can also present with recurrent episodes of sensory loss and ischemic infarctions.

   Systemic disease entities that can mimic ischemic stroke include mitochondrial myopathy (e.g., MELAS), hypertensive encephalopathy, symptomatic hypoglycemia, and hyperventilation.

Treatment. The most effective treatment is intravenous (IV) or intra-arterial (IA) thrombolysis which requires rapid diagnosis and introduction of the thrombolytic agent within 3–6 hours. The primary goal is to administer thrombolytics as quickly as possible; time is, neuron'.

Imaging

The goals of imaging in the setting of acute ischemic stroke are to determine the location and size of the infarct (irreversible damage), the size of hypoperfusing but viable brain tissue (penumbra), and the status of blood vessels. With this information, treatment can be tailored and prognosis can be determined.

Imaging with Computed Tomography

Indications. When evaluating a patient within a time window feasible for thrombolytic therapy, a standard noncontrast computed tomography (CT) is obtained to exclude hemorrhage, tumor, or other structural lesions which can preclude thrombolytic therapy. The CT findings in stroke evolve with time. Within the first 6 hours, early signs of infarction can be identified only in 30–40% of cases. With time, infarcts become more conspicuous. After 24 hours most infarcts are visible. Posterior fossa and brain stem infarcts are difficult to identify on CT owing to their small size and prominent beam hardening artifacts.

Protocol. Standard evaluation includes noncontrast head CT, which must be reviewed in parenchymal, stroke, and subdural windows. Computed tomographic angiography (CTA) can be obtained to evaluate the intra- and extracranial cerebral vessels. CT perfusion is a robust technique that can be performed immediately after CTA. CT perfusion is currently limited—in that one cannot image the entire brain.

Possible Findings (Figs. 11-1–11-3)

- **Early infarct**
  - Normal: majority of patients within the first few hours.

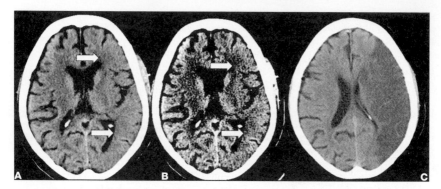

Figure 11-1. Left middle cerebral artery (MCA) infarct on noncontrast computed tomography (CT). **A:** Standard brain windows demonstrate loss of gray–white differentiation and sulcal effacement. **B:** These findings are much better seen on stroke windows. **C:** Infarct evolution 3 days later.

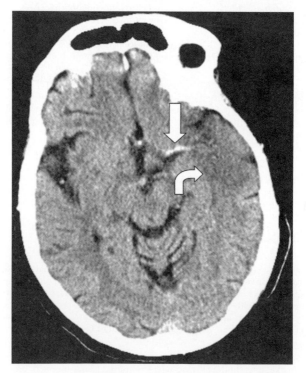

Figure 11-2. Acute right middle cerebral artery (MCA) infarct on noncontrast computed tomography (CT) with dense MCA sign (*straight arrow*), loss of gray–white differentiation and sulcal effacement in left temporal lobe (*curved arrow*).

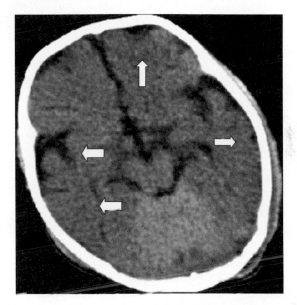

Figure 11-3. Global anoxic injury on noncontrast computed tomography (CT) with diffuse supratentorial hypodensity and loss of gray–white differentiation (*arrows*). Cerebellum is spared and has normal density.

- Subtle loss of gray–white differentiation: look at the insular ribbon and putamen.
- Subtle brain swelling: look for asymmetry of cerebral sulci.
- Hyperdense artery: indicates thrombus; look at the middle cerebral and basilar artery.

■ **Acute/subacute infarct**

- Well-defined hypoattenuation conforming to a vascular territory.
- Regional mass effect.
- Midline shift if a large area is involved.
- Hemorrhage into infarcted tissue.

■ **Chronic infarct**

- Tissue loss (encephalomalacia) and regional volume loss.

Imaging with Magnetic Resonance

Indications.   MRI provides a more comprehensive evaluation in the expense of time. Limited availability, longer study time, and artifacts limit the use of MRI in a stroke patient who is a candidate for thrombolysis. Diffusion weighted image (DWI) is the most sensitive and specific sequence for acute infarct. DWI becomes abnormal minutes after the ictus and stays abnormal for approximately 10 days. Perfusion weighted image (PWI) helps establish region of hypoperfusion and allows visualization of the penumbra which potentially can be salvaged. Magnetic resonance angiography (MRA) can establish patency/occlusion of a vessel which may directly affect treatment decisions.

Protocol.   Axial fluid-attenuated inversion recovery (FLAIR) and T2-weighted image (T2WI), DWI, PWI, and apparent diffusion coefficient (ADC) and perfusion maps.

Possible Findings (Fig. 11-4)

■ Increased signal on DWI with corresponding decreased signal on ADC maps.
■ Decreased perfusion within the DWI abnormality and often extending beyond the DWI abnormality.

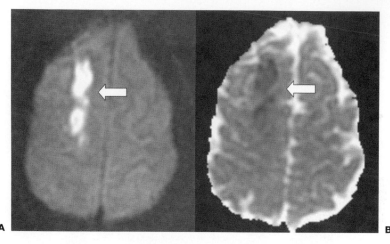

Figure 11-4. Acute infarct in right anterior cerebral artery/middle cerebral artery (ACA/MCA) watershed area on magnetic resonance imaging (MRI). Restricted diffusion with **(A)** high signal on diffusion weighted image (DWI) and **(B)** low signal on apparent diffusion coefficient (ADC) map (*arrows*).

- Increased signal on FLAIR and T2WI: appears hours after the ictus but generally before CT findings become abnormal.
- Sulcal effacement and local mass effect.
- Absence of flow voids on T2WI; indicates occlusion.
- Gyriform contrast enhancement in the subacute stage.

Protocol for MRA.   Time of flight (TOF) is the most frequently used technique. A three-dimensional (3D) TOF method is used for the intracranial vessels. For the neck vessels **2D or 3D TOF** can be used as well as 3D contrast-enhanced MRA. In general, the **3D TOF** sequence has better spatial resolution than 2D TOF. TOF overestimates the degree of stenosis.

Possible Findings for Magnetic Resonance Angiography

- Decreased vessel caliber and/or discontinuity of vessel with nonvisualization of distal branches.
- In many cases, MRA can detect the site of stenosis or occlusion and distinguish between these possibilities.

Issues After Imaging

Even when the clinical diagnosis of stroke has already been made, a positive finding on CT or magnetic resonance (MR) examination can still be valuable to clarify the extension and the mechanism of the infarction. Tissue plasminogen activator (tPA) is administered for stroke only if subjects meet strict criteria. Neurologists determine the time from the onset of the symptoms; if less than 3 hours, then IV tPA is considered; if less than 6 hours, then intra-arterial tPA is considered; if posterior circulation stroke, then longer time periods might be allowed. Treatment of stroke with heparin is indicated in only specific cases, for example, vascular dissection and atrial fibrillation.

 ARTERIAL DISSECTION

Arterial dissection represents an intimal tear and can result in luminal narrowing/occlusion or pseudoaneurysm development. Risk factors include trauma, hypertension, atherosclerotic disease, fibromuscular dysplasia, and connective tissue disorders. Patients usually present with neck pain and headache and may be otherwise asymptomatic, or may develop neurologic symptoms days to weeks after the onset. Clinical presentation can include ischemic stroke due to vascular compromise or embolic phenomena. Cervical carotid dissection can present with painful Horner syndrome because sympathetic nerves travel along the carotid arteries.

Imaging with Computed Tomographic Angiography

Indications. CTA is usually the first test for establishing the diagnosis of dissection and accessing the degree of luminal compromise because of its speed, high accuracy, and ready availability.

Protocol. CTA should be performed on a multislice scanner with the thinnest available slices. Bolus tracker (triggering at 120 HU in the aortic arch) or fixed delay (approximately 45 seconds) techniques can be used to minimize venous contamination.

Possible Findings

- Intimal flap/dissection.
- Vessel narrowing or occlusion.
- Pseudoaneurysm.
- Irregular vessel contour.
- Intramural hematoma.
- 3D reconstructions are often useful in establishing the diagnosis and in explaining imaging findings to the referring clinicians in a comprehensive manner.

Imaging with Magnetic Resonance

Indications. In the case of vascular dissection, combination of MRI and MRA is sensitive for detecting vascular injuries allowing assessment of vascular lumen, vessel wall, and tissues around the vessel.

Protocol. MRI/MRA protocol as discussed for ischemic stroke imaging. Additional axial fat-suppressed T1-weighted (T1W) images of the skull base and neck are necessary to visualize the intramural hematoma.

Possible Findings

- Intramural hematoma on unenhanced fat-suppressed T1W MR images.
- Narrowing and compromised flow.
- Pseudoaneurysms or aneurysmal dilatation of vessel.
- Vascular occlusion.
- Intimal flap.
- Retention of contrast in vessel wall.

Issues After Imaging

Dissections are usually treated with anticoagulation in order to prevent emboli formation. Luminal narrowing will usually improve over time. Angioplasty and stenting can be used to improve perfusion to vulnerable brain parenchyma.

 HEMORRHAGIC STROKE

Hemorrhagic stroke make up approximately 20% of all stroke cases. Two thirds of the hemorrhagic strokes are in the form of intracerebral hemorrhage (ICH). The remainder is subarachnoid hemorrhage which is discussed elsewhere. The overwhelming majority of ICH is secondary to hypertension. Other causes include vascular malformations such as AVM and cavernous angioma, coagulopathy, AA, underlying tumor, illicit drug use, venous occlusion, vasculitis, and encephalitis. Noncontrast CT is the modality of choice for initial evaluation. MRI is reserved for searching for an underlying cause. Cerebellar ICH is a neurosurgical emergency due to the danger of hydrocephalus, brainstem compression, and death. Hypertensive ICH at other locations is rarely treated surgically.

Hypertensive Intracerebral Hemorrhage

The most common locations of hypertensive ICH, in decreasing order of frequency, are the putamen, caudate nucleus, thalamus, lobe of a hemisphere (lobar), cerebellum, and pons. Clinical and imaging findings unusual for hypertensive ICH should invoke a workup for other potential causes which usually involves MRI/MRA and sometimes digital subtraction angiography (DSA). Intraventricular extension and large-sized hematoma are two imaging findings that predict a worse prognosis.

Arteriovenous Malformation

AVMs are congenital malformations of the cerebral vessels that develop as a result of failure of regression of the primitive connections between the arteries and veins. AVMs have a 2–4% annual risk of hemorrhage. AVMs are the leading cause of ICH in young adults. Hemorrhage can occur anywhere in the brain. Subarachnoid and intraventricular extension is common. Owing to compressive effect of the acute hematoma, AVMs may be difficult to diagnose on MRA and even on DSA in the acute phase. Follow-up may be needed to establish the diagnosis.

Amyloid Angiopathy

AA is a major cause of ICH in the normotensive elderly. The clinical hallmark of AA is repeated lobar ICH. MRI is critical in demonstrating old hemorrhages. Susceptibility weighted imaging shows innumerable small foci of hemosiderin deposition throughout the subcortical regions.

Brain Tumor

Primary brain tumors and metastases may present with hemorrhage. It may be difficult to realize the presence of an underlying mass lesion. Generally, the configuration of surrounding edema differs in that tumors have a fingerlike vasogenic edema whereas pure hematomas have a halolike edema. In tumor-related ICH, there may be a portion of the tumor that does not contain hemorrhage. On postcontrast images, an area of nodular enhancement implies underlying tumor.

Imaging with Computed Tomography

Indications.   Noncontrast CT is the test of choice for rapidly detecting the presence of intracranial hemorrhage.

Protocol.   Standard evaluation includes noncontrast head CT, which must be reviewed in parenchymal, stroke, and subdural windows. CTA can be obtained to evaluate the intra- and extracranial cerebral vessels.

Possible Findings (Figs. 11-5 and 11-6)

- Hematomas have high attenuation.
- Hematoma in a very anemic or coagulopathic patient may have less hyperattenuation.
- Hypoattenuation, representing edema and extracted serum, surrounding the hematoma that becomes larger and better defined over time.
- Mass effect, midline shift, intraventricular extension, and hydrocephalus.
- Serpentine tubular structures in the vicinity of hematoma in case of AVM rupture.
- Fluid–fluid levels in hematoma imply coagulopathy.

Imaging with Magnetic Resonance

Indications.   MRI provides a more comprehensive evaluation in the expense of time. MRI is primarily used for evaluation of underlying etiology of hemorrhage. It is highly

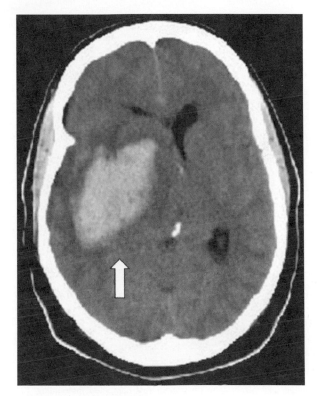

Figure 11-5. Hypertensive hemorrhage on noncontrast computed tomography (CT) with hematoma in right putamen (*arrow*). The hematoma is causing mass effect with midline shift and trapping of the left lateral ventricle.

sensitive to acute ICH, although the appearances are complex and depend on multiple factors. These include the paramagnetic form of hemoglobin present, clot matrix formation, changes in erythrocyte hydration, and changes in the degree of red blood cell packing.

Protocol.   MRI/MRA protocol as discussed for ischemic stroke imaging.

Possible Findings

■ There is a characteristic sequence of signal changes as the ICH forms and evolves. This sequence is listed in the subsequent text, and is most characteristic of intraparenchymal hemorrhage (Table 11-1).
■ Gradient echo T2*-weighted sequences highlight changes in magnetic susceptibility, and are very sensitive to acute and chronic hemorrhage.

Issues After Imaging

Medical therapy is centered on management of blood pressure, intracranial pressure, and seizure control. Surgical evacuation may be needed to relieve significant mass effect.

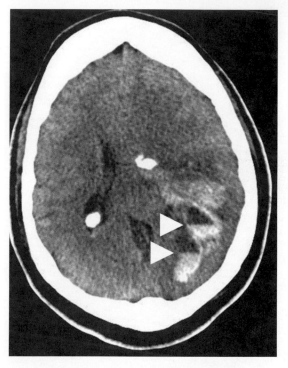

Figure 11-6. Intracranial hemorrhage on noncontrast computed tomography (CT) in a patient on warfarin (Coumadin). There is impaired clot formation with fluid–fluid levels in the hematoma (*arrowheads*) characteristic of coagulopathy.

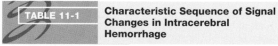

TABLE 11-1	**Characteristic Sequence of Signal Changes in Intracerebral Hemorrhage**	
	T1WI	**T2WI**
Hyperacute (0–3 h) (intracellular oxyhemoglobin)	Isointense	Hyperintense
Acute (3 h–3 d) (intracellular deoxyhemoglobin)	Isointense	Hypointense
Early subacute (3–7 d) (intracellular methemoglobin)	Hyperintense	Hypointense
Late subacute (1–4 wk) (extracellular methemoglobin)	Hyperintense	Hyperintense
Chronic (mo–yr) (hemosiderin)	Hypointense	Hypointense

T1WI, T1-weighted image; T2WI, T2-weighted image.

Further Readings

Davis DP, Robertson T, Imbesi SG. Diffusion-weighted magnetic resonance imaging versus computed tomography in the diagnosis of acute ischemic stroke. *J Emerg Med* 2006;31(3):269–277.

Grossman RI, Yousem DM. *Neuroradiology—the requisites*, 2nd ed. Philadelphia: Elsevier Science, 2003.

Lovblad KO, Baird AE. Actual diagnostic approach to the acute stroke patient. *Eur Radiol* 2006;16(6):1253–1269.

Muir KW, Buchan A, von Kummer R, et al. Imaging of acute stroke. *Lancet Neurol* 2006;5(9):755–768.

Osborn AG. *Diagnostic imaging brain*, 1st ed. Salt Lake City: Amirisys, 2004.

Schaefer PW, Copen WA, Lev MH, et al. Diffusion-weighted imaging in acute stroke. *Neuroimaging Clin N Am* 2005;15(3):503–530.

Srinivasan A, Goyal M, Al Azri F, et al. State-of-the-art imaging of acute stroke. *Radio graphics* 2006;26(Suppl 1):S75–S95.

Wintermark M. *Brain perfusion-CT in acute stroke patients*. *Eur Radiol* 2005;15(Suppl 4): D28–D31.

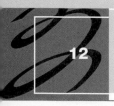

SUBARACHNOID HEMORRHAGE
12
Bradley R. Foerster and Myria Petrou

Etiology and Epidemiology. Intracranial aneurysm ruptures are responsible for approximately 80% of nontraumatic subarachnoid hemorrhage (SAH). Saccular aneurysms are the most common type and occur in regions of high mechanical wall shear stress like branch points (circle of Willis, etc.). Fifteen to 20% of patients with SAH have no aneurysm and typically have a perimesencephalic distribution of the clot. The source of hemorrhage is venous in these patients. Other causes of SAH include trauma (most common cause), intracranial and spinal arteriovenous malformation (AVM), hemorrhagic tumor, blood dyscrasias, amyloid angiopathy, moyamoya disease, and secondary leakage of blood from primary intraparenchymal hemorrhage.

Approximately 15–30% of patients die from their aneurysm rupture before reaching the hospital. Up to 25% of patients with an aneurysm have a second aneurysm. Between 0.5 and 1% of patients undergoing cerebral angiography for other reasons are incidentally found to have an aneurysm. The risk of aneurysm rupture in a person with no history of aneurysm rupture varies from 0.05–2% per year depending on the size and site of the aneurysm.

Risk factors for intracranial aneurysm include increasing age, female gender, hypertension, alcohol, smoking, and family history. Intracranial aneurysms are associated with fibromuscular dysplasia, autosomal dominant polycystic kidney disease, connective tissue disorders, congenitally anomalous vessels, AVMs, tumors, vasculitis, and infections.

CLINICAL INFORMATION

Symptoms and Signs. Classically, the symptoms of an intracranial aneurysm rupture include "worst headache of life," loss of consciousness, photophobia, meningismus, nausea, and vomiting. Only 10–15% of patients who complain of "worst headache of life" will have SAH. Sentinel headaches occur in approximately one half of patients before rupture, presumably caused by transient small leak of the aneurysm. Localized headache may occur from expansion of an aneurysm before rupture, requiring imaging to exclude this diagnosis even in the absence of blood in the cerebrospinal fluid. Expanding aneurysms can also cause focal neurologic deficits including visual field cuts, oculomotor paresis, and focal weakness. Classically, an aneurysm of the posterior communicating artery can cause third cranial nerve palsy with a dilated and relative fixed pupil.

Differential diagnosis includes stroke, migraine, meningitis, and sinusitis.

Complications

- Hydrocephalus can be either acute (20% of patients) or delayed. Acute hydrocephalus is related to amount of ventricular blood and usually appears within 3 days of the SAH, requiring immediate treatment. Delayed hydrocephalus occurs after 10 days and is related to amount of SAH.
- Seizures occur acutely in 3–5% of patients. Fifteen percent of patients can develop epilepsy following an SAH, usually within the first 18 months.
- Rebleeding occurs in up to 4–20% of patients with aneurysms.
- Delayed cerebral ischemia is caused by vasospasm and usually occurs 5 days from the initial hemorrhage. Vasospasm can affect any or all of the major branches of the circle of Willis. Ischemic complications have been reported to occur in up to one third of patients, with the amount of blood on the initial head computed tomography (CT) correlating to the severity of the vasospasm.

- Neurogenic pulmonary edema and syndrome of inappropriate secretion of antidiuretic hormone (SIADH) are potential systemic complications of SAH.
- Overall mortality is high (one third to two thirds of cases). Most survivors have significant permanent disability.

IMAGING WITH COMPUTED TOMOGRAPHY

Indications. A noncontrast head CT is the study of choice in the evaluation of a patient presenting with a severe headache in the emergency room setting. A noncontrast head CT is the fastest, easiest and most accurate test for detection of SAH. It has very high sensitivity (>96%) for the detection of SAH occurring within the last 24 hours. The sensitivity falls to 80% at 72 hours. Head CT is important for risk stratification (more blood = more complications), identification of the potential location of the aneurysm (where most blood is located), and detection of complications which can include hydrocephalus, mass, ischemia, and herniation. Occasionally, a noncontrast CT can identify a calcified aneurysm.

The use of computed tomographic angiography (CTA) in the setting of acute SAH is evolving. CTA has a comparable sensitivity to digital subtraction angiography (DSA) for aneurysm detection, but a negative CTA requires follow-up DSA. Many surgeons will request DSA for preoperative assessment, limiting the practicality of CTA in the setting of acute SAH.

Protocol. Routine noncontrast head CT is typically performed with 5-mm axial images. Thin slices (1 mm or less) can be very helpful in difficult cases. CTA should be performed with bolus tracking on multidetector CT to ensure optimal visualization of intracranial vessels. Images should be reviewed on a three-dimensional (3D) workstation.

Possible Findings (Figs. 12-1 and 12-2)

- **Noncontrast CT**
  - High attenuation (blood) within the cisterns, subarachnoid spaces, and ventricles can be subtle!
  - Look for predisposing causes: masses, trauma, and so on.
  - Complications including hydrocephalus, herniation, and infarction.
- **CTA**
  - Abnormal outpouching of vessel representing aneurysm. Occasional calcified aneurysm.

Pitfalls

- Aneurysms near the skull base may be difficult to see on CTA with 3D or thick maximum intensity projection (MIP) visualization techniques.

IMAGING WITH MAGNETIC RESONANCE

Indications. The sensitivity of T1-weighted imaging(T1-WI) and T2-weighted imaging (T2-WI) sequences for acute SAH is low. Fluid attenuation inversion recovery (FLAIR) sequence imaging is critical for detection of subarachnoid blood. Magnetic resonance imaging (MRI) is more sensitive than CT to subacute SAH. MRI can also help identify the culprit aneurysm in a patient with multiple aneurysms by localizing blood by-products. Magnetic resonance angiography (MRA) can be useful for the detection of intracranial aneurysms; however, it is inferior to CTA and DSA.

Protocol. FLAIR sequence is critical for detection of subarachnoid blood. Circle of Willis MRA is usually performed using 3D time-of-flight technique.

Possible Findings (Fig. 12-3)

- **MRI**
  - FLAIR: acute and subacute blood appears bright in the subarachnoid space.

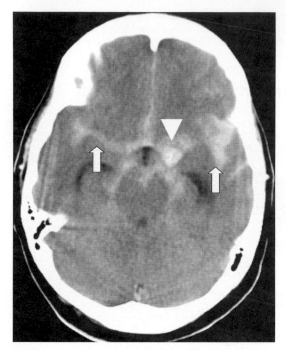

Figure 12-1. Noncontrast computed tomography (CT) scan demonstrating subarachnoid hemorrhage (*arrows*) due to ruptured left posterior communicating aneurysm and the clot at the rupture site (*arrowhead*).

- Potential causes for SAH (other than aneurysm): tumors, AVMs, vasculitis, and infection.
- Complications including hydrocephalus, herniation, and infarction.

■ **MRA**
- Abnormal outpouching of vessel representing aneurysm.

Pitfalls

■ FLAIR is nonspecific: bright signal in the subarachnoid space can represent elevated protein from meningitis, elevated oxygen tension in ventilated patients, or artifact.
■ Insensitive to small aneurysms.

 IMAGING WITH DIGITAL SUBTRACTION ANGIOGRAPHY

Indications.   Four-vessel DSA is the gold standard in the evaluation of SAH. If the initial angiogram is negative, a repeat angiogram is performed to exclude the possibility of vasospasm that may have prevented the filling of the aneurysm.

Protocol.   All four intracranial vessels must be injected separately using multiple projections depending on the vessel being interrogated.

Possible Challenges in Interpretation

■ Vascular loop versus aneurysm: a vascular loop has the same wash-in and wash-out as the parent vessel compared to the aneurysm which has different flow dynamics.

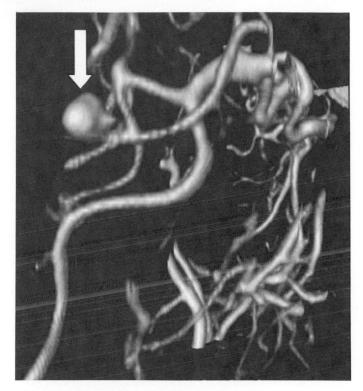

Figure 12-2. Three-dimensional (3D) rendering of brain computed tomographic angiography (CTA) demonstrating left middle cerebral artery (MCA) aneurysm *(arrow)*.

- Infundibular dilatation versus aneurysm: typically occurs at the origin of the posterior communicating artery. Infundibular dilatation lacks an aneurysmal neck or irregularity. Infundibulum is tentlike or cone-shaped rather than saccular. Size of an infundibulum is less than 3 mm.
- Multiple aneurysms found: correlate with prior head CT for localization of blood products. Look for adjacent vasospasm, most irregular aneurysm, largest aneurysm, and demonstration of contrast extravasation (rare).
- Patients with a negative angiogram and blood localized anterior to the brainstem and adjacent areas such as the interpeduncular fossa and ambient cistern are thought to have a perimesencephalic hemorrhage, caused by venous bleeding. There should not be significant extension of blood into the Sylvian fissure or interhemispheric fissure. These patients tend to have a more benign course.

 ISSUES AFTER IMAGING

A history suspicious for SAH, where the CT scan result is negative, requires lumbar puncture to exclude SAH. In the setting of SAH and identified intracranial aneurysm, early intervention minimizes the risks of rebleeding and infarction. A high-quality conventional angiogram is essential to enable the neurosurgeon/interventional neuroradiologist to plan the appropriate intervention, which depends on the aneurysm location and morphology. Patients with acute hydrocephalus need decompression. Calcium channel blockers to reduce risk of vasospasm and seizure prophylaxis are standard measures. Fluid administration with

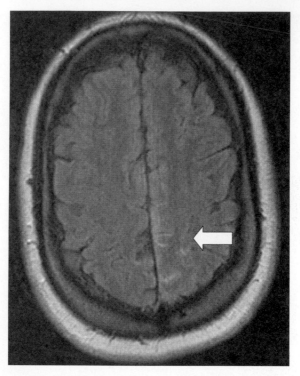

Figure 12-3. Subarachnoid hemorrhage on magnetic resonance imaging (MRI) with increased signal in left parietal sulci on fluid attenuation inversion recovery (FLAIR) sequence (*arrow*).

pulmonary wedge pressure monitoring is used to optimize cerebral perfusion to minimize potential impact of vasospasm.

Further Readings

Bradley GW, Daroff RD, Renichel GM, et al. eds. *Neurology in clinical practice*, 3rd ed. Woburn: Butterworth-Heineman, 2000.

Castillo M. *Neuroradiology*, 1st ed. Philadephia: Lippincott Williams & Wilkins, 2002.

Grossman RI, Yousem DM. *Neuroradiology: the requisites*, 2nd ed. Philadephia: Mosby, 2003.

Levy AD, Koeller KK, Chung EM, et al. eds. *Radiologic pathology*, 4th ed. Washington DC: Armed Forces Institute of Pathology, 2005.

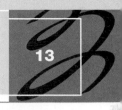

INTRACRANIAL VENOUS THROMBOSIS
Bradley R. Foerster and Myris Petrou

13

Etiology and Epidemiology.   Cerebral venous sinus thrombosis (CVST) is an uncommon condition with serious potential clinical consequences especially if the diagnosis is delayed. CVST has a 5–15% mortality rate and generally occurs in young or middle aged adults, accounting for 1–2% of strokes in these patients. Risk factors include pregnancy, oral contraceptive use, dehydration, adjacent infection (sinuses or mastoids), coagulopathy, malignancy and trauma. In 20% of patients, no underlying etiology is found. CVST is most common in the superior sagittal sinus, followed in decreasing frequency by the transverse and sigmoid sinuses, cerebral veins, straight sinus, and cerebellar veins. Septic cerebral venous thrombosis is relatively rare in developed countries and should be aggressively treated with antibiotics.

 ## CLINICAL INFORMATION

Symptoms and Signs.   Unfortunately, presentation of cerebral venous thrombosis is highly variable depending on the location and burden of the thrombosis and presence of venous collaterals. Headache is the most common, and sometimes the only, symptom occurring in up to 95% of cases and usually precedes the onset of other neurologic deficits by days or even months. Focal neurologic deficits are the next most common sign and include central motor and sensory deficits, seizures, aphasia, and hemianopia. These deficits may fluctuate and can alternate. Patients presenting with the syndrome of pseudotumor cerebri (headache, vomiting, visual changes, and papilledema) or unexplained hemorrhagic infarction (bilateral or not follow an arterial vascular distribution) must be evaluated for cerebral venous thrombosis.

    Septic cavernous sinus thrombosis has a distinct clinical picture with chemosis, exopthalmos, painful opthalmoplegia, third, fourth, and sixth nerve palsies. Complications include occlusion of the internal carotid artery and extension into dural sinuses or brain parenchyma. Because of its often rapidly fatal course, septic cavernous sinus thrombosis should be treated presumptively before imaging.

Differential Diagnosis.   Because of the highly variable presentation differential diagnosis includes arterial stroke, cerebral tumors, brain abscess, arteriovenous malformation, encephalitis, cerebral vasculitis, and seizure disorders.

Complications

- Infarction and hemorrhage occur in approximately 35–50% of patients. The venous thrombosis increases venous and capillary pressure, resulting in decreased blood flow to the brain parenchyma. Breakdown of the blood–brain barrier and diapedesis of erythrocytes are thought to contribute to the hemorrhagic infarct.
- Seizures can be focal or generalized and seen in 35–50% of patients and up to 75% in peripartum females.
- Obstructing hydrocephalus can occur with cerebellar vein thrombosis, causing cranial nerve palsies and life-threatening hydrocephalus.
- Encephalopathy and coma are seen in patients with extensive thrombosis or involvement of the deep venous system with bilateral thalamic involvement. Severe alteration of consciousness is the strongest predictor of poor clinical outcome.

IMAGING WITH COMPUTED TOMOGRAPHY

Indications. A noncontrast head computed tomography (CT) should be performed as the initial study for evaluation of patients presenting with acute neurologic symptoms. Unfortunately, noncontrast head CT is neither sensitive nor specific for the diagnosis of CVST but can help to exclude other life-threatening diseases. Computed tomographic venography (CTV) is a rapid and widely available modality for direct visualization of the intracerebral venous system to diagnose thrombosis. It is equal to magnetic resonance venography (MRV) for diagnosing CVST, but inferior to magnetic resonance imaging (MRI) in establishing other potential etiologies of the patient's symptoms.

Protocol. Routine noncontrast head CT should be performed first. CTV is performed after a short delay (~60 seconds) following contrast administration with acquisition of thin slices for review on a three- dimensional (3D) workstation.

Possible Findings (Fig. 13-1)

■ **Noncontrast head CT**
- Infarction which can be hemorrhagic and does not conform to typical vascular territories. This is one of the most helpful noncontrast CT signs in suggesting this potential diagnosis.
- Cord sign representing a high density clot in the affected vein (inconsistent sign).

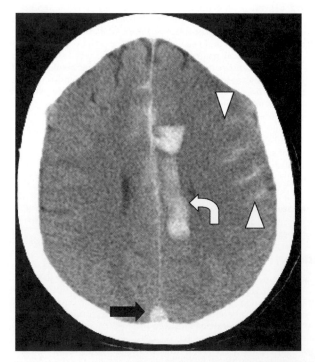

Figure 13-1. Cerebral venous sinus thrombosis (CVST) on computed tomography (CT) noncontrast axial head CT presenting with parenchymal (*curved arrow*) and subarachnoid (*arrowheads*) hemorrhage. There is increased density of the superior sagittal sinus secondary to thrombus (*straight arrow*).

- Dense triangle sign which represents hyperdensity of the superior sagittal sinus from acute clot (inconsistent sign).
- Localized brain swelling which is caused by elevated venous pressure. Edema is usually localized to the parenchyma near the thrombosed sinus. Bilateral involvement can occur in the medial frontoparietal regions in superior sagittal sinus thrombosis and in the thalami in internal cerebral vein/vein of Galen thrombosis.

■ **CTV**
- Segmental absence of enhancement or filling defect.
- Sinus wall enhancement and collateral venous drainage are secondary signs indicating obstruction/thrombosis of primary venous drainage pathways.

Pitfalls

■ Normal venous sinus is hyperdense to brain parenchyma and should not be confused with thrombosis. This is particularly pronounced in patients with dehydration or high hematocrit.

IMAGING WITH MAGNETIC RESONANCE

Indications.   MRI/MRV is generally considered the best tool for evaluation of cerebral venous thrombosis due to high accuracy and ability to detect other potential etiologies of the patient's symptoms. Diffusion-weighted MRI can detect infarction and other parenchymal abnormalities, which are seen in 40–70% of patients with cerebral venous thrombosis.

Protocol.   Routine enhanced brain MRI is used including pre- and postcontrast T1, T2, and fluid attenuation inversion recovery (FLAIR) images. Diffusion-weighted imaging is essential for detection of early infarcts. Gradient echo images are the most sensitive for hemorrhage. Blood flow can be evaluated using MRV techniques including phase contrast, time of flight, and gadolinium-enhanced MRV techniques.

Possible Findings (Fig. 13-2)

■ **Conventional MRI**
- Acute venous thrombosis (days): isointense on T1 and hypointense on T2.
  - Subacute venous thrombosis (first month): hyperintense first on T1 and then later on T2-weighted images.

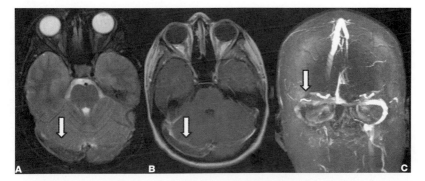

Figure 13-2. Cerebral venous sinus thrombosis (CVST) on magnetic resonance imaging (MRI). **A:** Axial T2 image shows hypointense thrombus expanding the right transverse sinus (*straight arrow*). **B:** Axial postcontrast T1 demonstrates isointense thrombus expanding the right transverse sinus with peripheral enhancement (*straight arrow*). **C:** Three-dimensional (3D) reconstruction time of flight—magnetic resonance venography (TOF–MRV) shows loss of signal on TOF imaging in the right transverse sinus (*straight arrow*) representing the clot burden.

- Chronic venous thrombosis: variable depending on level of recanalization. Usually isointense on T1 and hyperintense on T2.
- Infarction which can be hemorrhagic and does not conform to typical vascular territories.

■ **MRV**
  - Loss of signal seen on 2D or 3D time of flight imaging due to absence of flow.
  - Filling defect seen on gadolinium-enhanced MRV depicting the thrombus. May have enhancement of the sinus walls indicating collateral venous channels.

Pitfalls

■ Flow-related enhancement refers to paradoxical enhancement of slow blood flow perpendicular to the imaging plane and can mimic thrombus. It is therefore important to look at two orthogonal planes to distinguish between the two: thrombus will retain high signal in all planes and blood flow will only have high signal in a single plane. In addition, it is important to correlate the conventional MRI findings with the MRV portion of the examination.

■ Subacute thrombus may not be identified on time of flight venography because both subacute thrombus (methemoglobin) and normal blood flow will have high signal. Phase contrast venography can be helpful as the signal from the methemoglobin will be suppressed so that only flow signal is seen.

 IMAGING WITH CONVENTIONAL ANGIOGRAPHY

Indications.   Four-vessel angiography has traditionally been the gold standard for establishing the diagnosis of cerebral venous thrombosis. However, advancements in less invasive CTV and MRV techniques have led to its decline and it is only performed in ambiguous cases.

Protocol.   Images are taken in the delayed venous phase.

Possible Findings

■ Indirect signs are often more important than the direct signs and include dilated collateral veins with corkscrew appearance, delayed venous emptying, and collateral circulation.
■ Nonvisualization of thrombosed sinus or vein.

 ISSUES AFTER IMAGING

Controlled trials support the use of anticoagulation for cerebral venous thrombosis with improved outcomes. Even in the setting of intracranial hemorrhage, intravenous heparin use is recommended as untreated patients have an increased chance of further hemorrhage and death compared to anticoagulated patients. Thrombolysis therapy is controversial and perhaps should only be considered in comatose patients who have the highest risk of mortality even with heparin therapy. After the acute symptoms resolve, the patient is transitioned to oral anticoagulation warfarin (Coumadin) with an international normalized ratio (INR) goal of 2.0–3.0. Patients are treated for 3–12 months depending on their predisposing (if any) conditions.

In the acute phase, the patient's additional symptoms and predisposing conditions should be treated. Venous infarctions can be extremely epileptogenic and seizures should be treated with antiseizure medication. Elevated intracranial pressure should also be appropriately managed although it is important to remember to keep these patients well hydrated to avoid increasing the blood viscosity.

Further Readings

Bradley GW, Daroff RD, Renichel GM, et al. eds. *Neurology in clinical practice*, 3rd ed. Woburn: Butterworth-Heinemann, 2000.

Connor SEJ, Jarosz JM. Magnetic resonance imaging of cerebral venous sinus thrombosis. *Clin Radiol* 2002;57:449–461.

Grossman RI, Yousem DM. *Neuroradiology: the requisites*, 2nd ed. Philadephia: Mosby, 2003.

Masuhr F, Mehraein S, Einhaupl K. Cerebral venous and sinus thrombosis. *J Neurol* 2004;251:11–23.

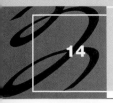

HYDROCEPHALUS AND SHUNT
Monica D. Watkins

*H*ydrocephalus may be life threatening and require emergency surgical treatment. It is subdivided into "communicating" hydrocephalus which is characterized by dilation of the entire ventricular system due to impaired cerebrospinal fluid (CSF) reabsorption versus "non-communicating" hydrocephalus which is due to a focal obstruction of a ventricle, foramina, or aqueduct.

In the pediatric population, most cases of hydrocephalus occur due to communicating hydrocephalus following intraventricular hemorrhage (~35% of all cases) or an episode of meningitis. Noncommunicating hydrocephalus due to aqueductal stenosis or brain mass is less common.

Causes of hydrocephalus in the adult population include communicating hydrocephalus following subarachnoid hemorrhage or meningitis. Normal pressure hydrocephalus (NPH) is a form of communicating hydrocephalus occurring in the elderly population. The diagnosis is suggested when the ventricular system is dilated out of proportion to the amount of sulcal dilatation due to atrophy. The patients tend to have clinical symptoms of dementia, gait ataxia, and urinary incontinence (the three W's: wacky, wobbly, and wet). Noncommunicating hydrocephalus due to tumor is less common.

Patients may become symptomatic from hydrocephalus due to increased intracranial pressure (ICP).

 INTRAVENTRICULAR SHUNT

In most cases of hydrocephalus, treatment requires placement of a shunt. One end of the catheter is placed in the ventricular system and the distal end is placed either in the peritoneal cavity (ventriculoperitoneal shunt) or the right atrium (ventriculoatrial shunt). The ventriculoperitoneal shunt is by far the most common type and is the treatment of choice for a pediatric patient. Typically, an extended tube length of 120 cm is placed within the peritoneal cavity in infants to allow for growth of the patient.

In the case of NPH, patients may receive a trial of repeated lumbar tap and if symptoms do improve, a ventricular peritoneal shunt may be placed.

 COMPLICATIONS OF SHUNTING

Shunt failure resulting in increasing hydrocephalus has been reported extensively in the pediatric population, where between 17 and 40% of ventriculoperitoneal shunts will fail within the first year.

There are many causes of shunt failure of which the most common is obstruction of tubing due to blood, proteinacious material, or even talc from surgical gloves. Obstruction is more common within the proximal end than the distal end. Mechanical failure due to broken or kinked tubing or valve malfunction is also common.

A rare cause of distal obstruction (6–8% of shunt failures) is the formation of abdominal pseudocyst in which a collection of CSF is surrounded by nonepithelial tissue and is usually associated with infection. Other uncommon complications include migration of the catheter out of the ventricular system or distal tip out of the peritoneal cavity. There are a few reported cases of the distal shunt catheter becoming entangled in the bowel and resulting in necrosis. A patient can be overshunted leading to "intracranial hypotension syndrome." Instead of enlarging ventricles, patients may present with headache, slitlike ventricle, and possibly subdural hematomas. This is rare as many shunt systems have antisiphoning devices to prevent overshunting.

 ## CLINICAL SIGNS AND SYMPTOMS OF HYDROCEPHALUS

Symptoms are mainly due to worsening hydrocephalus with resulting increased ICP.

- Mild increase in ICP
  - Headache, nausea, vomiting, ataxia.
  - In infants: apnea, bradycardia, and seizure.
- Moderate increase in ICP
  - Papilledema, altered mental status, upgaze palsy (setting sun sign), changes in vision due to optic nerve injury.
  - In infants: bulging fontanel, swelling around shunt tube.

  Differential diagnosis of shunt failure includes trauma, infection, and infarction.

 ## IMAGING WITH RADIOGRAPHS

Indications.   Radiographs are used to visualize the radiopaque portions of the shunt catheter from cranium to abdomen. Radiographs are insensitive and may be misleading as portions of the catheter are often radiolucent.

Protocol.   Shunt series usually includes lateral skull, anteroposterior (AP) neck, frontal chest, and AP abdomen.

Possible Findings

- Discontinuity or kink in tubing.
- Peritoneal tube in the exact same location as previous film, displaced bowel loops or calcified mass near the distal tip may suggest fibrosis at the tip or pseudocyst. Further evaluation may be needed with ultrasonography or computed tomography (CT) of the abdomen to rule out a pseudocyst.

 ## IMAGING WITH COMPUTED TOMOGRAPHY

Indication.   Noncontrast head CT is also the initial study of choice for any patient presenting with neurologic symptoms. Any patient with a shunt catheter who has signs or symptoms of increased ICP should be quickly imaged with a noncontrast head CT to assess for changes in ventricular size.

Protocol.   Routine noncontrast head CT.

Possible Findings of Shunt Failure

- Increasing hydrocephalus since prior examination—enlargement of the temporal horns is most sensitive.
- Periventricular hypodensity representing transependymal flow of CSF.
- Fluid tracking along the intracranial portion or the subcutaneous portion of the shunt.
- Change in shunt position.
- Effaced sulci.

Possible Findings of Overshunting

- Marked decrease in size of ventricle or slitlike ventricles.
- Subdural hematoma/hygroma.

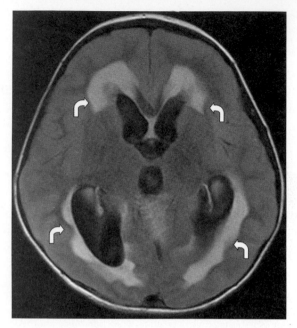

Figure 14-1. Hydrocephalus on magnetic resonance imaging (MRI) with high signal on fluid attenuated inversion recovery (FLAIR) sequence (*arrows*) in periventricular white matter due to transependymal cerebrospinal fluid (CSF) flow.

 IMAGING WITH MAGNETIC RESONANCE

Indication.   Magnetic resonance imaging (MRI) is often used as a secondary study to evaluate the underlying causes of hydrocephalus. It can be useful to further delineate location of a mass or confirm signs of acute infection. Artifact often prevents evaluation of the catheter and reservoir integrity.

Possible Findings of Shunt Failure (Fig. 14-1)

- Similar to CT: increasing hydrocephalus, fluid tracking along shunt.
- Periventricular T2 or FLAIR hyperintensity representing transependymal flow of CSF.

Possible Findings of Overshunting

- Dural thickening.
- Marked decrease in size of ventricle or slitlike ventricles.
- Subdural hematoma/hygroma.
- Inferior displacement of the cerebellar tonsils.

 IMAGING WITH NUCLEAR MEDICINE

Indications.   Nuclear medicine imaging is the most sensitive test for shunt patency.

Protocol.   Using sterile technique, 0.5–1 mCi ^{99m}Technetium (^{99m}Tc)-DTPA or 0.5mCi ^{111}Indium (^{111}In)-DTPA is injected into the shunt reservoir or directly into the shunt tubing. Imaging is begun immediately after injection.

Possible Findings.   Shunt is patent when radiotracer activity is seen diffusely throughout the peritoneal cavity by 1 hour.

IMAGING TIPS

- Comparison with the old studies is the key to diagnosis of shunt failure, allowing evaluation for change in ventricular size and catheter position.
- Even subtle changes in ventricular size could be clinically significant.
- Normal or stable head CT does not rule out early shunt failure.

ISSUES AFTER IMAGING

Patient may require emergent surgery to decompress the ventricular system or correct overshunting depending on the clinical picture and radiologic findings.

Further Readings

Couldwell WT, LeMay DR, McComb JG. Experience with use of extended length peritoneal shunt catheters. *J Neurosurg* 1996;85:425–427.

Greenberg MS. *Handbook of neurosurgery*, 5th ed. Thieme Medical Publishers, 2000.

Grossman RI, Yousem DM. *Neuroradiology: the requisites*, 2nd ed. Philadelphia: Mosby, 2003.

Mobley LW III, Doran SE, Hellbusch LC. Abdominal pseudocyst: predisposing factors and treatment algorithm. *Pediatr Neurosurg* 2005;41:77–83.

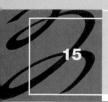

15 BRAIN HERNIATION
Joshua Smith

*B*rain herniation may occur across the falx cerebri, tentorium cerebelli, or through openings such as foramen magnum and craniectomy defects. Any process that causes an elevation in the intracranial pressure can result in brain herniation. Space-occupying lesions (e.g., tumor, abscess, hematoma, and stroke), diffuse processes (e.g., edema, encephalitis, and subarachnoid hemorrhage), or increased cerebrospinal fluid (CSF) (e.g., hydrocephalus) are examples. Herniations of the brain are classified into five categories: (1) transtentorial, (2) subfalcine, (3) tonsillar, (4) alar, and (5) extracranial (Fig. 15-1).

Imaging findings related to herniation have a similar appearance on both computed tomography (CT) and magnetic resonance imaging (MRI) although they are better depicted on MRI due to multiplanar capability and superior soft tissue contrast. Each category of herniation may occur in isolation or conjunction with other categories.

Each category of herniation may be associated with a specific neurologic syndrome, described subsequently. Early, nonspecific signs of herniation reflect elevated intracranial pressure and include headache, nausea, vomiting, vision disturbance, papilledema, altered level of consciousness, and Cushing's triad (alteration in respiration, bradycardia, and systemic hypertension). Late signs of herniation include decorticate and decerebrate posturing. Each category of herniation may rapidly progress to death, and because of this, it is imperative that the clinician be promptly notified of any imaging findings suggestive of herniation.

 SUBFALCINE HERNIATION

Subfalcine herniation is the most common form of herniation and occurs when mass effect displaces brain medially and forces the cingulate gyrus underneath the falx cerebri. The falx cerebri is a sickle-shaped fold of dura mater which lies within the longitudinal fissure, separating the cerebral hemispheres. The paired pericallosal arteries, branches of the anterior cerebral artery (ACA), travel along the free edge of the falx.

Clinical Findings

The clinical syndrome associated with subfalcine herniation relates to compression of the ipsilateral ACA which may get pinned against the relatively fixed falx, leading to infarction in its vascular distribution and the clinical syndrome of contralateral leg weakness.

Possible Findings (Fig. 15-2)

- Best depicted on the coronal scan.
- Midline shift of septum pellucidum. Measurement of septum pellucidum midline shift is performed in two easy steps. First, draw a straight line from the anterior-most to the posterior- most aspects of the falx. This represents the expected normal location of the septum pellucidum. Next, draw a perpendicular line from the displaced septum pellucidum to this first line. Serial measurements should be performed at the same approximate level to accurately document change in midline shift over time.
- Compression of the ipsilateral lateral ventricle.
- Dilatation of contralateral ventricle due to foramen of Monro obstruction.
- Widened subarachnoid space on side of falx away from mass lesion.
- Displacement of lateral ventricle and corpus callosum away from mass lesion.

80

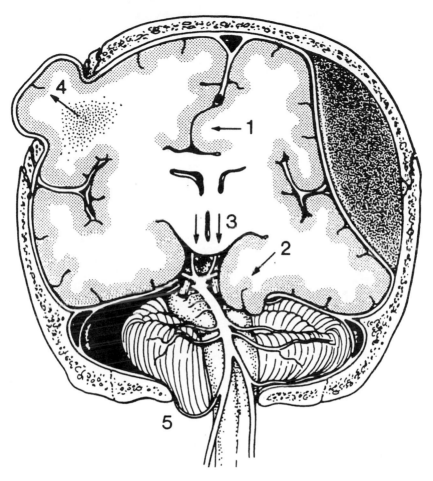

Figure 15-1. Major types of brain herniation. *1* Subfalcine herniation, *2* uncal herniation, *3* descending transtentorial herniation, *4* external herniation, *5* tonsillar herniation. (Barr R, Gean AD. Craniofacial trauma. In: Brant: WE, Helms CA, eds. Fundamentals of diagnostic radiology. Baltimore: Williams & Wilkins, 1994;52–84).

- Displacement of the ACA.
- Infarct in ACA distribution.

TRANSTENTORIAL HERNIATION

Transtentorial herniation occurs when mass effect displaces brain across the free edge of the tentorium cerebelli. The tentorium is an arched crescentic fold of dura mater that separates the occipital lobes from the cerebellum and is suspended by the falx cerebri. The tentorial incisure (notch) is an oval opening formed by the concave free edges of the tentorium and the dorsum sella. The tentorial incisure surrounds the midbrain and separates the middle and posterior cranial fossae. The medial temporal lobe lies along the free edge of the tentorium and is formed by the uncus and parahippocampal gyrus, with the uncus representing the medially curved anterior end.

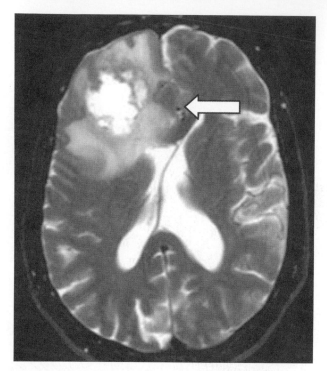

Figure 15-2. Subfalcine herniation on magnetic resonance imaging (MRI). Axial T2-weighted image (T2WI) demonstrates centrally necrotic right frontal lobe mass with surrounding vasogenic edema causing significant mass effect with subfalcine herniation (*arrow*).

Transtentorial herniation is subdivided into (1) unilateral descending, (2) bilateral descending, and (3) ascending. Unilateral descending transtentorial herniation is the most common subtype and occurs when mass effect arising within a hemisphere pushes the medial temporal lobe inferomedially through the tentorial incisure. Bilateral descending transtentorial herniation, also referred to as *central herniation*, occurs when severe uni- or bilateral mass effect displaces both cerebral hemispheres and basal nuclei downward. Ascending transtentorial herniation occurs when mass effect arising within the posterior fossa pushes the cerebellum superiorly through the incisure.

Clinical Findings

Understanding of the clinical syndromes associated with transtentorial herniation requires knowledge of anatomy of the suprasellar and perimesencephalic cisterns and their relationship with the medial temporal lobe and tentorium.

The anteriorly located suprasellar cistern is contiguous with the posteriorly located perimesencephalic cistern. The suprasellar cistern contains the circle of Willis and its major proximal branches and has been described as a six-pointed star (Star of David). The anterior interhemispheric cistern contains the proximal A2 segments and anterior communicating artery; the anterolateral Sylvian cisterns contain the proximal M1 segments; the postero-lateral ambient cisterns contain the proximal P2 segments; the posterior interpeduncular cistern contains the termination of the basilar artery which gives rise to the P1 segments. The anterior choroidal artery arises from the supraclinoid ICA after the takeoff of the posterior communicating artery and courses posteriorly along the uncus before entering the lateral ventricle temporal horn at the choroidal fissure.

The perimesencephalic cistern surrounds the midbrain and is bounded by the tentorium incisure. It is formed by the interpeduncular, ambient, and quadreminal plate cisterns. The oculomotor nerve passes through the interpeduncular cistern, between the posterior cerebral and the superior cerebellar arteries, and continues anteriorly between the posterior communicating arteries and medial temporal lobe before entering the cavernous sinus.

Transtentorial Herniation Can Cause

- Fixed, dilated pupil and impairment of extraocular movement (EOM).
- Infarct in posterior cerebral artery (PCA) distribution.
- Infarct in anterior choroidal artery distribution.
- Unilateral or bilateral motor weakness.

Motor weakness related to transtentorial herniation may be either unilateral or bilateral. In *unilateral* descending, transtentorial herniation, compression of the *contra*lateral cerebral peduncle (i.e., Kernohans notch on imaging) results in *ipsi*lateral motor weakness and is considered a false localizing sign as the hemiparesis is ipsilateral to the lesion. Bilateral motor weakness may occur when the bilateral cerebral peduncles are compressed as can be seen with either late unilateral or bilateral descending transtentorial herniation.

Possible Findings

Unilateral Descending Transtentorial Herniation (Fig. 15-3)
- Early findings
  - Medial displacement of medial temporal lobe.

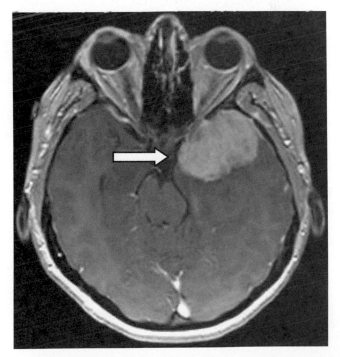

Figure 15-3. Unilateral descending transtentorial herniation on magnetic resonance imaging (MRI). Axial T1-weighted postcontrast image demonstrates a large left sphenoid wing meningioma causing medial uncal displacement (*arrow*), effacement of the ipsilateral suprasellar cistern and compression of the midbrain.

- Effacement of ipsilateral suprasellar cistern.
- Contralateral displacement of brainstem.
- Widening of ipsilateral ambient cistern.
■ Late findings
- Inferomedial displacement of the medial temporal lobe.
- Complete effacement of the suprasellar cistern.
- Effacement of ipsilateral ambient cistern.
- Downward displacement of brainstem.
- Compression of ipsilateral ventricle and dilatation of contralateral ventricle.
- Kinking of the contralateral cerebral peduncle (Kernohan's notch).
- Hemorrhage into the midbrain and pons tegmentum (Duret's hemorrhages).
- Infarct in PCA and/or anterior choroidal artery distributions.

Bilateral Descending Transtentorial Herniation

■ Inferomedial displacement of bilateral medial temporal lobes.
■ Complete effacement of basal cisterns.
■ Downward displacement of both cerebral hemispheres and basal ganglia.
■ Downward displacement of diencephalon and midbrain through the tentorial notch.
■ Transverse compression of brain stem with elongation in the anteroposterior (AP) dimension.
■ Downward shifting of the basilar artery and pineal gland.

Ascending Transtentorial Herniation

■ Superior displacement of vermis and cerebellum through tentorium incisure.
■ Effacement of quadreminal plate cistern.
■ Compression and distortion of the midbrain.
■ Effacement of cerebral aqueduct (of Sylvius).
■ Obstructive hydrocephalus.

 TONSILLAR HERNIATION

Tonsillar herniation occurs when mass effect displaces the cerebellar tonsils downward through the foramen magnum. This is most commonly due to a mass lesion within the posterior fossa although can occur with supratentorial mass lesions as well. Chiari I, a posterior fossa congenital malformation associated with low-lying cerebellar vermis and tonsils, may mimic tonsillar herniation. CSF leak from the spine may also cause inferior displacement of the cerebellar tonsils.

Clinical Findings

Acute cerebellar tonsillar herniation can be catastrophic resulting on obtundation and death.

Possible Findings

■ Best depicted on the midline sagittal scan. However, since typical CT is performed in the axial plane, it is important to be aware of signs of tonsillar herniation on axial scans.
■ Extension of tonsillar tips 5 mm in adults or 7 mm in children below level of the foramen magnum. The plane of the foramen magnum can be depicted by drawing a line connecting the foramen magnum anterior and posterior midpoints (i.e., basion and opisthion, respectively).
■ Visualization of cerebellar tissue in same image as dens on the axial scan.
■ Effacement of the cisterna magna.
■ Increased slope of tentorium.
■ Kinking of medulla.
■ Flattening of cervical cord.
■ Elongation of the cerebral aqueduct.

■ Compression of fourth ventricle.
■ Hydrocephalus.

Imaging Pitfalls

Ectopic cerebellar tonsils is a feature of Chiari I malformation. Therefore if cerebellar tonsilar "herniation" is discovered, every effort should be made to understand the underlying cause and to compare with prior studies.

 ## ALAR HERNIATION

Alar, or sphenoid, herniation occurs when brain herniates over the sphenoid wing and is subdivided into anterior and posterior herniation. In posterior alar herniation, a frontal lobe mass lesion causes brain parenchyma to extend posterior and inferior over the sphenoid ridge. In anterior alar herniation, a temporal lobe mass lesion causes brain parenchyma to extend anterior and superior over the sphenoid ridge. Imaging findings related to alar herniation are difficult to depict and the clinical findings are thought primarily related to other coexisting herniations.

 ## EXTRACRANIAL HERNIATION

Extracranial herniation typically occurs after either surgery or trauma, with brain extending through either a craniectomy or posttraumatic defect. The imaging findings related to extracranial herniation are generally readily evident.

Further Reading

Grossman RI, Yousem DM. *Neuroradiology: the requisites*, 2nd ed. Philadephia: Mosby, 2003.

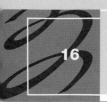

SPINAL CORD COMPRESSION
Azar P. Dagher and Andrew L. Holz

*S*pinal metastasis and epidural abscess are the most common entities that can cause spinal cord compression in addition to trauma and degenerative disease.

CLINICAL SIGNIFICANCE

Spinal Metastasis

Source. Approximately 70% of spinal tumors are metastatic in origin. The most common tumors associated with spinal cord compression are lymphoma and multiple myeloma (together accounting for approximately 19% of cord compression cases), metastatic lung cancer (17%), metastatic breast cancer (12%), metastatic genitourinary malignancies (11%), and metastases from an unknown primary (12%). Renal cell carcinoma and malignant melanoma also commonly metastasize to the spine and can cause spinal cord compression.

Location. Ninety percent of spinal metastases are extradural. Intramedullary metastases are rare. To cause cord compression, tumor typically invades the anterior epidural space from the adjacent vertebral body. Lung and breast cancer tend to metastasize to thoracic levels. Prostate cancer and renal cell carcinoma tend to metastasize to lumbosacral levels. Melanoma has no preference for spinal level.

Epidural Abscess

Source. Risk factors include age, IV drug abuse, spinal procedures, altered immune status (e.g., diabetes mellitus), and malignancy. *Staphylococcus aureus* is the most common organism, and is found in approximately 60% of cases. The incidence of epidural abscess is approximately 0.2–2.0 per 10,000 people.

Location. Most patients are infected through the hematogenous route. Most commonly the abscess begins as a focus of spinal discitis/osteomyelitis and enlarges to cause cord compression. Iatrogenically introduced bacteria can also cause these abscesses. The level of involvement is cervical in 25% and lumbosacral in 38%. The abscess is anterior in 50% and circumferential in 33%.

CLINICAL PRESENTATION

Symptoms and Signs. Early symptoms of spinal cord compression are back pain with or without a radicular component. Fast growth of tumor or abscess generally causes pain; slow growth causes weakness and other cord compressive signs. Hyperalgesia suggests nerve root involvement. In the evolution of symptoms and signs, motor loss occurs before sensory loss because of the anatomy of the tracts of the cord. Decreased strength results from compression of anterior horn cells. Posterior compression affects the posterior spinocerebellar and lateral spinothalamic tracts, manifesting as decreased posture appreciation, ipsilateral decreased vibration sensation, and contralateral decreased pain and temperature sensation. Incontinence occurs late in the course of cord compression, with urinary incontinence preceding rectal incontinence, and signifies that reversal of symptoms with therapy is unlikely.

If the cord compression is due to an epidural abscess, fever and obtundation are often present in addition to the neurologic deficits. When deterioration occurs rapidly, it is often secondary to the infection and inflammation causing venous thrombosis resulting in cord ischemia.

Level of Involvement.   The level of cord involvement can be predicted from the level of vertebral involvement and vice versa. Analysis of dermatomes is commonly used to determine the level of cord involvement.

 IMAGING WITH RADIOGRAPHS

Protocol.   Radiographs have limited sensitivity and do not suffice in the evaluation of a patient with symptoms of cord compression. In cord compression due to tumor, only two thirds of cases have significant bony abnormalities on radiograph. For those without the bony changes, invasion is likely through the intervertebral foramen from a paravertebral mass such as in lymphoma, neuroblastoma, or leukemia. In epidural abscess, the associated osteomyelitis is often not visualized on radiographs.

Possible Findings

Tumor
- Lytic lesion, blastic lesion, or compression fracture at a level corresponding to the cord symptoms.

Discitis/Osteomyelitis
- Bone destruction.
- Narrowing of intervertebral disc space with erosion of adjacent endplates indicates discitis.

 IMAGING WITH MAGNETIC RESONANCE

Protocol.   Typical protocol can include sagittal T1-weighted images (T1WI) and T2WI, axial T1WI and T2WI, postgadolinium axial and fat suppressed sagittal T1WI with phased array coil. Fat suppression techniques such as short T1 inversion recovery (STIR) increase sensitivity. Unenhanced T1WI are the most sensitive for bone metastases and a single sagittal T1WI sequence may suffice for both diagnosis and treatment planning. It is important to assure that bony landmarks such as C1 or S1 are included for potential subsequent radiation therapy or surgical planning. Care should be taken to include the potential radiation port (two vertebral bodies above and two below the lesion). Additional lesions may warrant a wider radiation port.

Possible Findings (Figs. 16-1 to 16-3)

Cord Compression
- Central canal diameter less than 10 mm.
- High T2 cord signal. This finding is only specific in the setting of actual compression as it can also be present with demyelinating disease, viral myelitis, infarct, tumor, venous congestion, and trauma.
- Cord thinning with chronic compression. This is typical with degenerative disease or slow-growing tumor.

Spinal Metastasis
- Compression fracture due to vertebral body metastasis
  - Complete marrow replacement, which is best seen as low signal on T1WI involving the entire vertebral body. Vertebral body metastases frequently have high T2 signal, unless heavily calcified. Contrast-enhanced images can confuse diagnosis because enhancing metastasis can appear similar to normal fatty marrow.

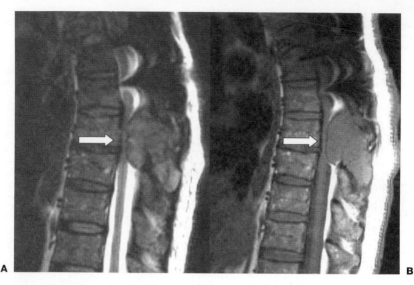

Figure 16-1. Cord compression by multiple myeloma on sagittal **(A)** T2-weighted images (T2WI) and **(B)** postcontrast T1-weighted images (T1WI) demonstrating large mass arising in posterior elements and causing severe narrowing of the central canal and cord compression (*arrows*).

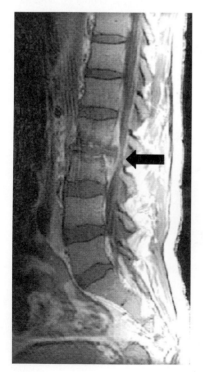

Figure 16-2. Epidural abscess (*arrow*) on postcontrast T1-weighted sagittal magnetic resonance imaging (MRI) at L2-3 level due to discitis/osteomyelitis.

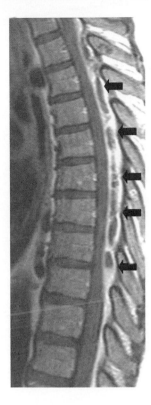

Figure 16-3. Large epidural abscess (*arrows*) on postcontrast T1W sagittal magnetic resonance imaging (MRI) extending along the posterior thoracic cord.

- Convex posterior border, unlike osteoporosis- or trauma-related compression fractures which tend to have sharp angles.
- Hematogenous metastases usually start in posterolateral corner of vertebral body extending to pedicles.
- Epidural extension of the tumor from vertebral body or adjacent tissues
  - Soft tissue mass that is best depicted on postcontrast fat suppressed T1WI.
- Pitfalls
  - Contrast-enhanced images can confuse diagnosis because enhancing metastasis can appear similar to normal fatty marrow on nonfat suppressed T1WI.
  - Vertebral body edema can be seen with osteoporosis- or trauma-related compression fractures; however usually does not involve the entire vertebral body.
  - Red marrow can have low T1 signal; however, it will be brighter then skeletal muscle unlike metastasis that is usually darker.

Epidural Abscess

- Epidural abscess is iso- to hypointense on T1 and hyperintense on T2WI. Enhancement varies from homogeneous to rimlike and is best visualized on fat-suppressed sequences.
- Discitis/osteomyelitis
  - Disc edema (high T2 signal), enhancement, and destruction. Disc can be spared with tuberculosis (TB) infection.
  - Vertebral endplate erosion.
  - Vertebral body marrow replacement (low T1 signal) and edema (high T2 signal).
- Differential diagnosis to consider for epidural abscess includes extradural metastasis, epidural hematoma, extruded/migrated disc, and epidural lipomatosis.

ISSUES AFTER IMAGING

Treatment of Spinal Metastases.   This depends on primary malignancy, affected level, and rapidity and duration of symptoms. If there is no other tumor site, obtaining tissue is necessary and treatment is decompressive laminectomy or corpectomy. Contraindications for surgery include complete transection of the cord, total paraplegia for more than 12 hours, loss of sphincter control greater than 24 hours, and a major sensory loss. Uncontrolled disease elsewhere is a relative contraindication.

Radiation treatment extends over 3 weeks. The radiation field includes two vertebral bodies above and two bodies below the known extent. Steroids are also given to decrease swelling and inflammatory response. Treatment is known to decrease pain, slow tumor growth, and save neurologic function. Complete neurologic recovery is unlikely when treatment is delayed beyond 12 hours of compression symptoms.

Cord radiation tolerance is limited by transient myelitis, demyelination, and necrosis. With 4,500 cGy the risk of these is approximately 5%. Transient myelitis occurs from 6 weeks to 5 months posttreatment. Delayed progressive myelopathy occurs from 6 months to 6 years posttreatment.

Treatment of Epidural Abscess.   Therapy is surgical drainage. Medical management carries the risk of venous thrombosis. Even with surgery, mortality and morbidity are high.

Further Readings

Grossman RI, Yousem DM. *Neuroradiology—the requisites*, 2nd ed. Philadelphia: Mosby, Elsevier Science, 2003.

Ross JS, et al. *Diagnostic imaging—spine*, 1st ed. Salt Lake City, Amirsys Inc., 2004.

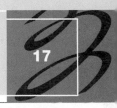
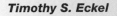

*H*eadache is purported to be the most common pain experienced by humans. Luckily, headache is only very rarely associated with significant pathology. Identifying pathologically significant lesions is the primary role of imaging in headache. For imaging purposes, headache is divided into two broad categories: acute and chronic. Computed tomography (CT) is usually chosen in the evaluation of acute cases, and magnetic resonance (MR) is usually chosen for chronic cases.

Acute Headache. Imaging in acute headache is most useful in situations of extreme severity, posttraumatic headache, or headache associated with other neurologic abnormalities. The primary reason for imaging these patients is to evaluate for pathology requiring emergent therapy—specifically, hemorrhage or other processes resulting in increased intracranial pressure. Owing to rapid availability and high sensitivity for acute hemorrhage, noncontrast CT is currently the imaging modality of choice.

Chronic or Recurrent Headache. As a general rule, imaging is not often useful in the evaluation of chronic headache. Only very few patients with chronic headache will have pathologically significant findings. Atypical characteristics of headache, associated neurologic deficits, and seizures may indicate the need for imaging. MR is the modality of choice for chronic headache due to the wide variety of pathologic conditions which may cause headache, and the increased sensitivity of MR in comparison with CT for small lesions and vascular anomalies.

 CLINICAL INFORMATION

Signs and Symptoms. A complete history is the most effective method for evaluating headache. Characterizing features of the pain (quality, severity, location, duration, time course, exacerbating and relieving factors) may be useful in arriving at an appropriate differential diagnosis; however, this is often not an adequate way to determine the pathologic significance of the symptoms and imaging will be necessary. In regard to severity, the degree of incapacitation caused by the symptoms is often a more reliable clinical sign than the subjective description of the intensity of the pain.

    Differential diagnosis of headache includes a wide variety of etiologies such as infectious diseases (viral illnesses, meningitis, sinusitis, and mastoiditis), trauma, subarachnoid hemorrhage (SAH), vascular malformations (hemorrhage), psychological factors (stress-related), referred pain (trigeminal neuralgia, temporomandibular joint [TMJ] pathology cervicogenic headache), neoplasms, vasculitis, and ocular problems. Migraine (numbness, weakness) and cluster headaches (Horner's syndrome) can present with focal neurologic findings. Postural headaches may result from cerebrospinal fluid (CSF) leak, and rebound headaches may occur when medications are discontinued. Headaches during pregnancy should elicit considerations of eclampsia, pituitary apoplexy, and dural venous sinus thrombosis. Stroke and transient ischemic attack (TIA) are uncommon causes for headache, and usually present with focal neurologic findings (see Chap. 11, "Stroke").

IMAGING WITH COMPUTED TOMOGRAPHY

Indications.   Evaluation of posttraumatic headache (± loss of consciousness). Evaluation of acute severe ("worst headache of life") or atypical headache (associated with neurologic findings on examination).

Protocol.   Noncontrast axial images.

Possible Findings

- High-attenuation material within subarachnoid space (cisterns) or within brain parenchyma, indicating hemorrhage.
- "Cord sign" due to thrombosed cortical veins or dural sinuses.
- Signs of increased intracranial pressure or impending herniation, such as obliteration of cisterns, midline shift, loss of gray-white differentiation.
- Signs of obstructive hydrocephalus, such as ventriculomegaly.
- Other findings: masses, cerebral edema.

Imaging Tips for Computed Tomography

- A negative head CT does not eliminate the need for lumbar puncture if clinical concern for SAH is high.
- CT is not indicated routinely before lumbar puncture except in clinical situations which are also indications for emergent CT (i.e., suspicion for elevated intracranial pressure).
- Positive findings should be communicated immediately to the referring physician and generally before lumbar puncture.

IMAGING WITH MAGNETIC RESONANCE

Indications.   Evaluation of chronic headache (generally with some associated neurologic deficit or other clinical history to increase level of suspicion for structural pathology).

Protocol.   Routine screening examination (sagittal T1, axial T2 and fluid attenuation inversion recovery [FLAIR], axial and sagittal postcontrast T1-weighted images) is usually adequate initially as the history is generally not specific enough for a focused examination. MR angiography may be useful if there is suspicion for possible aneurysm.

Possible Findings

- Region of hemorrhage or edema.
- Mass lesion.
- Vascular anomaly.
- Chronic subdural hematoma.
- Hydrocephalus.
- Pachymeningeal enhancement may be seen with infectious meningitis, meningeal metastatic disease, or reduced intracranial pressure and CSF leak.

Imaging Tips for Magnetic Resonance

If the clinical history includes positional headache, check for colloid cyst and positional obstruction of the foramen of Monro.

Further Readings

Bradley GW, Daroff RD, Renichel GM, et al. *Neurology in clinical practice*, 3rd ed. Woburn: Butterworth-Heinemann, 2000.
Grossman RI, Yousem DM. *Neuroradiology: the requisites*. 2nd ed. Philadephia: Mosby, Elesvier Science, 2003.

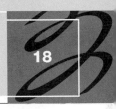

STRIDOR AND WHEEZING

David A. Weiland

18

 INSPIRATORY STRIDOR

Definition and General Workup.   Inspiratory stridor is defined as noisy breathing due to turbulent airflow through a partial upper airway obstruction (above the thoracic inlet). The most common causes of stridor in children include croup, epiglottis, and foreign body aspiration. Evaluation of inspiratory stridor should include anteroposterior (AP) and lateral soft tissue radiographs of the neck including the upper airway. If the cause of stridor is not evident from the radiographs, computed tomographic (CT) findings can identify the exact level of obstruction, and can oftentimes provide clues to the specific diagnosis.

Croup

Clinical Information
Croup affects children 6 months to 3 years of age. The patient typically presents with a characteristic "brassy, barking" cough. Hoarseness and inspiratory stridor are also common, and there is usually a history of a recent lower respiratory tract infection.

Etiology.   It is classically associated with the parainfluenza virus, but influenza and respiratory syncytial virus (RSV) can both cause an identical clinical presentation. The tracheal mucosa is loosely attached to the upper trachea. Inflammation and edema elevate the mucosa, which leads to narrowing just below the larynx. External restriction by the cricoid cartilage or complete tracheal cartilaginous rings can worsen the obstruction.

Radiography.   Given the correct clinical scenario, diagnosis is possible on AP and lateral radiographs of the upper airway (Fig. 18-1). The classic "steeple sign," seen on the AP view, represents symmetric subglottic narrowing. There is loss of the normal "shouldering" of the air column. The "steeple sign" is accentuated in expiration. The subglottic trachea is narrowed and indistinct on the lateral view; the epiglottis and aryepiglottic folds are normal.

Differential Diagnosis.   The aim of radiology in diagnosing croup is to exclude other causes of inspiratory stridor such as congenital or acquired subglottic stenosis, foreign body aspiration, epiglottitis, and subglottic hemangioma.

Epiglottitis

Clinical Information
The peak incidence of epiglottitis occurs in children 3–6 years old, who present with the abrupt onset of inspiratory stridor and severe dysphagia. The patient is usually febrile and appears ill. The classic description is that of a drooling patient who is sitting up and leaning forward in an effort to splint open the upper airway. The incidence of epiglottitis has become less frequent with the widespread immunization of children with the *Hemophilus influenza* type B (Hib) vaccine.

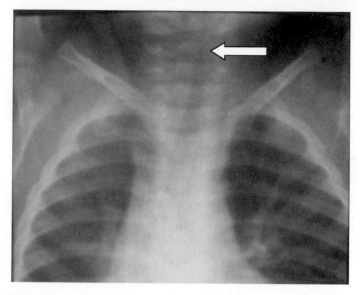

Figure 18-1. Croup on plain radiograph. There is narrowing of subglottic trachea (*arrow*) and absence of normal shoulders representing "steeple" sign.

Etiology.   *H. flu* had been by far the most common etiology, but is now rarely the cause of acute epiglottitis. Other organisms including group A *Streptococcus, Streptococcus pneumoniae*, and *Staphyloccocus aureus* have become more prevalent.

Radiography.   Patients with acute epiglottitis are in danger of suffocation as a result of complete airway closure (Fig. 18-2). The minimum examination should be performed to obtain the diagnosis, and the patient should always be accompanied by a physician experienced in endotracheal intubation. The lateral radiograph must be taken in the upright position and shows enlargement of the epiglottitis and the aryepiglottic folds. Thickening of the epiglottis and aryepiglottic folds results in airway obstruction. There is circumferential narrowing of the subglottic portion of the trachea during inspiration.

Differential Diagnosis.   Rare causes of epiglottic enlargement include omega-shaped epiglottis, hemophilia, angioneurotic edema, chronic epiglottitis, Stevens-Johnson syndrome, aryepiglottic cyst, chemical ingestion, thermal injury, and radiation.

Upper Airway Foreign Body

Upper airway foreign body, another cause of inspiratory stridor, is primarily a clinical diagnosis. However, radiographs of the chest and upper airway may demonstrate a radiopaque foreign body or hypoinflated lungs. (See Chap. 19, "Foreign Body Aspiration.")

 EXPIRATORY STRIDOR (WHEEZING)

Definition and General Workup.   Expiratory stridor or wheezing is the result of partial airway obstruction below the thoracic inlet. Radiographs are frequently obtained in a patient who is a "first-time wheezer." The evaluation of such a patient should include AP and lateral chest views. The most common causes of wheezing in this patient population are viral pneumonitis or bronchiolitis, reactive airway disease (RAD) or asthma, and foreign body aspiration.

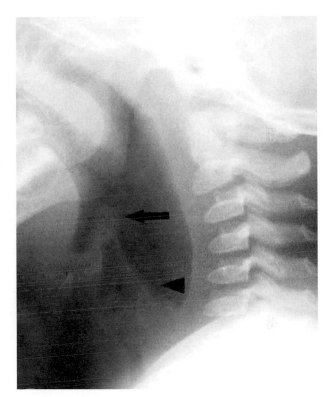

Figure 18-2. Epiglottitis on plain radiograph. There is marked thickening of epiglottis (*arrow*) and aeroepiglottic folds (*arrowhead*).

Viral Pneumonitis

Clinical Information
Patients often present with cough, fever, and wheezing.

Etiology.   Common causes include RSV, parainfluenza, adenovirus, and influenza virus. The inflammatory process affects the bronchi and bronchioles, causing airflow obstruction, but spares the distal alveoli.

Radiography.   Findings include hyperinflation, air trapping, and airway thickening. Bronchiolitis is often present in patients younger than 1 year.

Asthma

Clinical Information
Patients may present as a first-time wheezer or during an exacerbation of known asthma.

Etiology.   Antigens in the environment produce a hypersensitivity reaction that causes release of histamine, leading to increased vascular permeability, mucosal edema, and bronchial smooth muscle contraction. These effects cause partial airway obstruction and wheezing.

Radiography.   The chest radiograph in a patient with asthma typically demonstrates hyperinflation and airway thickening. These findings are similar to those seen in viral pneumonitis, so distinction from this entity must be made clinically. During an asthma exacerbation, a chest radiograph is obtained to exclude complications, such as atelectasis, obstructive emphysema, pneumomediastinum, pneumothorax, and pneumonia. Localized air trapping can be better demonstrated with fluoroscopy or expiratory chest radiographs.

Intrathoracic Foreign Body

An intrathoracic foreign body is another common etiology for a first-time wheezer. (See Chap. 19, "Foreign Body Aspiration.")

Further Readings

Gyepes MT, Nussbaum E. Radiographic-endoscopic correlations in the examination of airway disease in children. *Pediatr Radiol* 1985;15(5):291–296.

Rencken I, Patton WL, Brasch RC. Airway obstruction in pediatric patients. From croup to BOOP. *Radiol Clin North Am* 1998;36(1):175–187.

Rosenkrans JA. Viral croup: current diagnosis and treatment. *Mayo Clin Proc* 1998;73(11): 1102–1106.

Rotta AT, Wiryawan B. Respiratory emergencies in children. *Respir Care* 2003;48(3): 248–260.

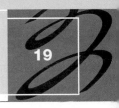

FOREIGN BODY ASPIRATION

Alexander M. Kowal

19

CLINICAL INFORMATION

Etiology and Epidemiology. Ingestions occur frequently with children and mentally handicapped adults. Foreign body aspiration represents 7% of lethal accidents in infants between 1 and 3 years. The mean age at presentation is 2 years with 98% of cases younger than 5 years. Boys outnumber girls 2:1. Younger children have smaller caliber airways and immature protective mechanisms, increasing the risk of morbidity and mortality. Careful medical history is the key to early diagnosis, but only 19–33% of events are witnessed and children may not volunteer the correct history. The correct diagnosis is only made within 24 hours of presentation in 59% of cases. Although negative imaging does not exclude foreign body aspiration, imaging is helpful when history is uncertain and the presentation is late. Complication rates greater than 95% have been observed with delays in diagnosis over 30 days, including pneumonia, lung abscess, granuloma, and bronchiectasis. Foreign body aspiration is rare in adults and associated with alcohol intoxication, traumatic intubation, psychosis, neurologic disorders with impaired swallow function, seizures, and dental procedures.

Symptoms and signs depend on the size, location, duration, and composition of the foreign body. The classic triad of cough, wheezing, and unilateral decreased breath sounds is present in 30–60% of cases of lobar bronchial foreign body aspiration. The most common presentation is choking followed by intractable coughing (72%). Other symptoms include prolonged, paroxysmal cough, dyspnea, recurrent pneumonia and fever, cyanosis, and intermittent hemoptysis. Laryngotracheal foreign bodies are more likely to be symptomatic and are commonly associated with apneic episodes, biphasic stridor, and hoarseness/dysphonia/aphonia. Symptoms may often subside spontaneously to a relatively asymptomatic state. Physical examination will be abnormal in 80% of cases. Symptoms include decreased unilateral air entry. Unilateral wheezing (60%) in the absence of prior pulmonary disease is highly suspicious for foreign body.

Differential diagnosis for the symptoms of foreign body aspiration include viral infection such as croup, asthma, cystic fibrosis, gastroesophageal (GE) reflux, mucus plugs, pneumonia, left to right shunt ("cardiac asthma"), hydrocarbon ingestion, allergic reactions, mediastinal tumors/adenopathy, and congenital/developmental anomalies such as tracheoesophageal fistula.

Location of Foreign Bodies. In general, the younger the age of the child, the higher the involved anatomic site. Approximately 60% lodge in the main stem bronchi and 35% in segmental bronchi. Although most cases are unilateral, there is no statistically significant difference when comparing the left and right main bronchus in children aged 1–3 years due to an equal angle of bifurcation. In adults, foreign bodies occur more often in the right bronchus, especially the bronchus intermedius. Foreign bodies can also lodge in the larynx (6–9%), trachea (5–17%), or esophagus.

Composition of Foreign Bodies. Most aspirated foreign bodies are foods (70%), especially peanuts (59%), sunflower seeds, popcorn, and hotdog fragments; therefore, most are radiolucent. In addition to causing obstruction, a foreign body will also elicit a local inflammatory response whose severity is dependent on the composition of the object. The most severe inflammation results from the oil content of vegetable substances, such as

97

peanuts, which increase local swelling further impeding airflow. In adults, the most common foreign bodies include aspirated denture and tooth fragments, animal bones, and tablets.

Valve Mechanisms.   The more proximal elastic airway tends to expand and permit air flow past the foreign body during inspiration, but the elasticity impedes air flow during expiration. This results in air trapping distal to the foreign body by a check valve mechanism. Reflex oligemia due to hypoventilation will also occur. If the object migrates more distally, complete obstruction with distal atelectasis occurs by a stop valve mechanism. The latter mechanism is less frequent, occurring in 10–25% of lobar foreign body aspirations.

 IMAGING WITH RADIOGRAPHS

Indications.   Radiographs should be used in the initial evaluation of all patients with suspected foreign body aspiration or chronic pulmonary symptoms. In 10–24% of cases, the foreign material is radiopaque and no further radiologic workup is necessary. Opaque foreign bodies may include metals, glass, and most animal bones. If radiolucent, indirect radiologic signs such as obstructive emphysema (44–64%) must be sought and other imaging modalities considered. Radiolucent foreign bodies can include aluminum, fish bones, plastic, wood, and vegetable products. Chest radiographs have 60–68% sensitivity and 37–71% specificity. A normal chest radiograph is present in 9–35% of cases.

Protocol.   Routine posteroanterior (PA) (inspiratory) and lateral views for cooperative children. Routine anteroposterior (AP) and cross-table lateral views for younger children. Other views: expiratory, lateral decubitus. Soft tissue AP and lateral views of the neck to identify upper airway foreign bodies.

Imaging Tips.   In infants and young children, obtaining an expiratory film may be very difficult. "Assisted expiratory" chest radiograph may be helpful in these instances. At the end of child's expiration, vigorous pressure is applied to the epigastrium, forcing diaphragm upward.

Possible Findings (Fig. 19-1)

Check valve mechanism:

- **On inspiration.** Hyperinflation with segmental or lobar hyperlucency (focal air trapping) distal to obstruction. Twenty-three percent of cases will demonstrate left lung hyperinflation, 11% right lung hyperinflation. Bilateral hyperinflation may also occur.
- **On expiration.** Mediastinal structures shift toward unobstructed side, caused by persistent hyperinflation of the obstructed side. The hemidiaphragm on the obstructed side may be low and flat and may fail to rise on expiration.
- **Decubitus view.** Obstructed lung remains hyperlucent even when in dependent position. Normally, the dependent lung on a lateral decubitus view is less well expanded because of compression by other structures in the chest.

Possible Findings

Stop valve mechanism:

- Distal atelectasis of obstructed segment or lobe (13%).
- Mediastinal shift toward obstructed side (11%).
- Hemidiaphragm elevation on obstructed side due to volume loss from atelectasis.

Other Findings.   Pneumomediastinum. Hyperinflation with atelectasis in the same hemithorax has been noted in 18% of cases and is not present in other pediatric respiratory diseases. Aeration within an area of atelectasis is also specific but occurs in only 6% of cases. Delayed presentations can lead to atelectasis in 10–33% of radiographs and consolidation secondary to pneumonia in 9–26%. Upper airway foreign bodies are often seen in lateral views of the neck in the subglottic region along with prevertebral soft tissue swelling and emphysema.

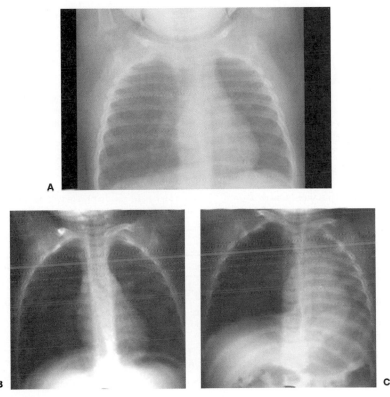

Figure 19-1. A: Posteroanterior (PA) chest radiograph demonstrating hyperinflation and hyperlucency of the right lung in a patient with known right main bronchus foreign body. **B:** Right lateral decubitus chest x-ray demonstrating persistent hyperinflation of the right lung despite dependent position. **C:** Left lateral decubitus chest x-ray showing volume loss of the left lung and persistent hyperinflation of the right lung. Courtesy of Visveshwar Baskaran, MD, Johns Hopkins Hospital.

 IMAGING WITH FLUOROSCOPY

Indications.   Nondiagnostic radiograph studies. Fluoroscopy works well for crying infants and has a sensitivity of 47% and specificity of 95%. Fluoroscopy will be normal in 53% of cases.

Protocol.   Videofluoroscopic study to observe diaphragmatic movement during normal respiration, full inspiration, and full expiration. Take spot films of each hemidiaphragm in full inspiration and expiration, with the spot film console locked in position.

Imaging Tip.   On the spot films, use the rib cage as a frame of reference to differentiate between chest wall motion versus true diaphragm motion.

Possible Findings

■ Normal diaphragmatic movement should be symmetric, with the right hemidiaphragm about one half rib interspace higher than the left. The individual findings are the same as those for the radiograph studies, except they should be more apparent. Paradoxical (opposite of expected) diaphragmatic movement can be seen in 16% of cases.

■ Mediastinal shift will be present in 31% of cases.

 ## IMAGING WITH COMPUTED TOMOGRAPHY

Indications. Computed tomography (CT) involves radiation exposure and is not considered initially in children. CT is often diagnostic of foreign body aspiration in adults referred for recurrent pneumonia and hemoptysis. CT may be useful when the foreign body is not localized on radiographs and fluoroscopy or is suspected in the larynx. In atypical cases, CT can rule out other diagnoses, including external or intraluminal obstructing tumors. In patients who are poor candidates for general anesthesia, CT may be considered to avoid needless bronchoscopy or when bronchoscopy is not immediately available.

Protocol. Thin slice noncontrast CT from the larynx to the diaphragm. With children, try to lower tube current (mAs) to reduce radiation exposure.

Possible Findings

■ Visualized foreign bodies. Foreign bodies that are radiolucent on plain radiography will be seen best on bone or lung window settings. Peanuts, unfortunately are not well visualized. Three-dimensional (3D) reconstructions and multiplanar views will help to identify smaller foreign bodies and to plan therapy.

■ Hyperaeration, atelectasis, infiltrates, and bronchiectasis will also be identified. Overall, CT has a sensitivity of 89% and specificity of 89%. The sensitivity and specificity are approximately 100% with 3D reconstructions and multiplanar views.

 ## IMAGING WITH NUCLEAR MEDICINE

Indications: not often considered. Ventilation-perfusion scanning can be done before bronchoscopy if the diagnosis cannot be confirmed by chest radiography or fluoroscopy. Documentation of changes in perfusion and ventilation may aid planning and timing of surgical intervention.

Protocol. Routine ventilation and perfusion scans with ^{133}Xenon (^{133}Xe) and ^{99m}Technetiumw (^{99m}Tc)-macroaggregated albumin (MAA).

Possible Findings

■ Ventilation defect equal to or greater than matched perfusion defect.
■ **Check valve obstruction.** Delayed ventilation washout from obstructed segment or lobe.
■ **Stop valve obstruction.** Absent radiotracer activity in obstructed segment or lobe on ventilation images.

 ## IMAGING WITH MAGNETIC RESONANCE

Indications. Magnetic resonance imaging (MRI) requires significant patient cooperation and is not routinely used. Of note, T1-weighted sequences may be helpful in detecting the high fat content of peanuts.

 ## ISSUES AFTER IMAGING

Treatment. Once a foreign body is localized, bronchoscopic removal is performed. If imaging findings are equivocal and foreign body is strongly suspected by history, bronchoscopy should not be delayed. However, complications of bronchoscopy can include pneumothorax, pneumomediastinum, tracheal laceration, and subglottic edema. Rarely, a thoracotomy is necessary to "milk" the object into a position where it can be removed by bronchoscopy. Lobectomy is occasionally required in cases of chronic vegetable foreign bodies.

Further Readings

Applegate KE, Dardinger JT, Lieber ML, et al. Spiral CT scanning technique in the detection of aspiration of LEGO foreign bodies. *Pediatr Radiol* 2001;31:836–840.

Bloom DC, Christenson TE, Manning SC, et al. Plastic laryngeal foreign bodies in children: a diagnostic challenge. *Int J Pediatr Otorhinolaryngol* 2005;69(5):657–662.

Chiu CY, Wong KS, Lai SH, et al. Factors predicting early diagnosis of foreign body aspiration in children. *Pediatr Emerg Care* 2005;21(3):161–164.

Girardi G, Contador AM, Castro-Rodriguez JA. Two new radiological findings to improve the diagnosis of bronchial foreign-body aspiration in children. *Pediatr Pulmonol* 2004;38:261–264.

Haliloglu M, Ciftci AO, Oto A, et al. CT virtual bronchoscopy in the evaluation of children with suspected foreign body aspiration. *Eur J Radiol* 2003;48:188–192.

Hunter TB, Taljanovic MS. Foreign Bodies. *Radiographics* 2003;23:731–757.

Kavanagh PV, Mason AC, Muller NL. Thoracic foreign bodies in adults. *Clin Radiol* 1999;54:353–360.

Kim TJ, Goo JM, Moon MH, et al. Foreign bodies in the chest: How come they are seen in adults? *Korean J Radiol* 2001;2(2):87–96.

Kosuco P, Ahmetoglu A, Koramaz I, et al. Low-dose MDCT and virtual bronchoscopy in pediatric patients with foreign body aspiration. *Am J Roentgenol* 2004;183:1771–1777.

Lea E, Nawaf H, Yoav T, et al. Diagnostic evaluation of foreign body aspiration in children: A prospective study. *J Pediatr Surg* 2005;40(7):1122–1127.

Orgill RD, Pasic TR, Peppler WW, et al. Radiographic evaluation of aspirated metallic foil foreign bodies. *Ann Otol Rhinol Laryngol Suppl* 2005;114(6):419–424.

Sersar SI, Hamza UA, AbdelHameed WA, et al. Inhaled foreign bodies: Management according to early or late presentation. *Eur J Cardiothorac Surg* 2005;28(3):369–374.

Swanson KL. Airway foreign bodies; what's new? *Semin Respir Crit Care Med* 2004;25(4):405–411.

Tokar B, Ozkan R, Ilhan H. Tracheobronchial foreign bodies in children: Importance of accurate history and plain chest radiography in delayed presentation. *Clin Radiol* 2004;59(7):609–615.

Zissin R, Shapiro-Feinberg M, Rozenman J, et al. CT findings of the chest in adults with aspirated foreign bodies. *Eur Radiol* 2001;11:606–611.

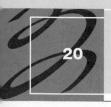

20 PULMONARY EMBOLISM
Krishna Juluru

CLINICAL INFORMATION

Epidemiology.   Although pulmonary embolism (PE) has been widely studied for many decades, its incidence, mortality, diagnosis, and treatment are still the subject of investigation. Incidence has been estimated to be 0.2 to 0.6 per 1,000 per year. Mortality rates as high as 30% have been reported in the older literature, although these studies are limited by use of clinical criteria for diagnosis of PE and by inclusion of patients with multiple comorbidities which may have independently contributed to death. The mortality in asymptomatic patients with PE and a low incidence of comorbid disease has been reported to be as low as 2.4%. Studies have shown that mild, untreated disease may have a low recurrence rate, arguing that clot burden should be a factor in determining management.

Risk Factors.   Most PE arise from clots within the venous circulation, and deep venous thrombosis (DVT) of the lower extremities is most common. Trauma and immobilization, cancer, and hypercoagulability comprise three broad categories of risk factors for DVT, with the latter two being most significant. The risk of recurrent thromboembolism is as high as 3.5 times greater in cancer populations than in those without cancer. Hypercoagulable states can exist due to genetic predisposition such as factor V Leiden mutation, prothrombin gene mutations, and deficiencies in protein S, protein C, and antithrombin III. Recently, blood types A and AB have been cited as additional risk factors. Certain medications, such as oral contraceptives, also increase risk.

Symptoms and Signs.   Clinical diagnosis of PE is unreliable. The most common symptom, dyspnea, is seen in only 73% of patients with angiographically proven PE. Other symptoms include pleuritic chest pain (66%), cough (37%), leg swelling (28%), leg pain (26%), and hemoptysis (15%). Angina, caused by right ventricular ischemia, and syncope have also been reported. Of note, patients with radiographic diagnosis of PE can be asymptomatic. The most common physical finding is tachypnea, seen in 70% of patients. Other findings include lung crackles on auscultation (55%), tachycardia (30%), and increased pulmonic component of the second heart sound (23%). The presence or absence of symptoms or signs should not exclusively influence a decision to proceed with further testing to diagnose PE.

Differential Diagnosis.   Owing to the lack of specific clinical findings, the differential diagnosis of PE is broad. Alternate considerations include pneumonia, congestive heart failure, acute myocardial infarction, exacerbation of chronic lung disease, aortic injury, and musculoskeletal inflammation/injury.

IMAGING WITH RADIOGRAPHS

Indications.   Chest radiography is a low-cost and low-radiation technique that, in most cases, is an appropriate start in the assessment of patients with chest symptoms. It can help identify other etiologies of the patient's symptoms and is used in conjunction with nuclear ventilation and perfusion imaging ($\dot{V}/\dot{Q}$) results, but it alone cannot help to include or exclude the diagnosis of PE.

Possible Findings. Radiographic signs of PE include prominent central artery (Fleischner sign), enlarged hilum, enlarged mediastinum, pulmonary edema, oligemia (Westermark sign), pleural-based areas of increased opacity (Hamptons hump), pleural effusion, and elevated hemidiaphragm. The highest sensitivity of any finding is 36% for pleural effusion. The highest specificity of any finding is 92% for oligemia. Entities that can be identified other than PE include pneumonia, pneumothorax, pneumomediastinum, heart failure, pleural effusion, lung mass, and fractures.

 IMAGING WITH COMPUTED TOMOGRAPHY

Indications. Computed tomographic pulmonary angiography (CTPA) performed on a multidetector computed tomographic (CT) scanner (four or more detectors) is the modality of choice for diagnosis of PE. Advantages include the ability to directly visualize pulmonary vessels and to diagnose diseases of the chest other than PE that may be contributing to the patient's symptoms. Renal insufficiency and allergy to contrast dye are the only major contraindications. Some patient cooperation in breath-hold is required. Using clinical outcome reference standards, the negative predictive value of computed tomographic angiography (CTA) ranges from 94–100% on scanners with less than four detectors. In comparison, studies performed on multidetector computed tomographic (MDCT) scanners demonstrate similar negative predictive values, but with reduced rates of respiratory and motion artifacts.

Protocol. CTA is performed following intravenous administration of 100–150 mL nonionic iodinated contrast agent at a rate of 3–4 mL/second. Power injection is considered unsafe through central lines, and therefore only peripheral venous access is used. The scan is performed from the lung apices to bases following live bolus tracking or a 23- to 28-second delay. Use thinnest possible (at most 1–2 mm) slice thickness. Multiplanar reconstruction of the pulmonary arteries from source data can be helpful in visualization of the pulmonary vessels.

Possible Findings (Fig. 20-1)

- Well-defined filling defects in a pulmonary artery seen on multiple sections are characteristic of PE (Fig. 20-1). Adjust the windows to make sure the pulmonary arteries

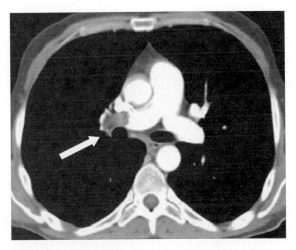

Figure 20-1. Computed tomographic pulmonary angiogram demonstrates a large pulmonary embolus in the right pulmonary artery (*arrow*).

are not too bright to detect subtle PE. These should be distinguished from flow-related artifacts and from masses, most notably in the mediastinum, that may be causing vascular compression.

■ Careful inspection of the scan may reveal other symptom-related findings such as pleural/pericardial effusion, pulmonary infiltrates, pulmonary masses, and fractures.

 IMAGING WITH NUCLEAR MEDICINE

Indications.   Nuclear $\dot{V}/\dot{Q}$ imaging scan can be used as a substitute for CTA, particularly in patients with renal insufficiency in whom iodinated intravenous contrast cannot be administered. Results are reported as normal, low, intermediate, or high probability. The sensitivity of a normal $\dot{V}/\dot{Q}$ scan is 98%, and the specificity of a high probability scan is 97%. A significant number of scans (39% in the Prospective Investigation of Pulmonary Embolism Diagnosis [PIOPED] study) fall into an intermediate probability category, limiting the strength of this imaging modality. Abnormalities on chest radiographs (e.g., infiltrates, masses) are associated with higher rates of intermediate probability scans, and when present, it is appropriate to let the ordering clinician know of this limitation.

Protocol.   Protocols vary by institution. The protocol at The Johns Hopkins Hospital is presented here. Ventilation imaging is performed before perfusion imaging because one of the energy peaks of the perfusion agent overlaps that of the ventilation agent. After the patient takes 1–2 normal breaths through a mask, 10–30 mCi (370–1,110 MBq) of ^{133}Xenon (^{133}Xe)-gas is introduced into the mask at end expiration. Images are traditionally obtained in anterior and posterior projections on a 128×128 matrix using a parallel-hole collimator centered at 80 keV. Some nuclear medicine departments prefer images in left posterior oblique (LPO) and right posterior oblique (RPO) projections. A single breath image is first obtained for 100,000 counts. Equilibrium images are then obtained for 300,000 counts after the patient breaths normally in the closed system for 3 minutes, followed by a series of 1-minute delayed washout images for 4–6 minutes.

Perfusion imaging is performed after intravenous injection of 4 mCi (300,000–500,000 particles) (111 MBq) of ^{99m}Technitium (^{99m}Tc)-macroaggregrated albumin (MAA). Images are obtained in anterior, posterior, and oblique projections. All images are obtained for a minimum of 600,000 counts on a 256×256 matrix using a parallel-hole collimator centered at 140 keV.

The MAA particle count should be decreased to 80,000 in patients with chronic obstructive pulmonary disease (COPD), pulmonary hypertension, or in those receiving mechanical ventilation, while maintaining a 4 mCi overall activity. Pregnant patients should first obtain perfusion imaging with a decreased dose of approximately 2 mCi ^{99m}Tc-MAA, followed by ventilation imaging only if there are perfusion abnormalities.

Possible Findings

The revised **PIOPED criteria** for interpretation of $\dot{V}/\dot{Q}$ scans are presented in Table 20-1. Determining the size of a defect can be difficult, and a knowledge of lung segmental anatomy is important (Fig. 20-2).

■ Small defects are defined as involving less than 25% of a segment, whereas large defects are defined as involving greater than 75% of a segment.

■ A normal $\dot{V}/\dot{Q}$ scan demonstrates uniform distribution of tracer to both lung fields, with clear definition of apices, diaphragms, and mediastinal contours (Fig. 20-3).

■ A high probability scan demonstrates mismatched defects (Fig. 20-4), defined as perfusion abnormalities that are larger or more severe than associated ventilation abnormalities.

■ A triple match, defined as a matching ventilation, perfusion, and chest x-ray (CXR) abnormality, should be interpreted as intermediate probability. There is insufficient data to show that triple matches in mid or upper lung zones are low probability.

■ One must be aware of the causes of false positive scans (Table 20-2).

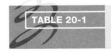

TABLE 20-1   The Modified Prospective Investigation of Pulmonary Embolism Diagnosis (PIOPED) Criteria for Interpretation of V̇/Q̇ Scans

High probability

- Two or more large (≥75% of a segment) mismatched segmental defects or equivalent with normal chest radiograph
- Any perfusion defect substantially larger than radiographic abnormality

Intermediate probability

- One moderate to less than two large mismatched segmental perfusion defects with normal CXR
- Solitary, moderate – large matched segmental defect with matching radiographic abnormality, regardless of lung zone (triple match)

Low probability

- Nonsegmental defects
- Matched V̇/Q̇ defects with normal chest radiograph
- Any perfusion defect with substantially larger radiographic abnormality
- Small, subsegmental perfusion defects
- Defects surrounded by normally perfused lung (stripe sign)

Normal

- No perfusion defects

CXR, chest x-ray; V̇/Q̇, ventilation/perfusion.

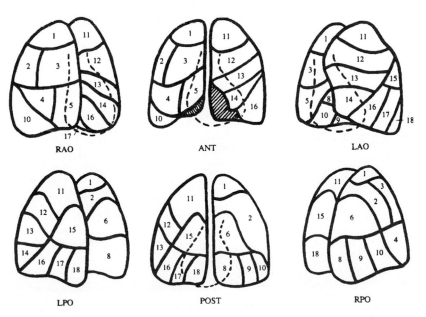

Figure 20-2. Anatomy of pulmonary segments. RAO, right anterior oblique; ANT, anterior; LAO, left anterior oblique; LPO, left posterior oblique; POST, posterior; RPO, right posterior oblique; RLAT, right lateral; LLAT, left lateral. (Dahnert W. *Radiology Review Manual*, 3rd ed. Baltimore: Williams & Wilkins, 1996;789.)

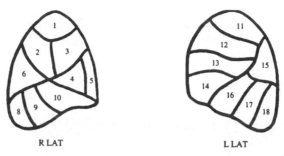

R LAT   L LAT

Figure 20-2. *(continued)*

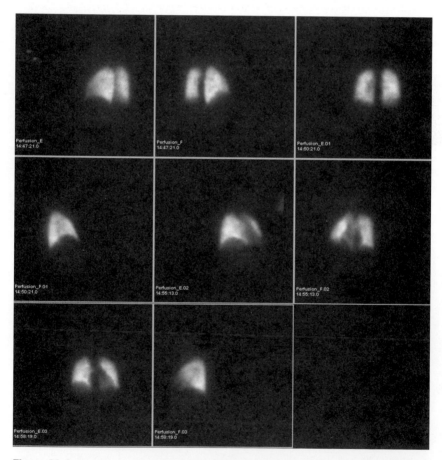

Figure 20-3. Normal nuclear medicine perfusion examination demonstrates uniform distribution of ^{99m}Technitium (^{99m}Tc) macroaggregrated albumin (MAA) in multiple projections. Normal nuclear medicine ventilation examination is shown in Figure 20-4B.

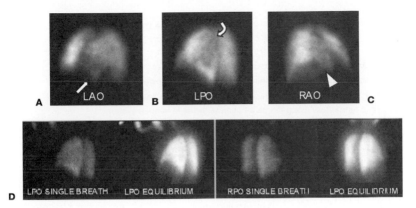

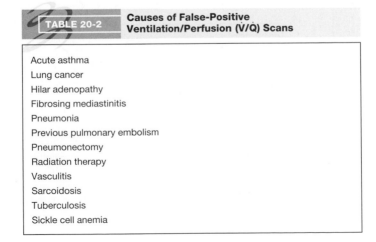

Figure 20-4. A: Left anterior oblique (LAO), **(B)** left posterior oblique (LPO), and **(C)** right anterior oblique (RAO) perfusion images demonstrate large perfusion defects in the anterior and basal segments of the left lower lobe (*straight arrow*), diminished perfusion in the superior segment of the left lower lobe (*curved arrow*), heterogeneous perfusion in the left upper lobe, and a moderate to large perfusion defect in the right lower lobe (*arrowhead*). **D:** Ventilation images following inhalation of ^{133}Xenon (^{133}Xe) gas demonstrate normal distribution of radiotracer throughout both lung fields. Multiple moderate to large perfusion defects in conjunction with normal ventilation images indicate high probability for pulmonary embolism.

■ A ventilation abnormality without an associated perfusion abnormality (reverse mismatch) is likely due to mucous plugging.

 ISSUES AFTER IMAGING

At present, there have been no known prospective, randomized trials that aim to distinguish clinically significant PE from those that are not clinically significant. Therefore, when even the smallest PE is detected with CTA, the current standard of care is a course of anticoagulation. However, this standard may change in the future as the significance of small subsegmental PEs is better understood.

TABLE 20-2	**Causes of False-Positive Ventilation/Perfusion (V/Q) Scans**
Acute asthma	
Lung cancer	
Hilar adenopathy	
Fibrosing mediastinitis	
Pneumonia	
Previous pulmonary embolism	
Pneumonectomy	
Radiation therapy	
Vasculitis	
Sarcoidosis	
Tuberculosis	
Sickle cell anemia	

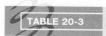

TABLE 20-3	Risk Factors/Clinical Features of Deep Venous Thrombosis (DVT)

Active cancer (treatment ongoing or within previous 6 mo or palliative)

Paralysis, paresis, or recent plaster immobilization of the lower extremities

Recently bedridden for more than 3 d or major surgery within 4 wk

Localized tenderness along the distribution of the deep venous system

Entire leg swollen

Calf swelling by more than 3 cm when compared with the asymptomatic leg (measured 10 cm below tibial tuberosity)

Pitting edema (greater in the symptomatic leg)

Collateral superficial veins (nonvaricose)

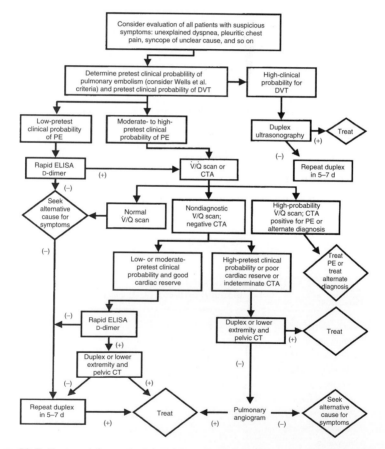

Figure 20-5. Proposed diagnostic algorithm for evaluation of pulmonary embolism (PE). DVT, deep venous thrombosis; ELISA, enzyme-linked immunosorbent assay; V̇/Q̇, ventilation/perfusion; CTA, computed tomographic angiography; CT, computed tomography. (Adapted from Laack TA and Goyal DG. Pulmonary embolism: an unsuspected killer. *Emerg Med Clin North Am* 2004;22(4): 961–983.)

Nondiagnostic CTA scans are rare, and usually occur due to poor bolus timing or uncontrolled respiration. Nondiagnostic $\dot{V}/\dot{Q}$ scans are more common. When either modality yields inconclusive results, the other modality may be used for further testing. If results remain inconclusive or if clinical suspicion remains high, pulmonary angiography may be performed. Because both PE and DVT are treated similarly, invasive testing can be avoided if a DVT is demonstrated using lower extremity Doppler ultrasound. DVT is unlikely in the absence of risk factors or certain clinical features (Table 20-3).

Anticoagulation may be safely withheld following either a negative CTA or normal $\dot{V}/\dot{Q}$ scan, given the high negative predictive value of these studies.

A diagnostic algorithm for acute PE is presented in Fig. 20-5. It is based on a clinician's pretest probability of PE, and includes D-dimer, CTPA, $\dot{V}/\dot{Q}$, lower extremity ultrasonography and pulmonary angiogram as part of the different diagnostic pathways.

Further Readings

Anderson FA, Wheeler HB, Goldberg RJ, et al. A population-based perspective of the hospital incidence and case-fatality rates of deep vein thrombosis and pulmonary embolism. *Arch Intern Med* 1991;151:933–938.

Calder KK, Herbert M, Henderson SO. The mortality of untreated pulmonary embolism in emergency department patients. *Ann Emerg Med* 2005;45:302–310.

Fedullo PF, Morris TA. Pulmonary thromboembolism In: Mason; Murray & Nadel's *textbook of respiratory medicine*, 4th ed, Elsevier Science, 2005:1425–1452.

Julurn K, Eng J. Imaging in the evaluation of pulmonary embolism. In: Medina LS, Blackmore CC, eds. *Evidence-based imaging*. New York: Springer-Verlag; 2005.

Laack TA, Goyal DG. Pulmonary embolism: an unsuspected killer. *Emerg Med Clin North Am* 2004;22(4):961–983.

Merli G. Diagnostic assessment of deep vein thrombosis and pulmonary embolism. *Am J Med* 2005;118:3S–12S.

Oger E. Incidence of venous thromboembolism: a community-based study in Western France. *Thromb Haemost* 2000;83:657–660.

The PIOPED Investigators. Value of the ventilation/perfusion scan in acute pulmonary embolism. Results of the prospective investigation of pulmonary embolism diagnosis (PIOPED). *JAMA* 1990;263(20):2753–2759.

Streiff MB, Segal J, Stuart GA, et al. ABO blood group is a potent risk factor for venous thromboembolism in patients with malignant gliomas. *Cancer* 2004;100:1717–1723.

Wells PS, Anderson DR, Bormanis J, et al. Value of assessment of pretest probability of deep-vein thrombosis in clinical management. *Lancet* 1997;350(9094):1795–1798.

Ziessman HA, O'Malley JO, Thrall JH. *Nuclear medicine, the requisites*, 3rd ed. St. Louis: Mosby, 2005.

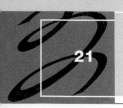

21

THORACIC AORTIC ANEURYSM AND DISSECTION

Paul D. Campbell, Jr. and Edward H. Herskovits

$\mathcal{B}$oth thoracic aortic aneurysm and dissection may constitute surgical emergencies, yet their diagnostic evaluations are fraught with difficulty due to the lack of specificity of clinical findings. Radiologic methods therefore assume a critical role in the evaluation for these conditions.

CLINICAL INFORMATION

Etiology and Epidemiology. Aortic aneurysm has a prevalence of approximately 10% in autopsy series. Morphologic types include saccular, fusiform, dissecting, false, and sinus of Valsalva. Although arteriosclerosis (saccular and fusiform aneurysms) is the major predisposing factor, trauma (false aneurysm), aortitis (e.g., syphilis, Takayasu arteritis), Marfan's syndrome, and infection (mycotic aneurysm) should be considered. The risk of aneurysm rupture is directly related to the wall tension, which in turn is a function of the diameter. In practice, the threshold for surgical repair is a diameter of 5 cm or greater, because these aneurysms have at least a 10% chance of rupture per year. A patient with chest pain and an aortic aneurysm must be considered to have a ruptured aneurysm until proved otherwise, and may require emergent surgical repair.

Thoracic aortic dissection is the most prevalent emergency involving the aorta; if untreated, it carries a mortality of approximately 70% during the first 2 weeks, and approximately 90% during the first 3 months; treatment may decrease the 3-month mortality to approximately 30%. The most common predisposing factors are hypertension and Marfan's syndrome.

Almost all dissections begin as an intimal tear in one of two locations where the aorta is relatively fixed: (1) the ascending aorta 2–5 cm above the aortic valve (the most common site) and (2) the descending aorta just distal to the origin of the left subclavian artery. Two classification systems are used to describe thoracic aortic dissection: the DeBakey and the Stanford systems. In the **DeBakey system,** type I dissections involve the ascending and descending aorta, type II dissections involve only the ascending aorta, and type III dissections involve only the descending aorta. In the **Stanford system,** type A refers to a dissection with any ascending aortic involvement, and type B refers to involvement limited to sites distal to the origin of the left subclavian artery. Dissection involving the aorta proximal to the arch (DeBakey types I and II, Stanford type A) is more worrisome, for it may lead to occlusion of the great vessels or coronary arteries, aortic insufficiency, and pericardial tamponade. For this reason, these dissections are treated surgically. Conversely, dissection restricted to that portion of the aorta distal to the aortic isthmus (DeBakey type III, Stanford type B) is usually treated medically with antihypertensive therapy, unless the renal arteries or other arterial branches are compromised. Involvement of the coronary arteries occurs in 10–20% of patients with thoracic aortic dissection. In the aorta, blood flow often dissects the portion of aortic wall where flow is greatest, that is, where the radius of curvature is greatest, which is the side of the aorta that is farthest from the heart. Therefore, dissections tend to be located anteriorly in the ascending aorta, superiorly at the level of the arch, and posteriorly and to the left in the descending aorta. Therefore, the left renal artery is in greater danger of occlusion by a dissection involving the descending aorta than is the right renal artery. The opposite would be true in a person with right aortic arch.

Symptoms and Signs. Symptoms include chest pain, particularly severe in patients with dissection, which may be indistinguishable from angina. The pain is usually of sudden onset, may radiate to the upper back, or to the lower back and flank. Physical examination of patients with aneurysm is often unrevealing, but in patients with dissection there may be an absent carotid pulse, a diastolic murmur, or difference between the blood pressures of the upper extremities or between the upper and lower extremities.

 IMAGING WITH RADIOGRAPHS

Protocol. Standard upright posteroanterior (PA) chest radiographs are much preferable to supine anteroposterior (AP) radiographs, but may not be possible due to the patient's condition. Chest radiography is highly sensitive for detecting aortic aneurysm, moderately sensitive for detecting aortic dissection from trauma, and nonspecific for either, thereby necessitating further evaluation when the radiograph is abnormal or when clinical suspicion is high.

Possible Findings. Relevant findings in the setting of aneurysm or dissection include the following:

- Widened mediastinum, especially if it increases with time. In cases of trauma, mediastinal widening is caused by injury and bleeding of mediastinal veins and serves as a marker of injury severity and is commonly associated with aortic dissection.
- Rightward displacement of the esophagus or nasogastric tube.
- Anterior displacement of the trachea and mainstem bronchi on lateral view.
- The false lumen may dissect arteriosclerotic mural calcification equal to or greater than 5 mm away from the aortic wall; although rare, this finding is relatively specific, and should be sought regardless of the modality employed.
- Either aneurysm or dissection may cause a left pleural effusion or apical pleural cap due to hemothorax.

Although these findings lack specificity, when more than one of them is present, further evaluation is almost always indicated. An aneurysm that is proximal to the descending aorta should alert the radiologist to consider nonarteriosclerotic etiologies, such as syphilis.

 IMAGING WITH COMPUTED TOMOGRAPHY

Indications. When adequate CT is performed, sensitivity for aortic aneurysm is approximately 100%, and specificity approaches 100%. Sensitivity and specificity for dissection are 90–100%. Multislice techniques have improved image quality and diagnostic accuracy compared to previous CT technology.

Protocol. Scanning the patient's chest, abdomen, and pelvis without intravenous (IV) contrast is useful to detect intramural hematoma. Choose as thin slice thickness as is possible on the scanner available. After excluding contraindications to contrast, inject 120 mL of nonionic contrast intravenously at 3 mL/second. Initiate scanning 30 seconds after the start of the injection or use bolus tracking. Depending on the type of CT scanner available, choose a slice thickness as low as 0.75 mm. Electrocardiography (ECG)-gated acquisition is preferable in order to eliminate motion artifacts in the ascending aorta, which can mimic aortic dissection. To further reduce the possibility of artifact, the patient's arms should be placed overhead, and motion should be reduced, as long as these measures are permitted by the patient's condition. Including the great vessels, abdominal aorta and iliac bifurcation in the aortic protocol is advised. Beware of IV contrast in a hypotensive patient as this can impair renal function. Protocols may vary with different types of CT scanners.

Possible Findings

Aneurysm
- Arteriosclerotic aneurysms are usually located in the descending aorta, and their prevalence decreases with a more proximal location. An aneurysm that is proximal to the descending aorta should alert the radiologist to consider nonarteriosclerotic etiologies.
- Mural thrombus seen on the luminal side of the intima (to be distinguished from intramural hematoma which is subintimal).
- Mural calcification.
- Mediastinal hematoma.
- Contrast extravasation (implying leakage or rupture).

Dissection or Intramural Hematoma (Figs. 21-1–21-4)
- The demonstration of true and false lumens and an intimal flap is pathognomic. Owing to the dynamics of flow in the thoracic aorta, the false lumen will usually be located anteriorly in the ascending aorta, superiorly in the arch, and posteriorly and to the left in the descending aorta.

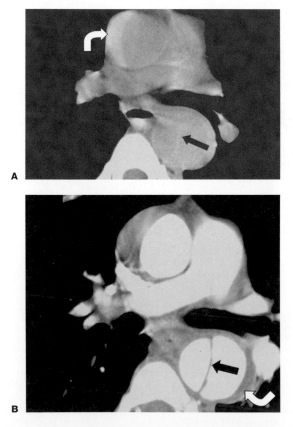

Figure 21-1. A: Precontrast and **(B)** postcontrast computed tomography (CT) demonstrates dissection of descending aorta and intramural hematoma of the ascending and descending thoracic aorta. The intramural hematoma (*arrow*) appears hyperdense to nonenhanced blood. Dissection flap (*black arrow*) is barely visible on noncontrast image but is well seen on contrast-enhanced image. Courtesy of Katarzyna Macura, MD, Johns Hopkins Hospital.

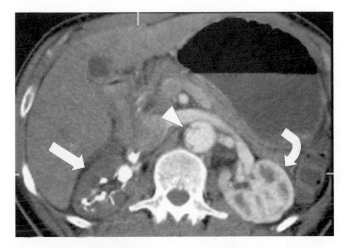

Figure 21-2. Aortic dissection (*arrowhead*) results in reduced perfusion of the right kidney (*straight arrow*) compared to the left (*curved arrow*). This is a common complication of dissection. Courtesy of Katarzyna Macura, MD, Johns Hopkins Hospital.

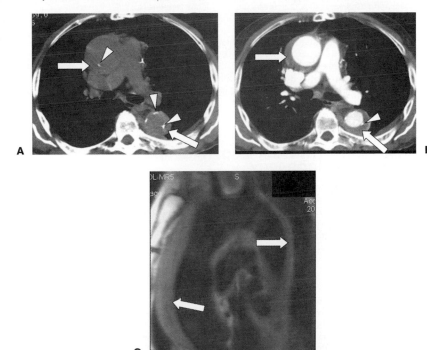

Figure 21-3. **A:** Precontrast computed tomography (CT), **(B)** postcontrast CT, and **(C)** black blood magnetic resonance imaging (MRI) results show intramural hematoma (*arrows*) of the ascending and descending thoracic aorta. Intimal calcifications (*arrowheads*) are best seen on noncontrast CT and help to differentiate intramural hematoma from mural thrombus. Courtesy of Katarzyna Macura, MD, Johns Hopkins Hospital.

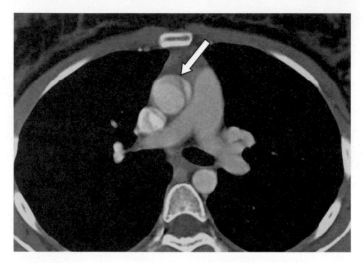

Figure 21-4. Contrast-enhanced computed tomography (CT) demonstrates a motion artifact, which simulates an intimal flap (*arrow*). This is a common problem with nongated imaging studies of ascending aorta. Courtesy of Katarzyna Macura, MD, Johns Hopkins Hospital.

- If there is differential enhancement of the two lumens, the true lumen usually manifests better enhancement, because flow in the false lumen is usually slower.
- Intramural hematoma is typically seen as subintimal (superficial to intimal calcifications) hyperdense material on the noncontrast scan.
- Although displacement of calcified plaque by the dissection or by intramural hematoma is rarely demonstrated on plain radiography, it is demonstrated on CT in approximately one third of patients with dissection.
- Pulsation artifact of the ascending aorta which often simulates dissection (Fig. 21-4).

 IMAGING WITH TRANSESOPHAGEAL ECHOCARDIOGRAPHY

Indications. Most studies demonstrate almost perfect sensitivity and specificity for transesophageal echocardiography (TEE) in evaluating the thoracic aorta for dissection or aneurysm. TEE is also excellent for evaluating complications of dissection, such as great vessel occlusion, aortic regurgitation, and cardiac tamponade. This examination is, however, highly operator dependent, and the necessary expertise, or in-house coverage may not exist at many medical centers.

Possible Findings. Aneurysm is readily demonstrated by TEE. The entry site will be demonstrated in approximately 80% of patients with dissection. An intimal flap that undulates with the cardiac cycle is virtually diagnostic of dissection. Similar findings allow the detection of extension of the flap into the coronary arteries. Doppler interrogation demonstrates velocities in the true and false lumens, reducing false-negative examinations due to slow flow in the false lumen. A false-positive examination is usually due to reverberation artifact caused by arteriosclerotic disease.

 IMAGING WITH MAGNETIC RESONANCE

The sensitivity of magnetic resonance imaging (MRI) for detecting aortic dissection is 95–100%, and the specificity is approximately 90–100%.

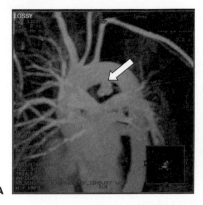
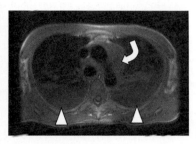

A **B**

Figure 21-5. **A:** Aortic magnetic resonance angiography (MRA) demonstrates a mycotic saccular pseudoaneurysm (*straight arrow*) arising from the aortic arch in a patient with a history of intravenous (IV) drug abuse. **B:** Black blood magnetic resonance imaging (MRI) shows a large mediastinal hematoma (*curved arrow*) and large bilateral pleural effusions (*arrowheads*). Courtesy of Katarzyna Macura, MD, Johns Hopkins Hospital.

Indications. MRI is most useful when contrast-enhanced CT cannot be performed (due to contrast allergy, renal failure, etc.) or when CT is inconclusive (due to motion artifact, etc.).

Protocol. Black blood axial and oblique (candy-cane view of the thoracic aorta) double inversion recovery (IR), bright blood (axial spoiled gradient-recalled echo [SPGR]), and 3D time of flight SPGR are performed followed by 3D time of flight SPGR after the administration of 0.2 mmol/kg of gadolinium at 2 mL/second. Extend axial images through the abdomen and pelvis.

Possible Findings

Aneurysm (Fig. 21-5)
- Aneurism.
- Mediastinal hematoma, implying leakage or rupture.

Dissection or Intramural Hematoma (Fig. 21-3)
- Intimal flap. Flowing blood (in the true and false lumens) will manifest signal void on spin-echo sequences, and as high signal on black blood sequences. It may be difficult to distinguish thrombus from slowly flowing blood in the false lumen, a distinction that has implications for surgical management; flow-sensitive techniques increase sensitivity under these circumstances and increase the accuracy of evaluation of the coronary arteries and great vessels.
- Intramural hematoma.
- Mediastinal hematoma, implying leakage or rupture.
- Contrast extravasation, implying leakage or rupture.

IMAGING WITH ANGIOGRAPHY

Indications. In patients with aortic dissection and aneurysm, aortography has been considered the "gold" standard for delineating the extent of involvement of the aorta and great vessels. When assessing for aortic dissection, false negatives can occur because of a thrombosed false lumen, simultaneous equal opacification of both lumens, or because of an intimal flap that is viewed en face rather than on edge. Aortography has sensitivity and sensitivity that approach 100% for aneurysm. However, because of the high sensitivity and specificity of computed tomographic angiography (CTA) and magnetic resonance angiography (MRA), aortography is typically only performed when these tests are nondiagnostic. One of the primary benefits of aortography is that treatment with stent grafting or fenestration can often be instituted by the interventional radiologist.

Possible Findings

- Aortic aneurysm manifests as focal dilation, by definition at least 4 cm in diameter.
- Dissection may manifest as an intimal flap with no contour abnormality. Both true and false lumens may be demonstrated, especially if the false lumen is not thrombosed.
- Aortic regurgitation, if present, is also easily demonstrated.

 DIAGNOSTIC ALGORITHM

Currently CT is the preferred initial diagnostic imaging modality due to its availability, speed, and high sensitivity and specificity. When contrast-enhanced CT is inconclusive or cannot be performed, TEE or MRI can be performed and offer benefits as outlined in the preceding text. Angiography remains the "gold" standard in the evaluation of thoracic aortic aneurysm and dissection but typically is only performed when previous testing is inconclusive or as part of a therapeutic endovascular procedure.

 ISSUES AFTER IMAGING

Ascending aortic dissections and intramural hematomas represent surgical emergencies. Descending aortic dissections and intramural hematomas are managed medically (if distal to left subclavian), surgically, or endovascularly. Aneurysms larger than 5 cm in diameter can be treated with surgery or endovascular therapy.

Further Readings

Khan IA, Nair CK. Clinical, diagnostic, and management perspectives of aortic dissection. *Chest* 2002;122:311–328.

Matsunaga N, Hayashi K, Okada M, et al. Magnetic resonance imaging features of aortic diseases. *Top Mag Reson Imaging* 2003;14:253–266.

Qanadii SD, El Hajjam M, Mesurolle B, et al. Motion artifacts of the aorta simulating aortic dissection on spiral CT. *J Comput Assist Tomogr* 1999;23:1–6.

Ravenel JG, McAdams HP, Remy-Jardin M, et al. Multidimensional imaging of the thorax. *J Thorac Imaging* 2001;16:269–281.

Yun KL. Ascending aortic aneurysm and aortic root disease. *Coron Artery Dis* 2002;13: 79–84.

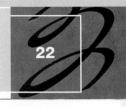

THORACIC AORTIC INJURY

Jens Vogel-Claussen and Edward H. Herskovits

22

*A*cute thoracic aortic injury accounts for 10–20% of fatalities in high-speed deceleration accidents. Aortic rupture is highly lethal if untreated: there is a bimodal distribution of mortality, with more than 88% dying within 4 hours and 90% of undiagnosed survivors dying in the 4 months after presentation. Thoracic aortic injuries include aortic dissection, aortic intramural hematoma, traumatic aortic rupture, and aneurysm (see Chap. 21, "Thoracic Aortic Aneurysm and Dissection.") The most frequent deceleration injury is at the aortic isthmus, near the ligamentum arteriosum and aortopulmonic window. Therefore, evaluating the mediastinum, particularly the aorta, great vessels, and mediastinal fat, is the radiologist's central role in this setting.

 CLINICAL INFORMATION

Mechanism of Injury.   The most common mechanism of injury is a high-speed motor vehicle accident, or one in which the victim is ejected from the vehicle; other settings include a pedestrian or cyclist struck by a motor vehicle, and fall from a height. Common to all of these mechanisms of injury is sudden deceleration in the anteroposterior (AP) or superoinferior axis, leading to traction on the aorta at the ligamentum arteriosum, and compression of the aorta between the thoracic spine posteriorly and the manubrium, first rib, and clavicle anteriorly. Mechanisms of dissection and intramural hematoma are discussed in Figures 22-1 and 22-2.

Symptoms and Signs.   Given these mechanisms of injury, it is not surprising that associated symptoms include back pain, subjective weakness or numbness in the extremities, and chest pain. Associated physical findings include fractures of the bony thorax, upper and lower extremity hypotension, return of frank blood from a pleural tube, shock, and extrathoracic injuries, including paresis or paraplegia. Significantly, signs of chest-wall injury are absent in one third of cases of traumatic aortic injury.

 IMAGING WITH RADIOGRAPHS

Indications.   Depending on the study quoted, the sensitivity of chest radiography for detecting aortic trauma is 80–85%, and the specificity is 45–62%. Although these numbers vary considerably with technique and other factors, they clearly confine the role of chest radiography to that of a screening technique to be incorporated with clinical information during rapid initial assessment of a trauma victim.

Protocol.   Standard upright posteroanterior (PA) chest radiographs are much preferable to supine AP radiographs, but may not be possible because of the patient's condition.

Possible Findings

Although these findings lack specificity, when more than one of them is present further evaluation is almost always indicated.

- Rightward displacement of a nasogastric tube.
- Left apical cap.

117

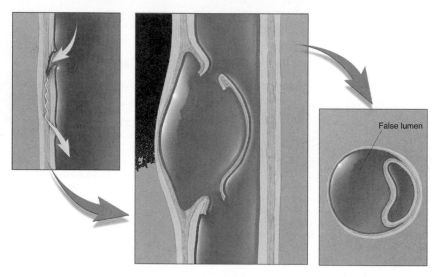

Figure 22-1. Diagram illustrates events leading to aortic dissection from formation of entrance tear and exit tear of intima to splitting of aortic media and formation of intimomedial flap. Blood under pressure dissects media longitudinally, and double-channel aorta is formed with blood filling both true and false lumens. (Macura KJ, Corl FM, Fishman EK, et al. Pathogenesis in acute aortic syndromes: aortic dissection, intramural hematoma, and penetrating atherosclerotic aortic ulcer. *AJR Am J Roentgenol* 2003;181:309–316.)

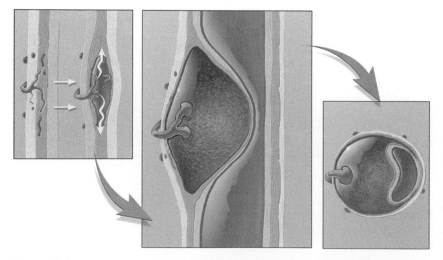

Figure 22-2. Diagram shows events leading to intramural hematoma, from rupture of vasa vasorum feeding aortic media to creation of intramedial hematoma with intact intimal layer. (Macura KJ, Corl FM, Fishman EK, et al. Pathogenesis in acute aortic syndromes: aortic dissection, intramural hematoma, and penetrating atherosclerotic aortic ulcer. *AJR Am J Roentgenol* 2003;181:309–316.)

- Fractures of ribs 1–3.
- Loss of the aortic knob outline.
- Widened mediastinum, which is caused by injury and bleeding of mediastinal veins and serves as a marker of injury severity and is commonly associated with aortic dissection.
- Wide paraspinal stripe.
- Loss of descending aorta outline.
- Thick paratracheal line.
- Pneumothorax.
- Hemothorax.
- Pneumomediastinum.
- Pulmonary contusion.

 IMAGING WITH COMPUTED TOMOGRAPHY

Indications. Computed tomography (CT) is the modality of choice for the evaluation of acute aortic injury. When adequate CT is performed, sensitivity for aortic trauma is 95–100%, using aortography as the "gold" standard. CT can rule out acute thoracic aortic injuries with submillimeter resolution and 3D reconstructions can be used to accurately describe aortic injuries. Therefore clinically stable patients with low, intermediate, or high suspicion for aortic trauma should undergo a contrast-enhanced CT examination. Unstable patients need to be stabilized before the CT examination or, if clinically indicated, triaged directly for emergency surgery. However, it is always helpful to establish the extent of the aortic injury on CT before surgery.

Protocol. (See Chap. 21, "Thoracic Aortic Aneurysm and Dissection.")

- Three-dimensional (3D) reconstructions are often useful in establishing the diagnosis and explaining imaging findings to the referring clinicians in a comprehensive manner.

Possible Findings

(See Chap. 21, "Thoracic Aortic Aneurysm and Dissection.")

- Intimal flap/aortic dissection.
- Pseudoaneurysm.
- Irregular aortic contour.
- Pseudocoarctation.
- Intramural hematoma.
- Indirect signs include periaortic and mediastinal hematoma.
- Concomitant injuries such as hemopneumothorax, rib fractures, and traumatic diaphragmatic hernia may also be detected, and their presence increases the probability of injury of the great vessels or aorta.

 IMAGING WITH MAGNETIC RESONANCE

Indications. This modality is not practical for acute trauma due to logistical constraints, such as the need for rapid availability and the presence of patient monitoring equipment. Magnetic resonance imaging (MRI) demonstrates vascular anatomy and blood flow, and therefore it plays a role in postsurgical follow-up as well as in chronic traumatic injury. In postoperative patients with thoracic aortic reconstruction surgery or known aortic hematoma and clinical symptoms, MRI can be useful especially in evaluating the composition of blood products (i.e., acute versus chronic hematoma).

 IMAGING WITH AORTOGRAPHY

Indications. Aortography is still considered the "gold" standard for demonstrating injury to the aorta and great vessels, and like CT, it can determine whether a patient with suspected mediastinal vascular injury will be surgically explored. However, because computed tomographic angiography (CTA) is noninvasive, rapid, and approaches the diagnostic sensitivity and specificity of conventional angiography, aortography is typically only performed when CTA is nondiagnostic. One of the primary benefits of aortography, however, is that treatment can often be instituted by the interventional radiologist, with stent grafting or fenestration.

Protocol.   Thoracic aortography is described in detail in Chapter 53, "Arteriography Primer" Either a femoral or an axillary approach may be employed, but the former is associated with lower morbidity. A pigtail catheter is introduced gently using a soft, J-shaped guidewire to minimize the probability of further vascular injury. Digital subtraction is typically employed. Minimizing contrast load is important, especially when thoracic CT has already been performed as a screening study. Injection rates range between approximately 20 mL/second and 30 mL/second. A minimal study must include right posterior oblique and AP views of the aorta centered on the arch; in addition, the descending thoracic aorta and all of the great vessels must be evaluated.

Possible Findings.   Aortic laceration may manifest as an intimal flap with or without contour abnormality. In severe cases, pseudoaneurysm (contrast extravasation) or even complete transection (contour disruption) may be demonstrated.

 DIAGNOSTIC ALGORITHM

On the basis of the diagnostic characteristics of aortography, CT, and radiography in delineating the extent of injury to the aorta and great vessels, many authors have proposed algorithms for patient management in the setting of blunt thoracic trauma. If the clinical suspicion is intermediate or high, CT examination with intravenous contrast should be performed whether or not there are positive findings on the chest radiograph. If symptoms persist and the initial CT scan was normal, repeat CT within a few hours of the first examination is sometimes useful because of the possibility of a delayed development of intramural hematoma or dissection. In an unstable patient with a high suspicion of an acute life-threatening aortic injury, thoracotomy, or aortography with interventional treatment can be performed with or without prior noninvasive imaging.

 ISSUES AFTER IMAGING

Ascending aortic dissections and intramural hematomas represent surgical emergencies. Descending aortic dissections and intramural hematomas are managed medically (if distal to left subclavian), surgically, or endovascularly.

Further Readings

Alkadhi H, Wildermuth S, Desboilles L, et al. Vascular emergencies of the thorax after blunt and iatrogenic trauma: multidetector row CT and three-dimensional imaging. *Radiographics* 2004;24: 1239–1255.

Duhaylongsod FG, Glower DD, Wolfe WG. Acute traumatic aortic aneurysm: the Duke experience from 1970 to 1990. *J Vasc Surg* 1992;15: 331–343.

Macura KJ, Corl FM, Fishman EK, et al. Pathogenesis in acute aortic syndromes: aortic aneurysm leak and rupture and traumatic aortic dissection. *AJR Am J Roentgenol* 2003;181: 303–307.

Takahashi K, Stanford W. Multidetector CT of the aorta. *Int J Cardiovasc Imaging* 2005;21(1): 141–153.

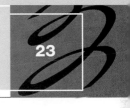

MYOCARDIAL ISCHEMIA AND INFARCTION

Jens Vogel-Claussen and Oleg M. Teytelboym

23

CLINICAL INFORMATION

Etiology and Epidemiology. Coronary artery disease is currently the number one cause of death of both men and women in the United States. Risk factors include smoking, diabetes, hypertension, dyslipidemia, and family history. It is caused by formation of atherosclerotic plaques within the walls of coronary arteries, which may impede vascular flow. Myocardial ischemia, like all tissue ischemia, results from excessive demand or inadequate supply of oxygen, glucose, and free fatty acids due to coronary artery luminal narrowing. Hemodynamically significant stenosis is present if there is a more than 50% luminal diameter narrowing of left main artery or a more than 70% narrowing of other vessels. As atherosclerotic plaque evolves, production of macrophage proteases and neutrophil elastases within the plaque can cause thinning of the fibromuscular cap that covers the lipid core. Increasing plaque instability coupled with blood-flow shear and circumferential wall stress can lead to plaque fissuring or rupture, especially at the junction of the cap and the vessel wall. Acute myocardial infarction results from a rupture of an unstable plaque and secondary thrombus formation which leads to occlusion of the lumen, most commonly occurring in the proximal portions of the coronary arteries. Unstable angina is characterized by rapid thrombolysis of this thrombus, which restores myocardial perfusion and prevents myocardial tissue death. Stable angina occurs due to significant luminal stenosis without plaque rupture and thrombosis.

Symptoms and Signs. Chest pain is the cardinal symptom of myocardial ischemia. The pain commonly radiates to the left arm or the jaw. Patients may also complain of dyspnea, nausea, diaphoresis, and chest pressure. However, particularly in patients with diabetes, myocardial ischemia may be asymptomatic. Stable angina manifests as increased myocardial demand due to exercise or emotional stress, and is relieved by rest or sublingual nitroglycerin. Unstable angina is characterized by increasing frequency and severity of chest pain (crescendo-angina), chest pain at rest, and increasing need of antiangina medication occurring in patients with a history of stable angina. Patients with unstable angina have a 20% risk of acute myocardial infarction. Acute myocardial infarction is characterized by sudden onset (typically occurring over 30 minutes) of intense chest pain and pressure. Electrocardiography (ECG) is the cornerstone of rapid diagnosis. Elevation of myocardial enzymes is used to confirm the diagnosis.

IMAGING

Clinical history, ECG changes, and cardiac enzyme analysis are sufficient for establishing the diagnosis of acute myocardial infarction in most cases. Imaging is primarily used to diagnose and evaluate stable and unstable angina in order to detect hemodynamically significant stenosis or to evaluate myocardial viability. Myocardial viability imaging can be used to distinguish scar from hypoperfused hibernating myocardium, in order to predict outcomes of revascularization.

Stress ECG has an approximately 80% sensitivity of detecting a critical coronary narrowing if the age-related target heart rate is obtained. Stress echocardiography has a sensitivity of approximately 90% in detecting wall motion abnormalities. However, this technique is operator dependent and has a limited field of view. Plain chest radiographs are quite insensitive in detecting coronary pathology. In patients with severe disease, heavy coronary artery calcifications may show up as "railroad tracks" on chest radiographs projecting over the heart silhouette. Also ventricular enlargement, cardiac aneurisms, pleural effusions, and pulmonary edema as sequela from myocardial infarction can be evaluated with chest radiographs.

In this chapter we focus on computed tomography (CT), magnetic resonance imaging (MRI), conventional coronary angiography, and nuclear medicine imaging techniques for detection of ischemic heart disease.

 IMAGING WITH COMPUTED TOMOGRAPHY

Indications. Rapid evolution of CT technology has brought cardiac CT to the forefront of cardiac imaging. Calcium scoring can be used for coronary heart disease screening and also typically performed as part of coronary computed tomographic angiography (CTA). CTA is excellent at accurately assessing the atherosclerotic burden and luminal narrowing, and has been shown to be superior to conventional coronary angiography in detection of nonobstructing plaque. Although the guidelines are rapidly evolving, currently coronary CTA is considered in patients with equivocal stress tests. Recently, however, some emergency rooms have started to use coronary CTA as a tool for rapid triage and management of patients with chest pain.

Protocol. A multislice CT scanner and heart rate control are the necessary prerequisites for performing an adequate cardiac CT. A 16-slice CT allows an adequate examination in 60–70% of patients, particularly if the heart rate can be maintained in the low 60s. A 64-slice CT achieves adequate results in more than 80–90% of patients, even if the heart rate is in the 70s. The new generation of dual source CT scanners should permit adequate cardiac CT with heart rates up to 100.

Heart rate control can be achieved with β-blockers: 50–100 mg of oral metoprolol 45–90 minutes before the scan or 5 mg metoprolol IV boluses, every 5 minutes up to 20 mg, with the patient on the CT table. Contraindications to β-blockers include second-degree Mobitz or third-degree arteriovenous (AV) block and severe chronic obstructive pulmonary disease (COPD).

Calcium scoring is obtained by performing a breath-hold noncontrast gated coronary CT, and is based on the Agatston scoring algorithm which was initially developed for electron beam CT. CT threshold density of 130 HU is used to detect coronary calcification in each of the four main coronary branches (left main, left anterior descending, circumflex, and right coronary arteries). The score is computer generated by measuring the volume of coronary calcification and multiplying it by a factor (between 1 and 4) based on the peak attenuation value of the lesion.

Coronary CT angiography is obtained by performing a breath-hold gated CT after injection of 80 mL of iodinated contrast bolus, injected at 4 mL/second, followed by 40 mL saline chaser (this requires a dual head injector) to reduce high-density artifacts in the superior vena cava and right heart (mixing 5 mL of contrast with the saline bolus can significantly improve septal visualization, without significant artifact). The image acquisition delay for each patient is usually determined by live bolus tracking in the descending aorta and triggering the scan when contrast density is 180 HU. Alternatively, a small test bolus can be used to determine peak contrast density time and adding 4–6 seconds to allow for larger volume of the actual bolus.

High radiation dose is the main drawback of the current 64-slice techniques (~9.8–16.3 mSv for males and 13.5–22.6 mSv for females versus 3–10 mSv for cardiac catheterization). Radiation dose can be reduced by using prospective ECG gating in order to scan only during diastole; however, this technique may significantly degrade examination quality in patients with even mildly irregular heart rate. Dose modulation by reducing the dose during the systole can decrease the total radiation dose by 40%.

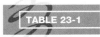

| TABLE 23-1 | Calcium Score Interpretation |

Calcium score	Evaluation	Risk of coronary artery disease
0	Normal	Very low, less than 5%
1–10	Minimal calcification	Low, less than 10%
11–100	Mild calcification	Mild or minimal coronary narrowing is likely
101–400	Moderate calcification	Possible significant coronary narrowing
401 or higher	Extensive calcification	High likelihood of atleast one significant coronary narrowing

Possible Findings

■ Calcium scoring (Table 23-1)
- Zero calcium score has a very high negative predictive value for presence of significant atherosclerotic disease.
- Poor correlation between the value of significant calcium score and the severity of disease, necessitating further evaluation.
- Patients with very high calcium scores may not be good candidates for coronary CT angiography because the high calcified plaque burden causes significant "blooming artifact," which makes the CT angiography study difficult to interpret. However, this may change with dual energy/dual source scanner technology.

Coronary Computed Tomograpic Angiography

■ Accurate interpretation of coronary CTA depends on user familiarity and comfort with the 3D workstation. It is necessary to use a combination of oblique multiplanar reconstruction (MPR), oblique maximum intensity projection (MIP), and 3D rendering techniques to achieve accurate results. It is impossible to be accurate with only axial or 3D images. When reporting the study, it is important to describe coronary anatomy (Fig. 23-1). Presence of major diagonal and marginal branches should be documented (terms *large* should be used when branch is large enough for bypass and *small* when it is not).

■ Normal study essentially excludes presence of coronary artery disease.

■ Look for congenital anomalies (Fig. 23-2), myocardial bridging, and AV malformations. A left coronary artery that arises from the right aortic sinus and passes between aorta and pulmonary artery significantly increases the likelihood of sudden death and should be treated with bypass surgery. Anomalous right coronary arteries that originate from left aortic sinus and pass between aorta and pulmonary artery increase the likelihood of sudden death, although to a lesser degree. Treatment is controversial and may include bypass, implantable defibrillator, and β-blockers. If myocardial bridging is present, dynamic stenosis can be detected by evaluating the vessel in systole and diastole.

■ If coronary artery disease is present, it is important to evaluate for more than 50% luminal diameter narrowing of left main artery or more than 70% narrowing of other vessels, because these lesions may require intervention with stenting or surgical bypass. Remember that degree of narrowing only refers to luminal diameter. External remodeling by plaque can significantly enlarge vessel size. Coronary CTA permits distinguishing between non-clacified and calcified plaque.

■ When critical stenosis is suspected, it is important to evaluate that segment with 0.5 mm MPR or MIP slices in order to accurately evaluate the stenosis because the lumen frequently appears narrower with thicker slices (use of thicker slices, up to 3.5 mm permits a more rapid survey of the coronary vessels).

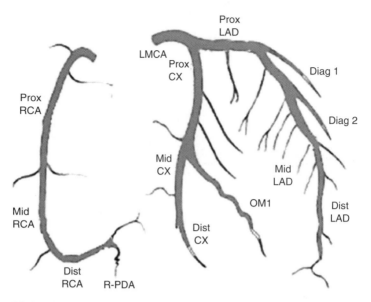

Figure 23-1. Diagram demonstrates classic coronary anatomy and nomenclature. Prox, proximal, LAD, left anterior descending, LMCA, left main coronary artery, RCA, right coronary artery, CX, circumflex, OM1, first obtuse marginal, R-PDA, right posterior descending artery.

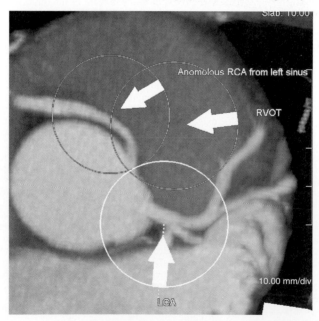

Figure 23-2. Coronary CTA oblique MIP shows right coronary artery (RCA) that originates from left aortic sinus and passes between aorta and pulmonary artery. This congenital anomaly is associated with increased likelihood of sudden death. CTA, computed tomographic angiography, MIP, maximum intensity projections, RVOT, right ventricular outflow tract, LCA, left coronary artery. Courtesy of Daniel Schwartz, MD, Summit Medical Group, NJ.

- **Approximate stenosis quantification:** (some rules of thumb; these do not apply to left main because of its size)
  - Less than 50% luminal narrowing if any view through suspected stenosis shows good flow (Fig. 23-3).
  - Seventy percent luminal narrowing if minimal flow seen in one view and all other views show plaque (Fig. 23-4).
  - Ninety percent luminal narrowing if no flow or practically no flow seen on any views; however, good distal flow is seen.

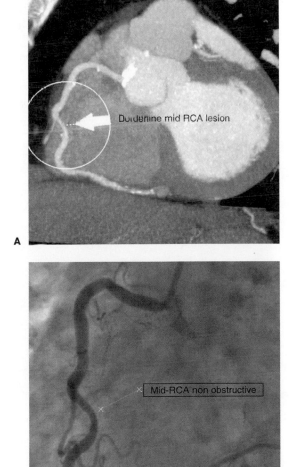

A

B

Figure 23-3. A: Coronary CTA oblique MIP shows 40–50% narrowing of right coronary artery (RCA) by soft plaque. CTA, computed tomographic angiography, MIP, maximum intensity projections. **B:** Catheter angiogram confirms the finding. RCA, right coronary artery. Courtesy of Daniel Schwartz, MD, Summit Medical Group, NJ.

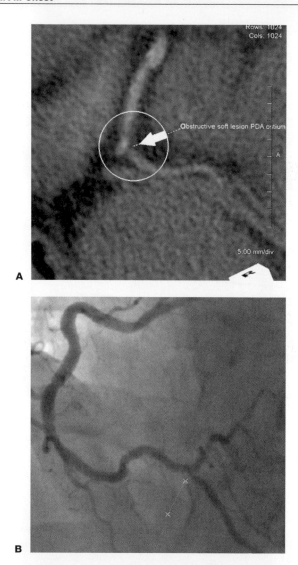

Figure 23-4. A: Coronary CTA oblique MIP shows 70% narrowing at the origin of posterior descending artery (PDA) by soft plaque. CTA, computed tomography, MIP, maximum intensity projections. **B:** Catheter angiogram confirms the finding. Courtesy of Daniel Schwartz, MD, Summit Medical Group, NJ.

- More than 95% luminal narrowing versus occlusion if no or only minimal distal flow present. Cardiac catheterization may be required for definitive answer (Fig. 23-5).
- 3D images should not be used to quantify degree of stenosis.
- CTA is excellent at determining coronary graft patency; however, it is important to note that up to 15–30% of grafts may become occluded after surgery without causing symptoms. Therefore accurate interpretation may require a baseline study.
- Coronary artery stent patency can be sometimes evaluated.

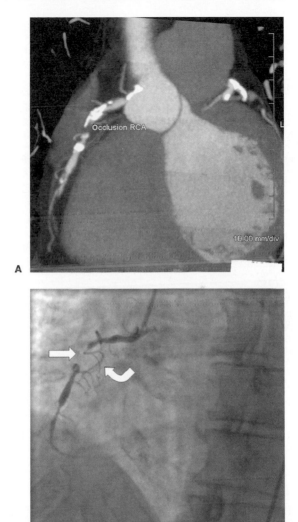

Figure 23-5. **A:** Coronary CTA oblique MIP shows occlusion of right coronary artery (RCA) by soft and calcified plaque. CTA, computed tomography, MIP, maximum intensity projections. **B:** Catheter angiogram confirms the finding and demonstrates the collateral branch that reconstitutes the right coronary artery. These findings suggest longstanding occlusion. Courtesy of Daniel Schwartz, MD, Summit Medical Group, NJ.

Four-dimensional Cardiac Computed Tomography

- Cardiac CT acquired with retrospective gating (scan during entire cardiac cycle) allows assessment of myocardial function, wall motion, chamber size, and to some degree valve function.
- Incorporation of wall motion information enables better assessment of true physiologic significance of observed coronary arterial narrowing.

■ 4D cardiac CT is very accurate at calculation of ejection fraction; however, unlike conventional echocardiography, current software excludes papillary muscle volume from chamber volume calculations, thereby reducing the ejection fraction by 10%.

 IMAGING WITH MAGNETIC RESONANCE

Indications.   Cardiac magnetic resonance imaging (MRI) is capable of accurately delineating nonviable or infarcted myocardium from potentially salvageable myocardium. This is particularly important for coronary bypass planning. Advantages of cardiac MRI compared to nuclear, echocardiographic, or positron emission tomography (PET) methods include high spatial resolution, lack of pharmacologic stress requirement, and short examination time. Disadvantages include reduced image quality in patients with arrhythmias and MRI safety exclusions (i.e., pacemaker, metal in orbit).

Protocol.   Viability MRI is performed after an intravenous injection of a gadolinium-based contrast agent, by acquiring immediate perfusion and delayed scans (10–20 minutes after contrast injection). MRIs are optimized so that normal myocardium is "suppressed" on gradient echo images. MRI can be performed with free-breathing technique, which does not require breath-hold.

Possible Findings

■ On delayed images 10–20 minutes after contrast injection, myocardial scar ("nonviable tissue" from prior infarct) retains the gadolinium contrast agent producing bright signal, whereas washout of the contrast agent occurs in viable myocardium.
■ High spatial resolution of MRI enables identification of subendocardial and transmural infarction.
■ Thinning of the ventricular wall can be observed due to old myocardial infarction, particularly in transmural infarction. In addition, thrombus or aneurysm formation can be identified.
■ Myocardial scar/fibrosis involving more than 50% of myocardial wall thickness by cardiac MRI is unlikely to recover contractile function following coronary revascularization.
■ After acute myocardial infarction, first pass MR perfusion images demonstrate lack of enhancement at the region of microvascular obstruction. This is typically at the "core" of the area of myocardial necrosis. Lack of enhancement of this infarct core, or microvascular obstruction, is related to poor patient prognosis with increased incidence of congestive heart failure, recurrent infarction and chest pain.

 IMAGING WITH CONVENTIONAL CORONARY ANGIOGRAPHY

Indications.   Conventional coronary angiography is considered to be the gold standard for detection of significant coronary artery disease and plays a key role in management of the disease. Contraindications include allergies to iodinated contrast agents, impaired renal function, and bleeding disorders.

Protocol.   Percutaneous access is usually gained through the common femoral artery using the Seldinger technique. The coronary artery origins are selected and iodinated contrast is injected through the intraluminal catheter. Digital subtraction angiography (DSA) sequences are then performed of the right and left coronary arteries. A spatial resolution of 0.1–0.2 mm can be obtained, which is superior to available CT angiography technology.

Possible Findings

■ Conventional coronary angiography can reliably detect significant coronary artery narrowing along the full length of the coronary arteries.

- "Lumenography"technique, therefore the wall structure cannot be evaluated unless intravascular ultrasonography is used.
- Ability to treat as well as to diagnose significant coronary artery disease is a significant advantage of conventional coronary angiography. A wide variety of coronary stents is available, some of which are coated with drugs or are radioactive in order to prevent in stent restenosis.

 IMAGING WITH NUCLEAR MEDICINE TECHNIQUES

Indications. Nuclear medicine stress testing is widely used to assess for obstructive coronary artery disease. It allows detection of physiologically significant coronary stenosis and enables evaluation of myocardial viability. Most studies are performed with single photon emission computed tomography (SPECT) technology; however PET has shown promising results in evaluating and differentiating viable, hibernating, stunned, and infarcted myocardium with better image quality. Increasing availability of PET technology indicates that this modality may play a more significant role in the evaluation of ischemic heart disease in the near future.

Protocol

1. ^{201}Thallium (^{201}Tl) or ^{99m}Technetium (^{99m}Tc) SPECT scintigraphy is performed at rest to establish a baseline. ^{201}Tl enables performing the stress phase during the same day (different photopeak from ^{99m}Tc. It has high extraction during transit through the capillary bed and imaging is performed 10 minutes after injection. ^{99m}Tc requires performing stress portion of the examination on a different day; however, it produces better quality images and is therefore required in very obese patients. Imaging is usually delayed up to 2 hours to allow time for washout from liver.
2. Patients can be stressed with treadmill exercise or by pharmacologic agents which increase cardiac inotropy and chronotropy such as dobutamine. Alternatively, vasodilatating agents such as adenosine can detect perfusion difference depending on degree of coronary stenosis (preferred in patients with atrial fibrillation).
3. Myocardial ischemia can only be demonstrated if the radiotracer (usually ^{99m}Tc) is injected during the period of ischemia; therefore, the tracer is injected during peak exercise. This tracer localizes in the mitochondria of viable myocardial cells with significantly delayed washout (several hours). Imaging can be performed as soon as 15 minutes after exercise, but usually delayed up to 2 hours to reduce breathing artifacts and allow time for washout from the liver.
4. Viability imaging relies on ^{201}Tl redistribution following second dose administration.

Possible Findings

- Accuracy is highly dependent on the degree of stress, usually measured by age-predicted peak heart rate.
- Significant physiologic coronary narrowing is detected based on decreased radiotracer activity during stress, with reversal of the defect at rest.
- Fixed radiotracer defects at stress and rest are areas of infarcted myocardium/scar tissue.
- Wall motion and the left ventricular ejection fraction should be evaluated and correlated with the radiotracer uptake.
- Common limitations and pitfalls include relatively low spatial resolution, with poor sensitivity for subendocardial reversible ischemia, and falsely decreased tracer activity due to breast or diaphragmatic attenuation.

Further Readings

Clark AN, Beller GA. The present role of nuclear cardiology in clinical practice. *Q J Nucl Med Mol Imaging* 2005;49(1):43–58.

Machac J. Cardiac positron emission tomography imaging. *Semin Nucl Med* 2005;35(1): 17–36.

Mollet NR, Cademartiri F, van Mieghem CA. High-resolution spiral computed tomography coronary angiography in patients referred for diagnostic conventional coronary angiography. *Circulation* 2005;112(15):2318–2323.

O'Rourke RA, Brundage BH, Froelicher VF, et al. American College of Cardiology. American heart association expert consensus document on electron beam computed tomography for the diagnosis and prognosis of coronary artery disease. *Circulation* 2000;102:126–140.

Thomson LE, Kim RJ, Judd RM. Magnetic resonance imaging for the assessment of myocardial viability. *J Magn Reson Imaging* 2004;19(6):771–788.

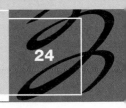

24

*I*ntra-abdominal abscesses occur most commonly after bowel perforation, surgery, trauma, pancreatitis, and in immunocompromised patients. Mortality can reach 30%. Intra-abdominal abscesses can be divided according to location: intraperitoneal, retroperitoneal, and visceral.

CLINICAL INFORMATION

Symptoms and Signs. Development of an abscess is often insidious, and the clinical picture is often confusing and nonspecific. Patients with abdominal abscesses usually present with fever, leukocytosis, and an elevated erythrocyte sedimentation rate. Secondary findings include pain near the abscess, anorexia, weight loss, nausea, vomiting, altered bowel habits, and occasionally a palpable mass. However, few signs and symptoms may be present if the patient is immunosuppressed, taking steroids or antibiotics, or has a chronic, walled-off abscess.

Causes and Locations

Intraperitoneal Abscesses
- Most commonly due to generalized peritonitis.
- Form most frequently within the pelvis (66% of intra-abdominal abscesses).
- Subphrenic and subhepatic spaces are the next most common sites. Subphrenic abscesses occur three times more often on the right than the left due to the natural flow of intraperitoneal fluid.
- Other sites include infracolic and paracolic gutters, lesser sac.

Retroperitoneal Abscesses
- Anterior pararenal space between the posterior peritoneum and anterior renal fascia caused by pancreatitis or perforated retroperitoneal bowel.
- Perinephric space between the anterior and posterior layers of the renal fascia due to rupture of renal parenchymal abscesses through the renal capsule.

Visceral Abscesses
- **Hepatic abscesses** can be due to bacterial seeding from diverticulitis, appendicitis, or endocarditis. Direct extension of cholecystitis-causing hepatic abscess can also occur. Fungal infections of the liver or spleen are often small and have a target appearance. Echinococcal or amebic abscesses may also occur.
- **Splenic abscesses** are uncommon and when present they are often the result of uncontrolled, widespread infection. They may also be sequela of splenic infarct or trauma. Ultrasonography can help differentiate a splenic infarct from a true abscess.
- **Pancreatic abscesses** are usually the sequela of acute pancreatitis and occur at sites of pancreatic necrosis.
- **Renal cortical abscesses** often occur as a result of hematogenous spread of *Staphylococcus*.
- **Renal medullary abscesses** are most frequently a complication of acute pyelonephritis.

Differential Diagnosis.   Any low-attenuation or cystic mass may mimic an abscess including a cyst, pseudocyst, loculated ascites, hematoma, urinoma, lymphocele, biloma, thrombosed aneurysm, or necrotic neoplasm. Normal structures such as stomach, bowel, and bladder can also be confused with abscesses.

IMAGING WITH RADIOGRAPHS

Indication.   Initial examination for generalized abdominal pain of unknown etiology. If localizing symptoms are present, patient is acutely ill, or there is a high clinical suspicion for abscess, the patient should have a computed tomographic (CT) scan.

Protocol.   Routine upright and supine abdominal views. Decubitus views or cross-table lateral for patients unable to sit upright.

Possible Findings

Radiographs have poor sensitivity for detecting abdominal abscess. Look for extraluminal air and air-fluid levels. If an abscess is suspected, additional imaging is usually required to confirm location and extent.

IMAGING WITH COMPUTED TOMOGRAPHY

Indications.   Study of choice for identifying and localizing most abdominal abscesses. CT is 95% sensitive, fast, and easily accessible. CT should be the initial examination in the acutely ill or patients with localized clinical findings. Ultrasonography is the initial study to examine the female pelvis and may be the first choice for right upper quadrant pain.

Protocol.   Administer oral and IV contrast if not contraindicated. Wait at least 2.5–3 hours after administration of oral contrast to ensure bowel opacification.

Possible Findings (Figs. 24-1 and 24-2)

- An acute abscess often appears as a soft tissue density mass.
- A chronic abscess often has the appearance of a fluid collection with a well-defined enhancing, irregular wall/capsule.
- There is significant overlap of the density of an abscess and cystic/low density solid masses.
- One third of abscesses contain air.
- Inflammation of adjacent fat.
- False-positive diagnoses are usually due to mistaking unopacified fluid-filled stomach, bowel, or bladder for an abscess.

IMAGING WITH ULTRASONOGRAPHY

Indications.   Preferred initial examination for possible abscess in the female pelvis, and is typically the initial examination for right upper quadrant pain. The accuracy of detecting abscesses is approximately 90% and most effective in the right upper quadrant, perinephric space, and pelvis. Ultrasound is a bedside examination that can be performed in patients unable to be moved. However, ultrasound is less useful for visualizing within or near structures with large amounts of gas, such as stomach and bowel and for the evaluation of the middle/lower abdomen and areas of the retroperitoneum. May be of limited value in obese patients.

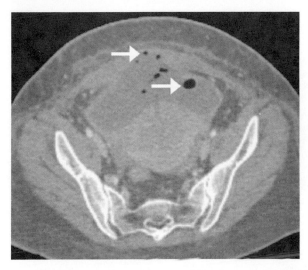

Figure 24-1. Pelvic abscess on computed tomography (CT) scan, containing multiple gas bubbles (*arrows*).

Protocol.   Real-time ultrasonography is used to examine the area of interest in sagittal and transverse planes. Doppler ultrasound should be used to investigate for internal flow and surrounding hyperemia.

Possible Findings (Fig. 24-3)

- Complex fluid-filled lesions with mixed echogenicity or hypoechoic solid lesions.
- Increased pain when pressure applied with transducer over suspected abscess.

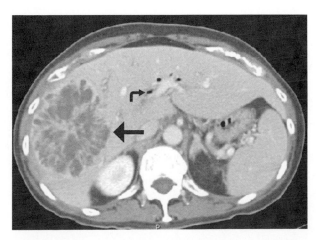

Figure 24-2. Hepatic abscess on computed tomography (CT) scan (*straight arrow*) with rim enhancement and innumerable loculation. Pneumobilia (*curved arrow*) is secondary to prior hepati-cojejunostomy, which is a significant risk factor for development of hepatic abscess.

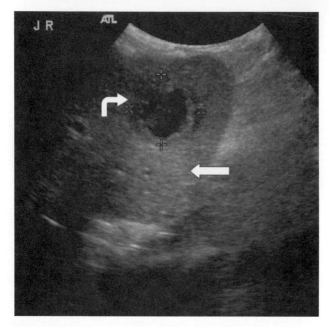

Figure 24-3. Hepatic abscess on ultrasonography (US) (*curved arrow*). It has echogenic rim, internal debris, and demonstrates enhanced through transmission (*straight arrow*).

■ No blood flow within abscess by Doppler examination.
■ Lack of abscess wall movement helps differentiate possible abscess from a peristaltic fluid-filled bowel loop.

 IMAGING WITH MAGNETIC RESONANCE

Indications.   Magnetic resonance imaging (MRI) has a limited role in evaluation of intra-abdominal abscesses because of availability, cost, and scanning time. However, MRI is superior to CT for detection of abscesses involving visceral organ and pelvis.

Protocol.   To examine the abdomen with no target organ, the following protocol may be used:

■ Use torso coil if small to average height person or a body coil for tall person.
■ Coronal scout image.
■ Axial T2-weighted imaging (T2WI) fast spin echo (FSE) with fat saturation (Fat Sat) from diaphragm to symphysis pubis with 8 mm thick sections and a 2 mm gap.
■ Axial in phase T1WI fast multiplanar spoiled gradient echo (FMPSPGR) from diaphragm to symphysis pubis with 8 mm thick sections and 2 mm gap.
■ Axial postgadolinium in phase T1WI FMPSPGR with Fat Sat with 70-second scan delay through the liver; 8 mm thick/2 mm gap.
■ Axial postgadolinium in phase T1WI FMPSPGR with Fat Sat through the remainder of abdomen and pelvis; 8 mm thick/2 mm gap.

Possible Findings

■ Rim enhancement.
■ High T2 signal of internal contents.

IMAGING WITH NUCLEAR MEDICINE

Indications.   Occult abdominal abscess in patients who are not acutely ill and have no localizing abdominal signs because whole body images are acquired If abnormal, another imaging study such as CI or MRI ultrasound is required to provide anatomic localization. Sensitivity of nuclear medicine studies for abdominal abscess is 80–92%.

¹¹¹Indium (¹¹¹In)-labeled Leukocytes

- Study time is shorter than gallium.
- More specific than gallium—does not accumulate in tumors and is not excreted by the colon.
- Chronic abscesses may not have a significant inflammatory response and therefore may not be detected.
- Upper abdominal abscesses may be obscured by normal high tracer activity within the liver and spleen.

⁶⁷Gallium (⁶⁷Ga) Citrate

- Requires 48–72 hours before interpretation.
- Accumulation is nonspecific; tracer accumulates in any area of inflammation and in certain tumors.
- Excretion by the colon makes differentiation between normal colon and adjacent abscess difficult, and limits its use for the evaluation of infectious processes in the abdomen.

 PERCUTANEOUS ABSCESS DRAINAGE

Indications.   The criteria for performing percutaneous drainage of an abscess with ultrasonography or CT guidance are as follows:

- Pus that is thin enough to be evacuated through a catheter.
- Few abscess cavities or loculations.
- Drainage route that does not traverse bowel, uncontaminated organs, or sterile pleural or peritoneal spaces.

Abscess drainage catheters usually remain in place for 7–10 days and the success rate is approximately 70%.

Further Readings
Brandt WE, Helms CA. *Fundamentals of diagnostic radiology*, 2nd ed. Philadelphia: Lippincott Williams & Wilkins, 1999.
Middleton WD, Kurtz AB, Hertzberg BS. *Ultrasound: the requisites*, 2nd ed. St. Louis: Mosby, 2004.

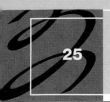

ABDOMINAL AORTIC ANEURYSM AND DISSECTION

25

Valerie A. Pomper and Paul D. Campbell, Jr.

*A*n abdominal aortic aneurysm (AAA) is defined as a focal widening of the aorta of more than 3 cm in anteroposterior (AP) diameter.

CLINICAL INFORMATION

Etiology. AAAs are most commonly caused by atherosclerosis (73–80%) and result from atrophy and fibrous replacement of the vessel media and adventitia. Other types of aneurysms are uncommon, including mycotic aneurysms (usually associated with intravenous drug abuse (IVDA), steroid therapy, or the immunosuppressed) or traumatic aneurysms. Even rarer are syphilitic aneurysms, which usually affect the ascending aorta and arch.

Location. Seventy-five percent of AAAs are confined to the abdomen; the remaining 25% also involve the descending thoracic aorta. AAAs occur in an infrarenal position in 95–98% of cases with extension into iliacs in 66% of cases.

Rupture. Rupture is the major complication of AAA, and the risk is related to the size of the aneurysm. A small aneurysm (4.5–6 cm) ruptures in 20% of patients over a period of 3 or more years. An aneurysm more than 6 cm ruptures in 50% of patients within 1–2 years (Fig. 25-1).

Symptoms and Signs. The classic triad (actually seen in only 20% of cases) for a ruptured AAA is as follows:

- Central abdominal or back pain.
- Pulsatile abdominal mass.
- Shock/hypotension.

Note that a prominent abdominal aortic pulsation may be normally present in thin people and be mistakenly diagnosed as an AAA. On the other hand, pulsations from an AAA may not be palpable in patients who are obese. Risk factors for developing atherosclerotic AAA include hypertension, coronary artery disease, peripheral vascular disease, and AAA in a first-degree relative.

IMAGING WITH COMPUTED TOMOGRAPHY

Indications. Computed tomography (CT) is the study of choice for evaluating patients for suspected ruptured AAA. Ultrasonography is *not* indicated for evaluation in emergent settings for several reasons: (1) the ileus that occurs with a ruptured aneurysm is likely to preclude an adequate study, (2) ultrasonography is not as sensitive as CT to diagnose the characteristic perinephric fluid collections, and (3) simply identifying an aneurysm by ultrasonography does not exclude another cause for the patient's abdominal symptoms. Arteriography does not add to the CT findings and is not necessary, unless it is being performed as a percusor to endovascular therapy.

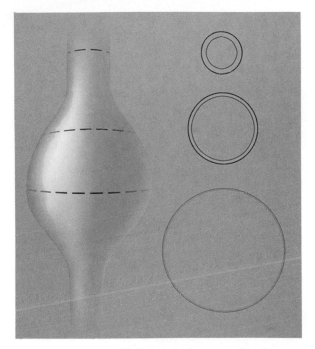

Figure 25-1. Drawing shows enlarging aortic aneurysm. First, wall tension is proportional to vessel radius, according to Laplace's law: $T = P \times r$, where T is circumferential wall tension, P is transmural pressure, and r is mean vessel radius. Second, increased tension stress from blood pressure results in progressive vessel dilatation and weakening of aortic media, which lead to enlargement of aortic aneurysm. Third, when mechanical stress on wall exceeds strength of wall tissue, aortic aneurysm ruptures. (Macura KJ, Corl FM, Fishman EK, et al. Pathogenesis in acute aortic syndromes: aortic aneurysm leak and rupture and traumatic aortic transection. *AJR Am J Roentgenol* 2003;181:303–307.)

Protocol. Scanning the patient without intravenous contrast is useful to detect intramural hematoma. After excluding contraindications to contrast, inject 120 mL of nonionic contrast intravenously at 3 mL/second. Initiate scanning 30 seconds after the start of the injection or use bolus tracking. Depending on the type of CT scanner available choose a slice thickness as low as 0.75 mm, if possible. If imaging both the thorax and abdomen, electrocardiography (ECG)-gated acquisition is preferable in order to eliminate motion artifacts in the ascending aorta, which can mimic aortic dissection. To further reduce the possibility of artifact, the patient's arms should be placed overhead, and motion should be reduced, as long as these measures are permitted by the patient's condition. Including the great vessels, thoracic aorta, abdominal aorta, and iliac bifurcation in the aortic protocol is advised. Beware of IV contrast in a hypotensive patient as this can impair renal function. Protocols may vary with different types of CT scanners.

COMPUTED TOMOGRAPHIC FINDINGS IN INDIVIDUAL CLINICAL SITUATIONS

Ruptured Aneurysm

Location. Rupture may occur into retroperitoneum (commonly on the left side), into the GI tract with massive GI hemorrhage (most commonly the duodenum), or into the inferior vena cava (IVC) with rapid cardiac decompensation.

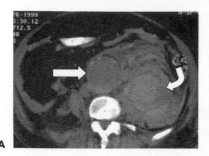 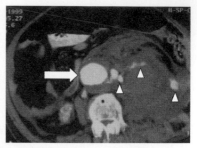

A   **B**

Figure 25-2. **A:** Precontrast and **(B)** postcontrast computed tomography (CT) scan demonstrates ruptured abdominal aortic aneurism (*straight arrows*). There is a large periaortic hematoma (*curved arrow*), which is hyperdense to nonenhanced blood. There is active contrast extravasation (*arrowheads*). Courtesy of Katarzyna Macura, MD, Johns Hopkins Hospital.

Possible Findings (Fig. 25-2)

- Large AAA with adjacent retroperitoneal hematoma.
- Obscuration or anterior displacement of the aneurysm by an irregular high density mass or fluid collection (hematoma) that extends into one or both perirenal spaces, left greater than right.
- Anterior displacement of the kidney by the hematoma.
- Enlargement or obscuration of psoas muscle.
- Focally indistinct aortic margin that corresponds to the site of the rupture (this is thought to be due to underperfusion of the disrupted wall by the vasa vasorum).
- High-attenuation "crescent" in the thrombus or wall of the aneurysm (on noncontrast scans, higher attenuation than the patent lumen; on contrast-enhanced scans, higher attenuation than psoas muscle). This finding has a high association with rupture, or at least should suggest that an aneurysm is at risk for rupturing. This sign may be seen without evidence of retroperitoneal blood and may represent the early CT manifestation of aneurysm rupture—a focal leak into the adjacent thrombus and aortic wall.

Chronic Aortic Pseudoaneurysm (False Aneurysm)

Definition. Complete disruption of aortic intima and media with vascular integrity maintained only by the adventitia, or other surrounding connective tissues, with subsequent hematoma formation. Pseudoaneurysms account for only 1% of all AAAs and 66% are due to penetrating trauma. Although pseudoaneurysm formation initially prevents a catastrophic event, rupture may occur at any time after the trauma; therefore, pseudoaneurysms should be resected.

Possible Findings

- Well-defined, round mass with attenuation value similar to or lower than that of native aorta on noncontrast studies.
- Laminated mural calcification due to focal, contained intra- and extramural hemorrhage from recurrent leaks.
- Enhancement of lumen of aneurysm and/or its communication to the aorta.

Aortic Dissection

Definition. A tear in the aortic intima with formation of a false channel within the media. Blood in the false channel may reenter the true channel through a second intimal tear, or it may rupture through the adventitia into periaortic tissues.

Location. Spontaneous dissection rarely originates in the abdominal aorta (1% of all aortic dissections). When it originates in the abdominal aorta, it is typically infrarenal.

Aortic dissection commonly begins in the thoracic aorta (ascending > descending) and may extend into the abdomen. (See Chap. 21, "Thoracic Aortic Aneurysm and Dissection.") If the dissection involves the origin of either renal artery, renal perfusion may be compromised.

Possible Findings

- Displaced intimal calcifications.
- Intimal flap.
- Enhancement of true and/or false lumen.

Traumatic Transection or Tear

Proper Workup.   Injuries to the abdominal aorta are rare, and most patients with this injury exsanguinate at the scene of trauma, or are hypotensive on arrival and go directly to the operating room. The infrarenal segment is most commonly involved. If there is suspected acute rupture (transection) of the aorta, CT should be performed immediately.

Location.   The site of most aortic damage resulting from blunt trauma is the descending thoracic aorta 1 cm from the origin of the left subclavian artery at the insertion of the embryonic ductus arteriosus. Most injuries at this site are complete transections. Less frequently, aortic injuries occur in the ascending aorta (including the arch), the distal descending aorta, and the abdominal aorta. (See Chap. 21, "Thoracic Aortic Aneurysm and Dissection.")

Postoperative Aorta

Surgical Anatomy.   CT appearance of aortic reconstruction is variable and depends on the type of surgical repair. The most common surgical repair involves an aortic, aortoiliac, or aortofemoral graft sutured in an end-to-end manner around which the aneurysm sac and thrombus are wrapped. Less commonly, the proximal anastomosis is end-to-side, which can be identified by a more anterior position of the graft in relation to the native, ultimately thrombosed, aorta.

Possible Findings

Normal Postoperative

- Aortic graft is slightly higher attenuation than unenhanced blood in the lumen. Visualization of an aortic graft may be extremely difficult on contrast-enhanced scans.
- Air is normally seen in the surgical bed in the immediate postoperative period (up to 10 days).
- Perigraft fluid collections, usually representing hematomas, are commonly seen, and resolve within 2–3 months.
- Fluid or soft tissue attenuation, corresponding to thrombus, normally separates aortic graft from native aortic wrap. Over time, this separation resolves and should not be seen after approximately 3 months.

Aortic Graft Infection

- Air seen in graft more than 21 days postoperatively is probably abnormal, whereas air seen more than 7 weeks after surgery is pathognomonic for graft infection.
- Perigraft soft tissue or fluid or persistent separation of the graft and native aortic wrap lasting more than 3 months after surgery are also abnormal and strongly suggest infection. In the immediate postoperative period, diagnosis of infection may be very difficult to make. Postoperative air usually consists of a few bubbles located anteriorly, whereas air resulting from graft infection usually consists of multiple tiny air bubbles located posterior to or around the entire aortic graft.

Aortoenteric Fistula

- Graft infection is almost always associated with aortoenteric fistula.
- Perigraft fluid and extraluminal air may be present.

- Sixty-six percent of patients present with gastrointestinal bleeding.
- Duodenum is the most common site of fistula formation, but jejunum and ileum may be involved.
- Extravasation of oral contrast material around the graft or intravasation of IV contrast into bowel is rare.

Possible Findings in Anastomotic Pseudoaneurysm

- Late complication, on average 6 years after surgery, occurring in up to 50% of patients with grafts.
- Inguinal region more frequent than in the abdomen.
- Eccentrically located pouch or diverticulum at anastomotic site.
- Partially or totally thrombosed pseudoaneurysm.
- Thickening or calcification of the pseudoaneurysm.

 IMAGING TIPS

False Positive.   CT diagnosis of ruptured AAA is possible in certain situations:

- A variety of retroperitoneal masses—lymphadenopathy, perianeurysmal fibrosis, and psoas muscle masses—may be mistaken as retroperitoneal hemorrhage.
- Unopacified duodenum can sometimes be misdiagnosed as a small preaortic hematoma.
- Retroperitoneal hemorrhage may develop for an unrelated reason (trauma, recent biopsy, blood dyscrasia, anticoagulant therapy, retroperitoneal neoplasm) in patients with an AAA. CT may suggest that retroperitoneal hemorrhage has not resulted from rupture of an AAA when the aortic wall remains intact, well visualized, and when the adjacent periaortic fat is preserved.

 IMAGING WITH MAGNETIC RESONANCE

Indications.   Magnetic resonance imaging (MRI) is most useful when contrast-enhanced CT cannot be performed (due to contrast allergy, renal failure, etc.) or when CT is inconclusive (due to motion artifact, etc.). The sensitivity of MRI in detecting aortic dissection is 95–100%, and the specificity is approximately 90–100%.

Protocol.   Black blood axial and sagittal oblique double inversion recovery (IR), bright blood (axial spoiled gradient recalled echo [SPGR]), and 3D time of flight SPGR are performed followed by 3D time of flight SPGR after the administration of 0.2 mmol/kg of gadolinium at 2 mL/second. Extend axial images through the chest, abdomen, and pelvis.

Possible Findings (Similar to Computed Tomography)

- Aneurysm.
- Retroperitoneal hematoma implying leakage or rupture.
- Intramural hematoma.
- Contrast extravasation implying leakage or rupture.
- Intimal flap (sign of dissection or intramural hematoma). Flowing blood (in the true and false lumens) will manifest signal void on spin-echo sequences, and as high signal on black blood sequences. It may be difficult to distinguish thrombus from slowly flowing blood in the false lumen, a distinction that has implications for surgical management; flow-sensitive techniques increase sensitivity under these circumstances and increase the accuracy of evaluation of the coronary arteries and great vessels.

 IMAGING WITH ANGIOGRAPHY

Indications.   In patients with aortic dissection and aneurysm, aortography has been considered the "gold" standard for delineating the extent of involvement of the aorta and great vessels. When assessing for aortic dissection, false negatives can occur because of a thrombosed false lumen, simultaneous equal opacification of both lumens, or because of an intimal flap that is viewed en face rather than on edge. Aortography has sensitivity and sensitivity that approach 100% for aneurysm. However, because of the high sensitivity and specificity of computed tomographic angiography (CTA) and magnetic resonance angiography (MRA), aortography is typically only performed when the former tests are nondiagnostic. One of the primary benefits of aortography is that treatment with stent grafting or fenestration can often be instituted by the interventional radiologist.

Possible Findings.   Aortic aneurysm manifests as focal dilation, by definition at least 4 cm in diameter. Dissection may manifest as an intimal flap with no contour abnormality. Both true and false lumens may be demonstrated, especially if the false lumen is not thrombosed. Aortic regurgitation, if present, is also easily demonstrated.

 DIAGNOSTIC ALGORITHM

Currently CT is the preferred initial diagnostic imaging modality due to its availability, speed, and high sensitivity and specificity. When contrast-enhanced CT is inconclusive or cannot be performed, transoesophageal echocardiography (TEE) or MRI can be performed and offer benefits as outlined in the preceding text. Angiography remains the "gold" standard in the evaluation of thoracic aortic aneurysm and dissection but is typically only performed when previous testing is inconclusive or as part of a therapeutic endovascular procedure.

Further Readings

Hartnell GG. Imaging of aortic aneurysms and dissection: CT and MRI. *J Thorac Imaging* 2001;16:35–46.

Rydberg J, Kopecky KK, Lalka SG, et al. Stent grafting of abdominal aortic aneurysms: pre and postoperative evaluation with multislice helical CT. *J Comput Assist Tomogr* 2001;25:580–586.

Sakalihasan N, Limet R, Defawe OD. Abdominal aortic aneurysm. *Lancet* 2005;365:1577–1589.

Sharma U, Ghai S, Paul SB, et al. Helical CT evaluation of aortic aneurysms and dissection: a pictoral essay. *J Clin Imaging* 2003;27:273–280.

Willoteaux S, Lions C, Gaxotte V, et al. Imaging of aortic dissection by helical computed tomography (CT). *Eur Radiol* 2004;14:1999–2008.

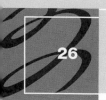

26

ABDOMINAL TRAUMA
Marcus W. Parker

$\mathcal{C}$omputed tomography (CT) is the primary modality for the evaluation of abdominal trauma of any cause. After presenting details about performing the study, possible findings will be discussed on an organ-by-organ basis.

IMAGING WITH COMPUTED TOMOGRAPHY

Indications.   CT should be performed on hemodynamically stable patients sustaining blunt or penetrating abdominal trauma in which there is suspicion for internal organ injury or inability to perform physical examination due to altered consciousness.

Protocol.   All patients should be given intravenous contrast unless creatinine is elevated or there is a significant allergy history. Intravenous (IV) contrast is critical for detection of solid organ injury. In the setting of significant trauma it is reasonable to give IV contrast even if the patient's renal function is unknown. Oral contrast can be helpful but frequently not practical in the setting of trauma.

ORGAN CHECKLIST OF COMPUTED TOMOGRAPHIC FINDINGS

HEMOPERITONEUM

Hemoperitoneum usually accompanies injury to the spleen, liver, mesentery, intestine, omentum, and occasionally the bladder.

Possible Findings

- Any unexplained area of nonenhancing hypodensity or inhomogeneity in the spleen, liver, pancreas, or kidneys is suspicious for laceration, especially in the presence of peritoneal fluid.
- Active bleeding should measure close to the HU density of IV contrast seen within a major artery. Clotted blood measures 40–70 HU, free blood measures 20–40 HU, and free fluid measures 0–15 HU. Note that blood and fluid are of lower attenuation than solid abdominal organs on contrast-enhanced CT. Hematoma may be isodense on unenhanced CT, making diagnosis difficult.
- Free abdominal fluid and blood will settle into dependent spaces within the abdomen. The most dependent region of the peritoneal cavity is Morrison's pouch—the hepatorenal fascia. Fluid or blood will also settle within the pelvic cul-de-sac, paracolic gutters, and perihepatic and perisplenic spaces and these regions should be examined carefully. Note that a small amount of free fluid within the pelvis of reproductive age women is physiologic.
- A "sentinel clot" indicates the source of abdominal hemorrhage on a noncontrast enhanced CT. The finding consists of a region of increased attenuation seen within lower attenuation peritoneal fluid, and represents acute hematoma adjacent to the site of injury.

SPLEEN

The spleen is the most commonly injured organ.

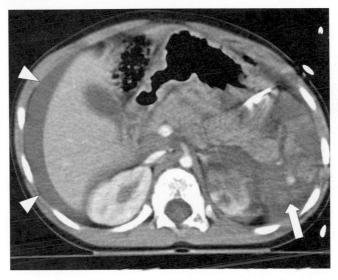

Figure 26-1. Contrast-enhanced computed tomography (CT) scan demonstrates severe splenic laceration (*arrow*) with disruption of blood supply. Hemoperitoneum is seen around the liver (*arrowheads*).

Possible Findings (Fig. 26-1)

- **Subcapsular hematoma.** Sharply defined, lenticular, hypodense collection that flattens or indents the splenic parenchyma. Peritoneal hemorrhage is usually not present.
- **Splenic laceration.** Irregular, jagged splenic fracture plane, altered contour, and/or nonhomogenous parenchymal enhancement. Peritoneal hemorrhage is present in almost all cases. Subcapsular hematoma may or may not be present.
- **Intrasplenic hematoma.** Focal nonenhancing area of low attenuation; a less common finding.
- **Splenic infarction.** Area of hypodensity with well-demarcated, linear borders caused by injury to the splenic artery intimal wall leading to thrombosis.
- **Associated fractures** of the left lower ribs are seen in 50% of adults, but rib fractures are rarely seen in children.

Imaging Tips

- Mottled enhancement of the spleen early in the arterial phase can be a normal finding and should not be confused with laceration. Splenic clefts, lobulations, and accessory spleens might also be mistaken for lacerations. True lacerations occur mostly along the lateral border and are jagged in appearance.
- Splenic vascular contrast extravasation has been shown to be highly predictive of a need for angiographic or surgical intervention.

Liver

The liver is the second most frequently injured abdominal organ. The right lobe is more frequently involved.

Possible Findings (Fig. 26-2)

- **Laceration.** Jagged line of hypodensity.
- **Subcapsular hematoma.** Peripherally located, crescentic, low-density collection that compresses hepatic tissue.

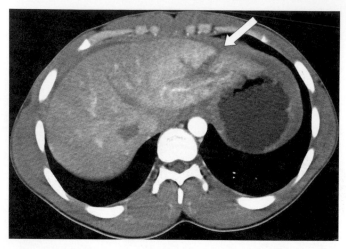

Figure 26-2. Contrast-enhanced computed tomography (CT) scan demonstrates hepatic laceration (*arrow*) extending to the liver capsule.

- **Contusion.** Ill-defined areas of decreased attenuation compared with normal enhancing liver.
- **Intrahepatic hematomas.** Focal, well-defined areas of decreased attenuation when compared with enhanced liver; areas of isodense or increased attenuation on noncontrast scans.

Imaging Tips

Lacerations can be simulated by artifacts from beam hardening caused by adjacent ribs. Bile ducts and unopacified venous structures may be confused with lacerations on noncontrast scans.

PANCREAS

The pancreas is uncommonly involved in abdominal trauma (<2% of blunt abdominal trauma patients). However, trauma is the most common cause of pediatric pancreatitis. Pancreatic trauma, when present, is usually the result of a motor vehicle collision due to compression of the pancreas against the lumbar spine.

Possible Findings

- **Lacerations.** Appear as regions of low attenuation perpendicular to the long axis of the pancreas.
- Deep laceration or transection (fracture) of the pancreas occurs, sometimes with disruption of the pancreatic duct.
- Focal enlargement of the pancreas and peripancreatic fat stranding or fluid are suggestive of injury.

Imaging Tips

- Unopacified bowel can simulate peripancreatic fluid.
- False negatives can be caused by an intrapancreatic hematoma that obscures margins of the fracture.
- Pancreatic trauma is associated with injuries to the liver, stomach, duodenum, or spleen in more than 90% of cases, so it is important to closely evaluate patients with pancreatic injury for other pathology.

BOWEL

Injury to the bowel is found in approximately 5% of blunt abdominal trauma and the findings can be subtle. The second and third portions of the duodenum are most commonly involved because of their fixed retroperitoneal position directly over the lumbar spine.

Possible Findings

- Mesenteric hematoma and/or mesenteric stranding are often seen.
- Peritoneal or retroperitoneal fluid.
- Pneumoperitoneum or retropneumoperitoneum—although this is often not seen.
- Sentinel clot—high density clot adjacent to involved bowel.
- Bowel wall thickening and/or extraluminal contrast.

Imaging Tips

- Use lung windows to evaluate for pneumoperitoneum or retropneumoperitoneum.
- Findings may be subtle. If clinical suspicion for bowel injury is high, consider a gastrointestinal (GI) fluoroscopic study using water-soluble contrast.

Kidney (Fig. 26-3)

The kidney is injured in 10% of patients with abdominal trauma and is often associated with trauma to other organs.

Possible Findings

- **Intrarenal hematoma.** A well-demarcated hypodensity within enhancing renal parenchyma. A renal contusion appears similar but is smaller and less well defined.
- **Renal laceration.** A low-density linear disruption of renal parenchyma.
- **Renal infarct.** Wedge-shaped region of hypoenhancement with absent excretion into the collecting system. Usually caused by renal artery or vein injury. Renal artery occlusion due to avulsion or intimal tear with resultant thrombosis.

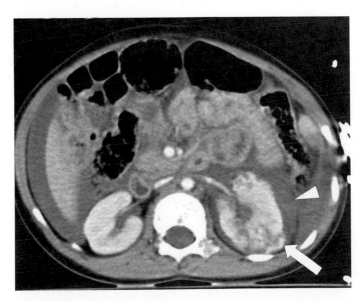

Figure 26-3. Contrast-enhanced computed tomography (CT) scan demonstrates laceration of the right kidney (*arrow*) with subcapsular hematoma.

Imaging Tips

- **The CT "rim sign" of renal artery occlusion.** Peripheral enhancement near a wedge-shaped hypodensity is not sensitive or specific.
- Renal motion can simulate a subcapsular hematoma so check for motion artifact on the abdominal wall.
- **Pseudofracture.** Parenchymal cortical lobulation or parenchymal invagination into the hilum. The renal contour is smooth and no perinephric fluid is seen.

Further Readings

Brandt WE, Helms CA. *Fundamentals of diagnostic radiology*, 2nd ed. Philadelphia: Lippincott Williams & Wilkins, 1999.

Miller LA, Shanmuganathan K. Multidetector CT evaluation of abdominal trauma. *Radiol Clin North Am* 2005;43(6):1079–1095.

Mirvis S, Shanmuganathan K. *Imaging in trauma and critical care*, 2nd ed. Elsevier Science, 2003.

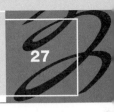

CLINICAL INFORMATION

Etiology and Epidemiology. Appendicitis is the most common cause of surgical abdomen affecting approximately 10% of the population. It can occur at any age; however, it is most common between the ages of 10 and 30 years. Appendicitis is caused by luminal obstruction from lymphoid hyperplasia, fecalith, foreign body, stricture, or tumor. In the United States, virtually every patient with suspected appendicitis is evaluated with computed tomography (CT) or ultrasonography.

Historically the diagnosis of acute appendicitis was primarily based on clinical information, and radiologic evaluation was performed only in ambiguous cases. This approach resulted in discovery of normal appendix at surgery in 10–20% of patients, and in 30–45% of young women, in whom numerous gynecologic processes may mimic the symptoms and signs of appendicitis. Appropriate imaging can significantly reduce rate of false-negative appendectomies to less than 4%.

Symptoms and Signs. Appendicitis usually begins with vague periumbilical or epigastric pain caused by distension of the appendix. As inflammation extends to anterior abdominal wall peritoneum, the pain shifts to the right lower quadrant and the physical examination should demonstrate presence of peritonitis with right lower quadrant rebound tenderness, guarding, and rigidity.

The presentation of appendicitis may vary considerably if the appendix is not in contact with anterior abdominal wall. Retrocecal appendicitis may cause flank pain and psoas sign on physical examination. Pelvic appendicitis can present with discomfort on pelvic examination. Urinary frequency, dysuria, microscopic hematuria, and pyuria will occur if the appendix is adjacent to bladder. Diarrhea may be present if the appendix is adjacent to sigmoid colon.

Nearly all patients experience anorexia and majority have nausea with few episodes of vomiting. Appendicitis is unlikely if the patient is hungry (look for full stomach on CT).

Low-grade fever is common. Leukocytosis and/or abnormal cell differential counts are found in 96% of patients. High fever and leukocytosis above 20,000 cells/μL suggest perforation.

These symptoms and signs may be very subtle in elderly or immunocompromised patients.

Differential Diagnosis. Appendicitis can be mimicked by a wide variety of disorders. The most common conditions discovered at surgery when acute appendicitis is erroneously diagnosed are nonspecific abdominal pain, mesenteric lymphadenitis, acute pelvic inflammatory disease, ruptured ovarian follicle or corpus luteum cyst, and acute gastroenteritis. Clinical differential diagnosis also includes inflammatory bowel disease, acute cholecystitis, perforated ulcer, acute pancreatitis, acute diverticulitis, strangulating intestinal obstruction, urolithiasis, pyelonephritis, and typhlitis in immunocompromised patients. In women, ectopic pregnancy and ovarian torsion should also be considered.

IMAGING WITH COMPUTED TOMOGRAPHY

Indications.   CT is very accurate and is the study of choice for evaluation of suspected appendicitis for most patients. Young children can initially be evaluated with ultrasonography (followed by CT if ultrasonographic findings are ambiguous). CT can accurately diagnose complications of appendicitis as well other pathologic conditions that may mimic appendicitis.

Protocol.   CT with intravenous (IV) contrast should be performed 2.5–3 hours after administration of oral contrast to fill distal ilium, cecum, and hopefully the appendix with oral contrast. Appendicitis can be diagnosed without oral or IV contrast; however both are very helpful, especially for diagnosis of other pathology. If the cecum is not yet opacified by contrast and findings are ambiguous, CT scan can be repeated after appropriate delay. Rectal contrast can be helpful in select cases as it may increase the likelihood of appendicial filling by contrast. Routine use of rectal contrast is not indicated due to patient discomfort and absence of clear advantage in accuracy of diagnosis.

Possible Findings (Figs. 27-1 to 27-3)

- Appendix distension (>6 mm), wall thickening, and periappendiceal inflammation are diagnostic of appendicitis.
- Appendicolith is seen in 25% of the cases and can be helpful for establishing the diagnosis. However, appendicolith can be seen incidentally in asymptomatic patients, possibly indicating increased risk of appendicitis.

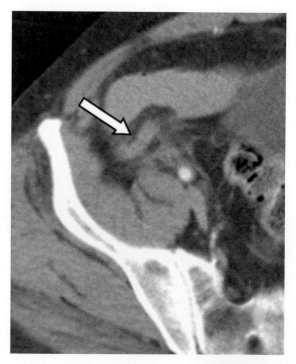

Figure 27-1. Early appendicitis with contrast-enhanced computed tomography (CT) demonstrating minimally thickened and distended appendix with mild stranding of the periappendiceal fat.

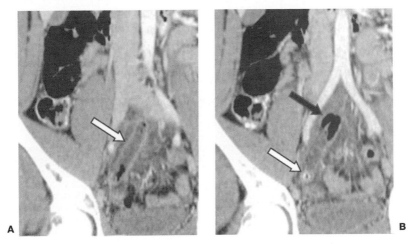

Figure 27-2. A: Appendicitis with contrast-enhanced computed tomography (CT) demonstrating thickened and distended appendix with haziness of the periappendiceal fat. **B:** *Black arrow* demonstrates perforation of the appendix with minimal amount of adjacent gas. Perforation was confirmed at surgery. *White arrow* shows an appendicolith which resulted in obstruction and appendicitis.

- Abscess or phlegmon indicate perforated appendicitis, occurring in 20% of patients, primarily the very old and the very young. Abscesses can be found adjacent to the cecum and in the dependent portion of the pelvis. Other possible complications include hepatic abscess, mesenteric vein thrombosis, small bowel obstruction, and adynamic ileus (Fig. 27-3).
- Nonvisualization of the appendix is unusual in acute appendicitis but may occur in very thin patients even despite coronal and sagittal reformats. If the appendix is not seen due to lack of fat planes, presence of free fluid in males and nonmenstruating females

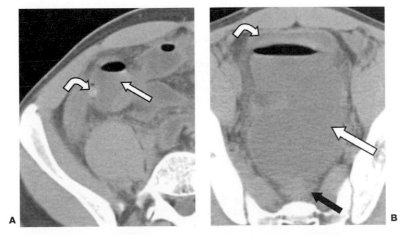

Figure 27-3. A: Contrast-enhanced computed tomography (CT) scan demonstrates an abscess (*straight arrow*) adjacent to the cecum resulting from perforated appendicitis caused by an appendicolith (*curved arrow*). **B:** Abscess (*white arrow*) in the dependent portion of the pelvis between bladder (*curved arrow*) and rectum (*black arrow*) occurred as a complication of perforated appendicitis.

should raise suspicion of peritonitis due to appendicitis in appropriate clinical settings. If adequate fat planes are present around the cecum, absence of pericecal stranding practically rules out appendicitis even if the appendix is not visualized.

- Appendicitis is excluded if appendix is completely filled by oral contrast. Gas in the lumen of the appendix does not rule out appendicitis.

IMAGING WITH ULTRASONOGRAPHY

Indications.   Ultrasonography is the study of choice in young children and pregnant women as it does not involve ionizing radiation. However, uterine enlargement during pregnancy makes ultrasonography very technically challenging, and ultrasonography is often nondiagnostic in the setting of altered anatomy. In women, ultrasonography has the advantage of being able to identify a number of the gynecologic conditions that can mimic appendicitis.

Thin patients and extensive experience are necessary for adequate evaluation of appendicitis with ultrasonography. The ability to identify normal appendix can serve as a useful marker of an institution's expertise and patient population. Recent studies by experienced operators report visualization of normal appendix in 60–80% of the patients without appendicitis.

Protocol.   Transabdominal right lower quadrant ultrasonography is performed with gradual pressure to displace and compress normal bowel loops, until iliac vessels and psoas muscle are visualized, because they are posterior to the appendix. Scanning should start with identification of the ascending colon by absence of peristalsis and gas and fluid in the lumen. Subsequently, terminal ileum can be identified by easy compressibility and active peristalsis. The appendix arises at the cecal tip approximately 1–2 cm below the terminal ileum.

In women, a routine transabdominal and endovaginal pelvic ultrasonography should also be performed if no evidence of appendicitis is found on the abdominal ultrasonography.

Possible Findings (Fig. 27-4)

- Visualization of a noncompressible, aperistaltic, blind-ending loop greater than 6 mm in diameter is diagnostic of appendicitis. Other possible findings do not significantly alter the accuracy of the examination.
- Fluid in the appendiceal lumen and flow in wall are specific but not sensitive findings.
- Peritoneal fluid is not sensitive or specific, and can be a normal finding in menstruating women.
- Nonvisualization of the appendix is probably the biggest problem associated with ultrasonographic evaluation for appendicitis. For an experienced sonographer, who is capable of visualizing the appendix in most normal patients, nonvisualization of the appendix has approximately 90% negative predictive value for appendicitis. In obese patients or for a less experienced sonographer, nonvisualization of appendix is not helpful toward establishing a diagnosis and CT should be performed for further evaluation.

IMAGING WITH RADIOGRAPHS

Indications.   Radiographs are not helpful in the workup of suspected acute appendicitis due to low sensitivity (50%) and specificity (<20%).

Protocol.   Supine and upright views of the abdomen. A left side down decubitus film may be substituted for an upright view in debilitated patients.

Possible Findings

- Normal findings are seen in approximately 50% of cases.
- Calcified appendicolith can be seen in 7–15% of cases and pathognomonic for appendicitis.

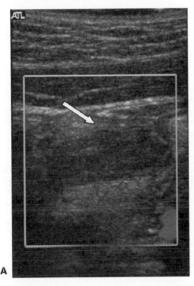
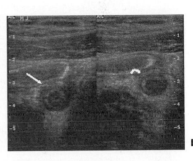

A
B

Figure 27-4. A: Appendicitis on ultrasonography with longitudinal image showing thickened and blind-ending appendix with increased flow in the wall. **B:** Cross-sectional image of the appendix demonstrating thickening of the wall and noncompressibility after application of pressure (*curved arrow*).

■ Other possible radiograph findings in appendicitis are nonspecific and include focal adynamic ileus (air–fluid levels in the right lower quadrant), soft tissue mass (displacement of bowel loops, distortion or partial loss of the psoas line or properitoneal fat line), or extraluminal gas bubbles in a periappendiceal abscess.

 IMAGING WITH MAGNETIC RESONANCE

Indication.   Magnetic resonance imaging (MRI) should be considered to aid in the diagnosis of acute appendicitis in the pregnant patient when ultrasound is nondiagnostic, and to avoid radiation exposure to a fetus (especially in the first trimester).

Protocol.   Written informed consent should be obtained, which is routine with all pregnant patients. The consent form should inform the patient of the method of MRI, current lack of approval from the U.S. Food and Drug Administration (FDA) for use in pregnant patients, unknown risk to patient or fetus, and unknown long-term biological effects on the fetus. Axial T1, T2 and sagittal and coronal T2 images should be performed. IV gadolinium should not be administered as it crosses the placenta and is not approved for use in pregnant patients.

Possible Findings

Similar to CT. Appendicoliths will not be as easily seen on MRI, as on CT, and may only appear as signal void.

 IMAGING WITH CONTRAST ENEMA

This study is not indicated for evaluation of suspected appendicitis because dense contrast limits subsequent CT scanning due to significant artifact. Contrast enema is helpful only if it is negative, demonstrating completely filled appendix. However, the appendix does not fill completely in 35% of normal patients, and it may be difficult to differentiate between complete and partial filling.

 ISSUES AFTER IMAGING

Acute appendicitis is treated with emergent surgery unless complicated by abscess or phlegmon. Percutaneous drainage should be performed for abscess due to perforated appendix. Antibiotics are used to treat appendicitis complicated by phlegmon. Interval appendectomy should be performed several months later.

Further Readings

Birnbaum RA, Wilson SR. Appendicitis at the millennium. *Radiology* 2000;215:337–348.

Brant WE, Helms CA, eds. *Fundamentals of diagnostic radiology*, 2nd ed. Philadelphia: Lippincott Williams & Wilkins, 1999.

Braunwald E, Fauci AS, Kasper DL, et al. *Harrison's principles of internal medicine*, 15th ed. New York: McGraw-Hill, 2001.

Kaiser S, Frenckner B, Jorulf HK. Suspected appendicitis in children: US and CT—a prospective randomized study. *Radiology* 2002;223:633–638.

Kessler N, Cyteval C, Gallix B, et al. Appendicitis: evaluation of sensitivity, specificity, and predictive values of US, Doppler US, and laboratory findings. *Radiology* 2004;230:472–478.

Urban BA, Fishman EK. Tailored helical CT evaluation of acute abdomen. *Radiographics* 2000;20:725.

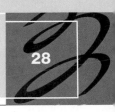

CHOLECYSTITIS
Oleg M. Teytelboym

28

CLINICAL INFORMATION

Etiology and Epidemiology. Acute cholecystitis is the most common cause of acute right upper quadrant pain. Most cases are caused by cystic duct obstruction from an impacted gallstone. Approximately one third of the patients with gallstones will develop cholecystitis. Acalculous cholecystitis accounts for 5–10% of acute cholecystitis cases and typically occurs in critically ill patients who have not been fed orally for a prolonged period of time. In patients with acquired immunodeficiency syndrome (AIDS), acute cholecystitis can be caused by infection with cytomegalovirus, cryptosporidium, or microsporidium.

Before widespread use of imaging, up to 22% of patients who were surgically explored for suspected cholecystitis did not have it. Imaging is also used to look for emergent complications of acute cholecystitis, such as gangrene (2–38% of cases) or perforation (3–15%).

Symptoms and Signs. Acute cholecystitis usually presents with sudden onset of right upper quadrant or epigastric pain and tenderness, frequently precipitated by a fatty meal. Most cases subside spontaneously due to antegrade or retrograde stone passage. Attacks lasting more than 1 day are unlikely to resolve spontaneously. Most patients experience nausea and vomiting. Fever and mild leukocytosis are common. Mild elevation of liver function tests is not unusual; however, persistent or significant elevation suggests choledocholithiasis.

Differential Diagnosis. Clinical presentation of acute cholecystitis can be mimicked by pancreatitis, appendicitis, peptic ulcer disease, gastroesophageal reflux, hepatitis, liver abscess, liver neoplasm, right lower lobe pneumonia, and cardiac disease.

Complications

- **Gangrenous or necrotizing cholecystitis** occurs when gallbladder distension impedes venous drainage, leading to ischemia and transmural necrosis. Clinical and imaging findings are frequently indistinguishable from uncomplicated acute cholecystitis and the diagnosis is often not made preoperatively. These patients commonly require an open cholecystectomy, with 8–75% conversion rates from laparoscopic to open cholecystectomy.
- **Emphysematous cholecystitis** results from infection with gas-forming bacteria, typically occurring in elderly or diabetic patients.
- **Gallbladder perforation** is a life-threatening complication of cholecystitis with up to 24% mortality. Perforation can lead to generalized peritonitis, pericholecystic abscess, or enterohepatic fistula, often to the duodenum or common bile duct (CBD). The presence of gangrenous and emphysematous cholecystitis significantly increases the risk of perforation.
- **Choledocholithiasis** results from gallstone passage into the CBD and may lead to biliary obstruction, pancreatitis, and ascending cholangitis.
- Mirizzi syndrome describes CBD obstruction by inflammation related to a gallstone impaction in the cystic duct.
- **Chronic cholecystitis** can result from repeated episodes of acute cholecystitis or from persistent gallbladder wall irritation by gallstones. Chronic cholecystitis may

153

be asymptomatic for years or may progress to acute cholecystitis or chronic symptomatic gallbladder disease.

IMAGING WITH ULTRASONOGRAPHY

Indications.   Ultrasonography is the preferred modality for evaluation of suspected acute cholecystitis because of ready availability and high accuracy. It can also provide additional information about nonbiliary pathology in cases where the gallbladder is found to be normal.

Protocol.   If possible, the examination should be performed after 6-hour fast to ensure adequate distension of the gallbladder. The gallbladder should be examined with the patient in supine and left posterior oblique positions. If cholelithiasis is present, every effort should be made to evaluate for stone impaction in the gallbladder neck or cystic duct by turning or standing the patient to determine if the gallstone is mobile.

Possible Findings (Fig. 28-1)

- Sonographic Murphy's sign (maximal tenderness over the sonographically localized gallbladder) is the most reliable finding for diagnosis of acute cholecystitis. In the presence of cholelithiasis, this sign is highly suggestive of acute cholecystitis with 92% positive-predictive value. Absence of significant gallbladder tenderness has 72% negative-predictive value for acute cholecystitis.
- Gallbladder wall hyperemia on Doppler ultrasound can be very helpful for diagnosis of acute cholecystitis with 98–100% specificity and 30–95% sensitivity.
- Less specific signs of acute or chronic cholecystitis include cholelithiasis, gallbladder dilatation, wall thickening (>3 mm), pericholecystic fluid, and sludge.
- Asymmetric gallbladder wall thickening or intraluminal membranes suggest gangrenous cholecystitis. The sonographic Murphy's sign may be absent, possibly due to denervation of the gallbladder wall by gangrenous changes.
- Hyperechoic foci with "dirty shadowing" in the gallbladder wall or lumen represent gas and are diagnostic for emphysematous cholecystitis. This appearance can be confused with gallbladder wall calcifications. Definitive diagnosis can be established with computed tomography (CT).
- Pericholecystic abscess or extraluminal stones suggest gallbladder perforation.
- In acalculous cholecystitis, ultrasonographic findings tend to be nonspecific because many of these patients are too ill or sedated to adequately evaluate for sonographic Murphy's sign. The gallbladder may be distended with a thickened wall and contain sludge. If ascites is absent, presence of pericholecystic fluid can help to confirm the diagnosis.

IMAGING WITH COMPUTED TOMOGRAPHY

Indications.   CT is frequently performed as the initial study in the evaluation of acute abdominal pain. CT findings of cholecystitis are very specific and approach the sensitivity of ultrasonography for evaluation of gallbladder disease. CT may be superior to ultrasonography for evaluation of complications related to acute cholecystitis such as gangrene, perforation, and emphysematous cholecystitis. CT is also excellent in detection of choledocholithiasis with sensitivity as high as 90% and specificity up to 97%.

Protocol.   Routine abdominal CT with IV contrast is usually adequate for evaluation of gallbladder and biliary disease. Dual phase CT with hepatic arterial and portal venous phases can better demonstrate increased enhancement of hepatic parenchyma adjacent to inflamed gallbladder. Dedicated protocols with 2–3 mm reconstructions can facilitate detection of cholelithiasis and choledocholithiasis. Oral contrast may help demonstrate presence of other pathology.

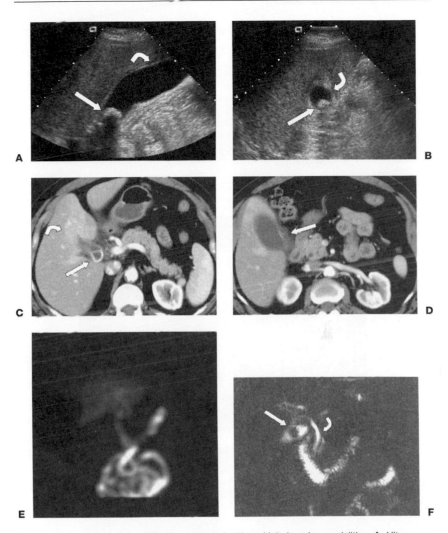

Figure 28-1. Acute cholecystitis demonstrated with multiple imaging modalities. **A:** Ultrasonography demonstrates a gallstone (*straight arrow*) in the gallbladder neck which did not move when patient stood up, indicating impaction. The sonographic Murphy's sign was positive suggesting acute cholecystitis. There is minimal fluid around the gallbladder (*curved arrow*). **B:** There is minimal thickening of the gallbladder wall (*curved arrow*) and other gallstones in the gallbladder (*straight arrow*). **C:** Contrast-enhanced computed tomography (CT) scan shows increased hepatic enhancement (*curved arrow*) around the inflamed gallbladder and a gallstone in the gallbladder neck (*straight arrow*). **D:** Fat haziness (*straight arrow*) around the gallbladder suggests pericholecystic inflammation. **E:** Nonvisualization of gallbladder on delayed images during hepatobiliary scan is compatible with acute cholecystitis. Common bile duct and small bowel are visualized. **F:** Magnetic resonance cholangiopancreatography (MRCP) obtained because of elevated liver function tests demonstrates cholelithiasis (*straight arrow*) and normal common bile duct (*curved arrow*).

Possible Findings (Figs. 28-1 and 28-2)

- Pericholecystic inflammatory changes with fluid and fat stranding are highly suggestive of acute cholecystitis.
- Focal increased enhancement of hepatic parenchyma adjacent to inflamed gallbladder is strongly suggestive of acute cholecystitis. This phenomenon probably occurs due to hepatic arterial hyperemia and early venous drainage.
- Gallstones can be visualized on CT with 80–85% sensitivity.
- Gallbladder wall thickening (>3 mm) and increased attenuation can be seen in acute or chronic cholecystitis. Gallbladder wall thickening can also occur in hepatitis, ascites, and hypoalbuminemia. Sometimes, low-density wall thickening (usually circumferential) can be mistaken for pericholecystic fluid (typically accumulates in the dependent areas).
- Gallbladder distension.
- Increased bile density (>20 H) due to biliary stasis, pus, blood, or debris.

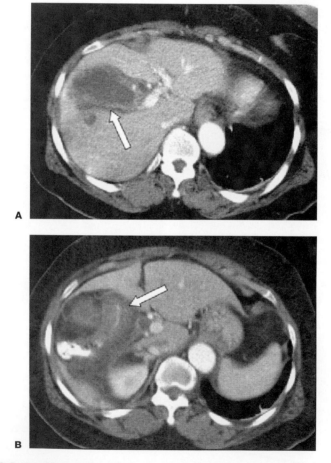

A

B

Figure 28-2. Necrotizing cholecystitis on computed tomography (CT) scan. **A:** Contrast-enhanced CT scan shows irregular thickening of the gallbladder wall (*arrow*) compatible with necrotizing cholecystitis. **B:** There is wall thickening of the hepatic flexure (*arrow*) secondary to pericholecystic inflammation, accounting for diarrhea.

■ Gas in the lumen or in the wall suggests emphysematous or gangrenous cholecystitis. Other findings with high specificity for gangrenous cholecystitis include intraluminal membranes, irregular or absent wall, and pericholecystic abscess.

■ Unremarkable gallbladder is a rare but possible finding in some patients with acute cholecystitis. Ultrasonography or nuclear hepatobiliary scan should then be performed if there is persistent clinical concern.

NUCLEAR MEDICINE IMAGING

Indications. Hepatobiliary scan is the gold standard for diagnosis of acute and chronic cholecystitis. However, if the nuclear medicine study result is negative, little information is provided about nonbiliary causes of the patient's symptoms. It is also rarely helpful in significant hepatic insufficiency (bilirubin >20 mg/dL) due to poor uptake and excretion of the radiotracer by the liver. Hepatobiliary scan is typically performed when CT or ultrasonographic findings are indeterminate or when chronic cholecystitis is suspected.

Protocol

1. The patient should be NPO for more than 4 hours. If the patient is NPO for more than 24 hours, administer sincalide (synthetic cholecystokinin [CCK]) 0.02 μg/kg IV over 5- 10 minutes. Routine CCK use can shorten the study by speeding up gallbladder visualization in patients with chronic cholecystitis.

2. Inject 3–10 mCi of ^{99m}Technetium (^{99m}Tc)-labelled iminodiacetic acid (IDA) derivative such as diisopropyl iminodiacetic acid (DISIDA) or mebrofenin (Choletec).

3. Obtain images for 30–60 minutes or until gallbladder and small bowel are visualized.

4. Delayed imaging up to 2–4 hours may be necessary if the gallbladder is not visualized, or in certain clinical circumstances (e.g., suspected bile leak, partial CBD obstruction, and hepatic insufficiency).

5. If the CBD and small bowel are visualized but the gallbladder is not, administer morphine 0.04 mg/kg IV. Morphine causes contraction of the sphincter of Oddi, stimulating reflux of radiotracer into the cystic duct if it is patent.

6. Left anterior oblique and right lateral views can help to separate radiotracer activity in the gallbladder from the adjacent duodenum. The gallbladder is anterior on both views.

7. Gallbladder ejection fraction for evaluation of chronic cholecystitis can be calculated by using a 30-minute IV infusion of CCK at a dose of 0.02 μg/kg.

Possible Findings (Fig. 28-1)

■ Visualization of the gallbladder during the first 4 hours postinjection almost entirely excludes the diagnosis of acute cholecystitis with accuracy greater than 95%.

■ Nonvisualization of the gallbladder within 4 hours, or 1 hour if CCK or morphine was given, in the presence of adequate hepatic uptake and transit into the small bowel establishes the diagnosis of acute cholecystitis with cystic duct obstruction.

■ "Rim sign" of increased hepatic radiotracer activity adjacent to the gallbladder is seen in approximately 20% of hepatobiliary scans with nonvisualization of the gallbladder. Approximately 40% of patients with this sign have a gangrenous or perforated gallbladder.

■ Absent or delayed (>60 minutes) visualization of small bowel suggests mechanical CBD obstruction or functional CBD obstruction with ascending cholangitis.

■ Chronic cholecystitis can be diagnosed if gallbladder ejection fraction is reduced to less than 35%. Delayed gallbladder visualization (2–4 hours) is suggestive of chronic cholecystitis.

■ In acalculous cholecystitis, gallbladder visualization is usually absent, but the obstruction can be partial, permitting delayed visualization.

■ Extrabiliary radiotracer activity, particularly in Morison's pouch or the peritoneal cavity, indicates perforation.

■ False positives (with gallbladder nonvisualization) for acute cholecystitis can be due to recent meal within 4 hours, fasting for more than 24 hours, hyperalimentation, chronic cholecystitis, hepatic insufficiency, cystic duct cholangiocarcinoma, and possibly alcoholism, and pancreatitis.

■ False negatives (with gallbladder visualization) for acute cholecystitis can be secondary to acalculous cholecystitis, duodenal diverticulum simulating a gallbladder, or visualization of an accessory cystic duct.

IMAGING WITH MAGNETIC RESONANCE

Magnetic resonance cholangiopancreatography (MRCP) is the noninvasive study of choice for evaluation of CBD pathology. It is not routinely indicated for evaluation of acute cholecystitis unless choledocholithiasis is suspected. MRCP is equal to endoscopic retrograde cholangiopancreatography (ERCP) and superior to CT and ultrasonography in detection of choledocholithiasis and CBD obstruction.

ISSUES AFTER IMAGING

Laparoscopic cholecystectomy is the treatment of choice for acute and chronic cholecystitis. In patients with acute cholecystitis who are at high surgical risk, percutaneous cholecystostomy can be performed to decompress the gallbladder.

Further Readings

Bennett GL, Rusinek H, Lisi V, et al. CT findings in acute gangrenous cholecystitis. *Am J Roentgenol* 2002;178:275–281.

Brant WE, Helms CA, eds. *Fundamentals of diagnostic radiology*, 2nd ed. Lippincott Williams & Wilkins, Philadelphia, 1999.

Braunwald E, Fauci AS, Kasper DL, et al. *Harrison's principles of internal medicine*, 15th ed. New York: McGraw-Hill, 2001.

Hanbidge AE, Buckler PM, O'Malley ME, et al. From the RSNA refresher courses: imaging evaluation for acute pain in the right upper quadrant. *RadioGraphics* 2004;24:1117–1135.

Harvey RT, Miller WT. Acute biliary disease: initial CT and follow-up US versus initial US and follow-up CT. *Radiology* 1999;213:831.

Majeski J. Gallbladder ejection fraction: an accurate evaluation of symptomatic acalculous gallbladder disease. *Int Surg* 2003;88(2):95–99.

Soyer P, Brouland JP, Boudiaf M, et al. Color velocity imaging and power Doppler sonography of the gallbladder wall: a new look at sonographic diagnosis of acute cholecystitis. *Am J Roentgenol* 1998;171:183–188.

Thrall JH, Ziessman HA. *Nuclear medicine: the requisites*, 2nd ed. St. Louis: Mosby, 2001.

Urban BA, Fishman EK. Tailored helical CT evaluation of acute abdomen. *Radio Graphics* 2000;20:725.

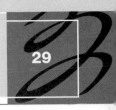

CLINICAL INFORMATION

Etiology. Diverticulosis is the most common colonic disease of Western society. It is seen in approximately 40–50% of people older than 50 years and approximately 80% of people older than 85 years. A diverticulum is an acquired herniation of mucosa through the muscularis layer of bowel.

Diverticulitis is a complication seen in 10–20% of patients with diverticulosis. It occurs when an inspissated piece of fecal material collects within and obstructs the lumen of a diverticulum. The vascular supply to the wall of the diverticulum becomes compromised and renders the diverticular wall susceptible to invasion by colonic bacteria. Obstruction and/or perforation of a diverticulum create a local inflammatory response which dissects into the adjacent pericolic fat causing a localized phlegmon or a discrete abscess, and occasionally generalized peritonitis.

Location. Diverticulitis most commonly affects the sigmoid colon, which is also the most common location of diverticulosis (the location of highest intraluminal pressure). Diverticula can be seen anywhere in the bowel except the rectum.

Symptoms and Signs. Potential symptoms and signs include fever, chills, leukocytosis, left lower quadrant colicky pain and tenderness, palpable mass, altered bowel habits, and local signs of peritoneal irritation.

Differential Diagnosis. Any process causing acute left lower quadrant pain can mimic diverticulitis. Differential diagnosis includes colon cancer, inflammatory bowel disease, radiation colitis, ischemic colitis, pseudomembranous colitis, appendicitis, epiploic appendagitis, ectopic pregnancy, ovarian torsion, endometriosis, salpingitis, ureteral colic, intestinal obstruction, psoas abscess, and leaking aortic aneurysm.

IMAGING WITH RADIOGRAPHS

Indication. Appropriate initial examination for abdominal pain is an abdominal radiograph. However, if localizing signs are present and diverticulitis is suspected, computed tomography (CT) is the imaging modality of choice.

Protocol. Routine upright and supine abdominal views.

Possible Findings

- Pneumoperitoneum if there is perforation of bowel.
- Ileus.
- Small or large bowel obstruction.
- Left lower quadrant mass.
- Bowel thickening.
- Pneumatosis.
- Portal venous air.

IMAGING WITH COMPUTED TOMOGRAPHY

Indications.   CT is the best modality for diagnosis of diverticulitis. CT is fast and accurate, with a reported sensitivity and specificity up to 99%. Furthermore, CT is particularly useful in evaluating atypical features and/or complications of diverticulitis, and identifying other abdominal and pelvic pathology. CT can also be also used for guiding drainage of a diverticular abscess.

Protocol.   Intravenous (IV) and oral contrast should be administered if not contraindicated (allergy or renal insufficiency). Oral contrast is given to help distinguish between fluid-filled bowel and potential intraperitoneal fluid collections. The patient should be imaged approximately 3 hours after oral contrast administration to allow the contrast to reach the sigmoid colon.

Possible Findings (Fig. 29-1)

- Bowel wall thickening and fat stranding.
- Diverticulosis.
- Long segment of colonic involvement (>10 cm).
- Pericolic abscess or phlegmon.
- Sinus tracts and fistulae involving bowel, bladder, and less commonly, vagina and uterus.
- "Arrowhead sign"—secondary to edema at orifice of an inflamed diverticulum.
- Colonic and/or ureteral obstruction.
- Free air and/or peritonitis.
- Gas and/or thrombus in mesenteric and portal veins.
- Liver abscesses.

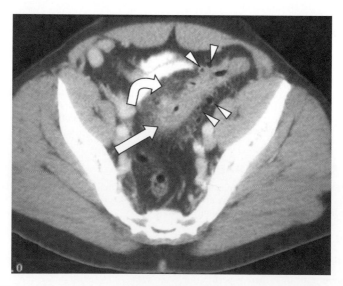

Figure 29-1. Diverticulitis on computed tomography (CT). Axial CT scan with oral and intravenous (IV) contrast demonstrates moderate wall thickening of sigmoid colon segment (*straight arrow*). There are multiple diverticula (*arrowheads*) present. There is moderate stranding of adjacent fat (*curved arrow*).

Further Readings

Ambrosetti P, Jenny A, Becker C, et al. Acute left colonic diverticulitis-compared performance of computed tomography and water soluble contrast enema: prospective evaluation of 420 patients. *Dis Colon Rectum* 2000;43(10):1363–1367.

Davis M. The colon and appendix. In: Juhl JH, Crummy AB, eds. In: *Essentials of radiologic imaging*, 6th ed. Philadelphia: JB Lippincott Co, 1993:619–637.

Federle MP, Jeffrey RB, Desser TS, et al. *Diagnostic imaging: abdomen.* Salt Lake City: Amirsys Inc., 2004:28–31.

Shrier D, Skucas J, Weiss S. Diverticulitis: an evaluation by computed tomography and contrast enema. *Am J Gastroenterol* 1991;86(10):1466–1471.

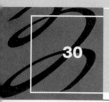

GASTROINTESTINAL HEMORRHAGE
Mandeep Dagli and W. Dee Dockery

*G*astrointestinal (GI) hemorrhage is a common, potentially life-threatening cause of acute hospital admission and often requires intensive care unit (ICU)-level care. Before radiologic evaluation, the clinical evaluation should focus on assessing patient stability and providing resuscitation. Once the patient is stable, the focus can turn to localization and therapy.

The initial diagnostic workup of GI bleeding involves answering two questions: Is the GI bleed acute or chronic? Is the bleeding source from the upper GI tract (mouth to ligament of Treitz) or the lower GI tract (jejunum to anus)? Acute GI bleed usually stops spontaneously; however in 25% of cases therapy is required. Chronic GI bleeds are often occult and do not require urgent therapy.

CLINICAL INFORMATION
Symptoms and Signs

Acute Upper Gastrointestinal Bleed
Patients usually present in middle or older age with a pertinent medical history (nonsteroidal anti-inflammatory agent [NSAID] therapy, peptic ulcer disease, alcoholism, prior upper GI surgery, recent vomiting, portal hypertension), "coffee ground" emesis (previous bleed), hematemesis (ongoing bleed), melena (shiny, pitch-black stool; occurs after blood has been in the GI tract for ≥4 hours), and possibly shock (massive bleed). Hemoptysis is a nonspecific complaint, often implicating tracheobronchial lesions.

Acute Lower Gastrointestinal Bleed
Although there may be some overlap of symptoms in upper and lower GI bleeding cases, patients with acute lower tract bleeding usually present in older age with maroon stools or bright red blood per rectum; melena is possible if the lesion is relatively proximal.

Chronic Gastrointestinal Bleed
Chronic upper and lower GI bleeds present with fatigue and anemia (nonspecific) and occult fecal blood (lower or upper GI bleed), and possibly with a history of previous bleed. Initial workup is nonemergent and usually involves endoscopy.

Differential Diagnosis

Upper Gastrointestinal Bleed
Pyloroduodenal ulcer, gastritis, esophageal varices, Mallory-Weiss tear, gastric ulcer (usually antrum or lesser curvature), esophagitis with or without hiatal hernia, carcinoma, and hemobilia (patients with biliary tract tumors and/or percutaneous biliary drain).

Lower Gastrointestinal Bleed
Lower GI bleed is usually colonic in origin; however, 10–25% may originate in the small bowel. Top three causes are colorectal cancer (first cause of chronic colorectal

bleed); diverticular disease (often the culprit in acute bleed; bleeding from right-sided diverticulum more common; resolves spontaneously in 80% of cases; however, rebleeds in 25%); and angiodysplasia (second cause of chronic, intermittent bleeding; 15% massive; often multiple and in ascending colon, easily missed on angiography; usually rebleeds and therefore requires resection). Other possibilities include hemorrhoids; inflammatory bowel disease; Meckel's diverticulum (consider in children and young adults); invasive enterocolitis (*Salmonella*, *Shigella*); vasculitis (e.g., polyarteritis nodosa); small bowel tumors (leiomyomas a common cause of episodic GI bleed in young adult, metastasis in older patients); trauma; vasculoenteric fistula; or brisk upper GI bleed.

Clinical Workup and Diagnostic Strategy (Fig. 30-1)

Before considering imaging studies, the patient should be resuscitated and stabilized if necessary. Patients who cannot be stabilized often require emergency surgery. Serial hematocrits should be drawn. Because most patients receive intravenous (IV) fluid resuscitation, a fall in hematocrit is often observed during the clinical course unless blood transfusions are given. If acute upper GI bleeding is a possibility, then a nasogastric tube (NGT) should be placed. Large-bore (34 F) oro- or nasogastric tube lavage sensitively and specifically identifies acute or subacute upper GI bleed (repeated pink or red aspirates after clots are evacuated). Rare false positives occur when there is massive lower GI bleed, and occasional false negatives occur with duodenal bleeds. NGT aspirate should be billous to reduce false negatives.

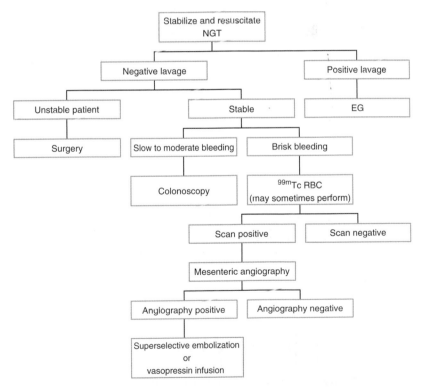

Figure 30-1. Gastrointestinal (GI) bleeding diagnostic algorithm. NGT, nasogastric tube; EGD, esophagogastroduodenoscopy; ^{99m}Tc RBC, ^{99m}Technetium red blood cell scan.

Upper Gastrointestinal Bleed. Patients with upper gastrointestinal (UGI) bleeding are referred for endoscopy, which identifies a source in more than 95% of patients and is the primary therapeutic measure. Treatment is with electrocautery, injection sclerotherapy, or banding. Advanced radiologic studies are usually not necessary for diagnosis or therapy. However, in situations where a UGI source cannot be identified with endoscopy or is difficult to reach (such as a duodenal ulcer), arteriography may be used.

Lower Gastrointestinal Bleed. The diagnosis and treatment of lower gastrointestinal bleed (LGIB) varies from institution to institution. In general, the initial choice of a localization test hinges upon the stability of the patient and the estimated rate of bleeding. For stable patients with minimal to moderate bleeding, endoscopy after a rectal washout can be used both for localization and therapy. Several studies have showed definitive site localization in 62–76%. Higher levels of bleeding or excessive feces can hinder visualization with endoscopy. In these situations, angiography may be necessary. A nuclear medicine tagged red cell scan is sometimes performed before angiography to localize the bleed because of its greater sensitivity for slow or intermittent bleeding. If the red cell scan is negative, arteriography is not performed in the acute setting; if positive, arteriography can be employed to deliver vasopressin or embolic agents selectively into the bleeding artery. Indications for emergent surgery (subtotal colectomy or hemicolectomy if bleeding can be localized) include inability to achieve hemodynamic stability, rapid clinical deterioration, transfusion requirements greater than six units, and persistent recurrent hemorrhage.

 IMAGING WITH NUCLEAR MEDICINE

Indications. Radionuclide scanning can detect bleeding at a rate as low as 0.1–0.2 mL/minute. The reported sensitivity for scintigraphy ranges from 41–94%. Two common indications for radionuclide bleeding scan are: (1) suspected mild to moderate level or intermittent LGIB before going to angiography; and (2) chronic bleeding resistant to attempts at localization by endoscopy and small bowel fluoroscopic studies (this situation is nonemergent). Because of the greater sensitivity of scintigraphy, it is thought that bleeding undetectable by scintigraphy will likely be undetectable by angiography as well. In addition, localization may help determine which mesenteric vessel to evaluate first. However, even after a positive result during a scintigraphic bleeding study, angiography has only been reported to be positive 44–54% of the time. In addition, several studies have reported a high incidence of positive angiographic results after a negative-tagged red blood cell (RBC) scan. Intermittent bleeding is one likely explanation for this discrepancy. For this reason, it is essential that before performing an RBC scan the interventional team be contacted to minimize the delay between scintigraphy and angiography. Patients who are bleeding profusely or are unstable rarely need a bleeding scan and should go straight to angiography or surgery. A bleeding scan has little role in the evaluation of upper GI bleeding because of the high accuracy of upper GI endoscopy.

A Meckel's scan, using free ^{99m}Technetium (^{99m}Tc)- pertechnetate to identify ectopic gastric mucosa, should be considered in a young patient with GI bleeding.

Protocol. No special patient preparation is needed. The most commonly used radiotracer is ^{99m}Tc-labeled RBCs. Once the RBCs are labeled, a large field of view γ-camera is placed over the anterior abdominal wall of the supine patient. Immediately after injection, flow images at 1 second/frame for 60 seconds are acquired followed by 1 hour of images at 1 minute/frame. If no bleed is seen, the study is continued for another hour. If a bleed is still not seen, the patient can return to the department up to 24 hours later for delayed scanning if bleeding recurs.

Possible Findings

Extravasation manifests as focal activity that appears during the blood pool phase, initially intensifies, and then moves antegrade or retrograde in a bowel-like trajectory on subsequent images. It is extremely important to view the study in cine mode, which can clarify difficult studies.

Imaging Tips. To differentiate bladder activity from a rectosigmoid bleed, obtain postvoid images and lateral views. Scrotal and penile activity is a common normal finding and should not be confused with a bleed. Although uncommon with modern *in vitro* labeling techniques, free ^{99m}Tc-pertechnetate may simulate gastric bleeding.

 IMAGING WITH ARTERIOGRAPHY

Indications. Endoscopy is the initial diagnostic and therapeutic maneuver for patients with UGI bleeding, slow to moderate acute lower gastrointestinal (LGI) bleeding, and chronic GI bleeding. Arteriography is indicated in cases of acute, brisk, and lower GI bleeding when visualization with endoscopy is difficult. Past medical and surgical history, creatinine, platelets, and coagulation studies are required to determine the risks of arterial puncture, IV contrast administration, vasopressin infusion, and embolotherapy. Patients with prior bowel surgery have altered collateral blood flow and are at increased risk of bowel infarction if vasopressin infusion or embolotherapy is attempted.

Protocol

■ **Upper Gastrointestinal Bleed.** Perform celiac arteriogram (see Chap. 53, "Arteriography Primer") If the result is negative, perform selective arteriography of the left gastric artery (LGA) and common hepatic artery. If the result is negative, selective arteriography of the proper hepatic artery, gastroduodenal artery (GDA), and pancreaticoduodenal artery (PDA) can be considered. Diagnosis of diffuse mucosal bleeds may require superselective arteriography.

■ **Lower Gastrointestinal Bleed.** Placement of a Foley catheter is helpful in preventing obscuration of the field of view by contrast accumulation in the bladder. If the location of the bleeding source is known or highly suspected, begin by selecting the most likely vessel. If the bleeding location is not known, perform an inferior mesenteric arteriogram (IMA) first, and then a superior mesenteric arteriogram (SMA) (see Chap. 53, "Arteriography Primer"). If these results are negative, then perform a celiac arteriogram because the middle colic artery can arise from the dorsal pancreatic artery in 1–2% of patients.

Possible Findings

Arteriography can detect bleeding at a rate as low as 0.5–1.0 mL/minute. Extravasation is recognized as a progressively dense blush of contrast that does not move during a given filming sequence; contrast may trickle down the bowel wall, outlining mucosal folds or simulating a vein. Although extravasation is the only direct proof of bleeding, indirect signs may be the only clues available. Neoplasms can manifest with neovascularity, arteriovenous shunting, mass effect, or vascular compression, obstruction, or thrombosis. Arteriovenous malformations, more common in the colon, manifest as a tangle of small vessels with an early draining vein. Varices and other signs of portal hypertension can be seen on the venous phase images; extravasation from varices is rarely visualized due to technical factors, and an ongoing bleed should be attributed to visualized varices only when other causes have been excluded.

Lower GI bleeds are detectable by arteriography in 52% of cases. The SMA supplies duodenal bulb to distal transverse colon; the IMA supplies the remainder of the colon and rectum. The inferior hemorrhoidal arteries, branches of the internal iliac artery, supply part of rectum and anus.

Imaging Tips. Avoid studies requiring oral contrast, especially barium, as they interfere with endoscopy, arteriography, and nuclear medicine scans. Arteriography should be performed while the patient is bleeding rather than delaying the study until a more convenient time. This strategy will increase the rate of positive studies and reduce the number of repeat studies.

INTERVENTION WITH ARTERIOGRAPHY

The main two options for therapeutic intervention during angiography for lower GI bleed are embolotherapy or vasopressin. The current availability of superselective microcatheters has significantly decreased the risk of bowel infarction, making, according to some authors, embolotherapy the treatment of choice.

Embolotherapy. Before the widespread use of superselective catheters, embolotherapy carried a risk for bowel infarction ranging from 0–15%. This risk has now been greatly reduced. Superselective embolization of LGIB has a reported 90% success rate, with rebleeding in 20% of patients. Recent studies using polyvinyl alcohol (PVA), microcoils, and gelatin sponge have had a 90% success rate with few incidences of bowel infarct. Currently, coils are the embolic agents of choice for embolization therapy. Despite this, it is essential that patients be closely monitored for ischemia. The postprocedure rebleeding rate is approximately 12%. Embolization of angiodysplasia can have a high frequency of rebleeding due to multiple feeding collaterals and surgical treatment may ultimately be necessary.

Vasopressin. Vasopressin causes smooth muscle contraction and has been shown to control bleeding due to diverticula or recent polypectomy in up to 90% of patients. Vasopressin is not recommended for bleeding secondary to arteriovenous malformations (AVM)s, ischemic bowel, and pseudoaneurysms. The bleeding recurrence rate is 50%. Because of its potent vasoconstrictive effects, vasopressin should be avoided in patients with significant atherosclerotic vascular disease. Patients should be monitored in the ICU for hypertension, myocardial and peripheral ischemia, arrhythmias, and hyponatremia (vasopressin causes free water retention).

Once bleeding has been localized, the catheter tip is placed in the proximal SMA or IMA. The following protocol can then be used.

1. Start vasopressin at 0.2 IU/minute using an arterial infusion pump.
2. Repeat arteriogram after infusing vasopressin for 20 minutes.
3. If arteriogram shows excessive vasoconstriction or if patient complains of unrelenting cramping, cut infusion rate to half and go to step 2.
4. If arteriogram shows continued bleeding and the vasopressin infusion rate is less than 0.4 IU/minute, increase the rate by 0.1 IU/minute and go to step 2. If the infusion rate is 0.4 IU/minute, or if the infusion rate is limited by patient symptoms, then alternative treatments need to be considered.
5. If arteriogram shows no bleeding, transfer patient to the ICU for monitoring, and continue infusion at same rate for 12 hours. After 12 hours decrease infusion by 50% and taper to normal saline over the next 12–24 hours, ultimately discontinuing the infusion if there is no clinical evidence of rebleeding.

Further Readings

Cotran RS, Robbins SL, Kumar V. *Robbins pathologic basis of disease*, 6th ed. Philadelphia: WB Saunders, 1999.

Hastings GS. Angiographic localization and transcatheter treatment of gastrointestinal bleeding. *Radiographics* 2000;20:1160–1168.

Hoedema RE, Luchtefeld MA. The management of lower gastrointestinal hemorrhage. *Dis Colon Rectum* 2005;48:2010–2024.

Kaufman JA, Lee MJ. *Vascular and interventional radiology: the requisites*. Philadelphia: Mosby, 2004.

Margulis AR, Burhenne HJ, Freeny PC, et al. *Alimentary tract radiology*, 5th ed. St. Louis: Mosby-Year Book, 1994.

McIntyre RC, Stiegman GV, Eiseman B. *Surgical decision making*. Philadelphia: WB Saunders, 2004.

Sabiston, DC, ed. *Textbook of surgery*, 13th ed. Philadelphia: WB Saunders, 1986:828–829.

Sleisenger MH, Fordtran JS, eds. *Gastrointestinal disease: pathophysiology, diagnosis, management*, 5th ed. Philadelphia: WB Saunders, 1993:162–192.

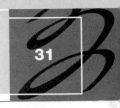

INTESTINAL OBSTRUCTION
Simon Bekker and D. Darrell Vaughn

31

*A*n appropriate imaging approach to bowel obstruction requires understanding a varied spectrum of diseases which can precipitate intestinal blockage. A categoric approach helps in formulating a useful and clinically relevant differential diagnosis. Ultimately, the goal in evaluating patients with suspected intestinal obstruction is to perform the following:

- Establish or exclude the diagnosis of obstruction.
- Identify the level and cause(s) of obstruction.
- Assess whether the obstruction is partial or complete (intestinal contents can or cannot pass beyond the point of blockage).
- Determine if there are any associated complications.

CLINICAL INFORMATION

Etiology and Epidemiology. Causes of intestinal obstruction vary between adult and pediatric patient populations (Tables 31-1 and 31-2). Intestinal obstruction can be categorized as to whether it involves the small or large bowel. In addition, bowel obstructions can be subdivided into those resulting from mechanical causes, those due to either intrinsic bowel abnormalities (e.g., rectal mass causing colonic obstruction), and those resulting from extrinsic pathologies (perforated appendiceal abscess causing terminal ileum and small bowel obstruction [SBO]).

Hypomotility disorders and adynamic bowel can also lead to obstruction, albeit functional. Although no true anatomic narrowing precipitates an adynamic, hypomotile obstruction, one must recognize the varied and numerous causes of adynamic ileus (Table 31-3).

In adults, approximately 80% of intestinal obstructions occur in the small bowel, whereas the remaining 20% involve the large bowel. Adhesions, hernias, and neoplasms account for most SBOs, in order of decreasing frequency. Inflammatory bowel disease (i.e., Crohn's disease) has been demonstrated as an increasingly common cause of SBO, possibly more frequent than hernias and neoplasia. Colorectal carcinoma, diverticulitis, and volvulus are the most common causes of large bowel obstruction (LBO), in order of descending frequency.

In children, intussusception is responsible for most SBOs, whereas adhesions and inguinal hernias are responsible for most LBOs (Table 31-2).

Complications of intestinal obstruction include strangulation and perforation. SBO can be either partial or complete (no bowel contents can pass beyond the point of obstruction), and can be either simple or strangulated (compromised blood supply). Strangulated obstructions with bowel ischemia are surgical emergencies. If not diagnosed and properly treated, vascular compromise can lead to bowel infarction with further morbidity and mortality.

In general, the cause of obstruction can often be deduced from the location of the obstruction, the patient's age, and the pertinent clinical history.

Before discussing relevant radiologic and imaging workup, a few diagnostic entities deserve additional comment: specifically, closed-loop obstruction, gallstone ileus, and internal hernias.

- **Closed-loop obstruction** occurs when bowel becomes occluded at two sites, resulting in a locked-in (i.e., "closed") segment of bowel. The most common cause of closed-loop

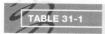

TABLE 31-1	Common Causes of Bowel Obstruction in Adults

Level	Differential diagnosis
Small bowel (80% of bowel obstructions)	Adhesions (75% of SBO) Postsurgical Postinflammatory Incarcerated hernia Malignancy (usually metastatic) Intussusception Volvulus Gallstone ileus Parasites (ascaris) Foreign body
Large bowel (20% of bowel obstructions)	Colon carcinoma (50–60% of LBO) Metastatic disease (pelvic malignancies) Diverticulitis Volvulus Fecal impaction Amebiasis Ischemia Adhesions

SBO, small bowel obstruction; LBO, large bowel obstruction.
(Modified from Brant WE, Helms CA, 2nd ed. *Fundamentals of diagnostic radiology.*
Baltimore: Lippincott Williams & Wilkins, 1999:997–1023.)

obstruction is volvulus, occurring most often in the elderly. Other causes include ventral hernias, adhesions, congenital bands, and malrotation (the last two more often in a pediatric setting). Volvulus occurs anatomically in locations where bowel and mesentery are long, tortuous, and floppy, frequently in the cecum and sigmoid colon. Torsion of the mesentery can lead to strangulation. Cecal volvulus has a mortality rate of 20–40%, whereas sigmoid volvulus is fatal in 20–25% of cases.

■ **Gallstone ileus** refers to mechanical SBO caused by gallstone erosion through the gallbladder wall into adjacent bowel, often creating a cholecystoduodenal fistula. The stone commonly impacts and obstructs at the distal ileum. The term *ileus* is technically a misnomer, as a mechanical obstruction (i.e., the gallstone impacted in the

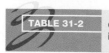

TABLE 31-2	Common Causes of Bowel Obstruction in Children

Level	Differential diagnosis
Small bowel	Adhesions Appendicitis Intussusception (most common cause) Incarcerated inguinal hernia Malrotation with volvulus or Ladd bands Meckel diverticulum
Large bowel	Adhesions inguinal hernia

(Modified from Donnelly LF. *Fundamentals of pediatric radiology.* Philadelphia: WB
Saunders, 2001: 97–140.)

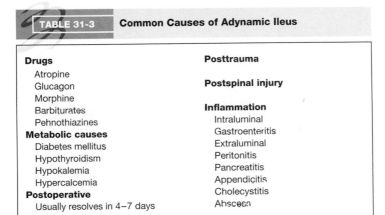

TABLE 31-3	Common Causes of Adynamic Ileus

Drugs	**Posttrauma**
Atropine	
Glucagon	**Postspinal injury**
Morphine	
Barbiturates	**Inflammation**
Pehnothiazines	Intraluminal
Metabolic causes	Gastroenteritis
Diabetes mellitus	Extraluminal
Hypothyroidism	Peritonitis
Hypokalemia	Pancreatitis
Hypercalcemia	Appendicitis
Postoperative	Cholecystitis
Usually resolves in 4–7 days	Abscess

terminal ileum) underlies the pathophysiology. The characteristic radiographic findings in approximately 50% of patients are referred to as *Rigler's triad*; it consists of mechanical SBO, pneumobilia, and an ectopic gallstone. Radiographically, the gallstone is usually obscured by overlying shadows or is nonopaque.

- **Internal hernias** consist of bowel herniation, usually small intestine, through a normal or abnormal aperture within the peritoneal cavity (as opposed to the external variety). Internal hernias may be congenital or acquired (postsurgical), and herniation may be either continuous or intermittent. Most internal hernias are paraduodenal, but others include transmesenteric, supra- or perivesicular, intersigmoid, hernias through the foramen of Winslow, and omental hernias. Internal hernias have become increasingly common as greater number of patients undergo surgeries which create new bowel anastamoses and/or openings in the mesentery (e.g., orthotopic liver transplants, Whipple's surgeries, and gastric bypass surgeries)

Symptoms and Signs

Patients with mechanical obstruction of the proximal small bowel usually present with vomiting and abdominal discomfort. If the obstruction is in the middle or distal small bowel, the patient will also have colicky abdominal pain, abdominal distension, constipation-obstipation, and peristaltic rushes. Similarly, colonic obstruction presents as constipation-obstipation, abdominal distension and pain, and nausea/vomiting (late).

 IMAGING WITH RADIOGRAPHS

Indications. Radiologic examination of suspected intestinal obstruction begins with abdominal radiographs.

Protocol

- Routine supine and upright abdominal radiographs.
- Left-side down decubitus or cross-table lateral view if the patient is unable to stand.
- Ideally a 5–10 minute pause after the decubitus and before the upright radiographs allows for extraluminal, intraperitoneal gas to percolate through abdomen.
- A prone abdominal film may be useful in distinguishing distal LBO from colonic ileus. In the latter, air will be seen in the rectum.

Possible Findings (Fig. 31-1)

Evaluation of radiographs for intestinal obstruction should be methodical. First, one should determine the presence of bowel dilatation, and if possible, a general level of obstruction

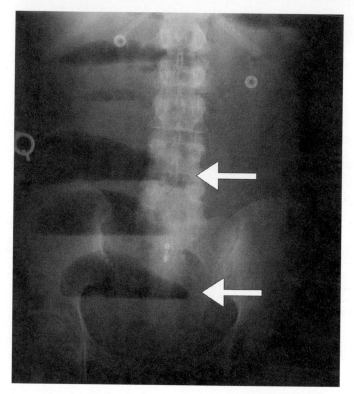

Figure 31-1. Small bowel obstruction with upright anteroposterior (AP) view of the abdomen demonstrating air-fluid levels in distended loops of small bowel (*arrows*).

(i.e., small versus large bowel). Ideally, the presence of haustra versus valvulae conniventes can discriminate between large and small bowel, respectively. Small bowel loops should be less than 3 cm in diameter, whereas large bowel caliber is usually less than 5 cm (Note: the cecum can measure up to 9 cm due to its intrinsically greater capacitance). Air-fluid levels can also indicate obstruction but are not entirely specific, as they can be seen with adynamic ileus. One should examine for presence of gas distal to a presumed site of obstruction—absence of distal gas supports the diagnosis of obstruction, but gas may be present in situations with incomplete distal evacuation. A rough guideline of increasing number of dilated small bowel loops reflecting a relatively more distal point of SBO can also be utilized.

In LBO, the appearance depends often on competency of the ileocecal valve. Specifically, a competent ileocecal valve results in strictly colonic distension, whereas an incompetent ileocecal valve allows gas to decompress proximally and retrograde into the ileum and small bowel. When complete obstruction is present, compensatory hyperperistalsis develops throughout the intestine and often results in clearing of gas distal to the site of occlusion. Presence of distal colonic air may reflect partial or early complete obstruction.

Normal Bowel Gas Pattern
- No dilated loops of bowel.
- Fewer than three small bowel air-fluid levels, with each air-fluid level not exceeding 2.5 cm in length.
- Obstruction is less likely if caliber of bowel is normal.

Excessive Gas in a Single Segment of Bowel

■ Closed-loop obstruction can be considered in cases of focal moderate-marked bowel distension.
■ Sentinel loop sign occurs when a focal, isolated loop of distended bowel results from a localized ileus secondary to nearby acute inflammatory processes (e.g., pancreatitis, cholecystitis, appendicitis, or diverticulitis).
■ "Double bubble" sign consists of an air-distended stomach and proximal duodenum and is characteristic of duodenal obstruction. Duodenal obstruction can occur at any age. In children, it usually indicates a congenital obstruction; in adults, it is usually acquired. Complete obstruction at birth or reflex hyperperistalsis results in a gasless abdomen distal to the obstruction.
■ Excessive gas in small bowel and none in the colon suggests SBO with evacuation of gas from the colon.
■ Excessive gas in colon and none in small bowel can indicate LBO with a competent ileocecal valve (no retrograde peristalsis of air).

Differential Diagnosis

■ Cecal volvulus. Classically, a "kidney-shaped" distended cecum directed toward the left upper quadrant (LUQ), often with a single air-fluid level.
■ Sigmoid volvulus: classically, a distended (often massively) large bowel loop arising from pelvis with a "coffee bean" appearance due to a prominent stripe representing opposing colonic walls.
■ Toxic megacolon suggested if transverse colon dilated more than 6 cm.
■ High risk for perforation if cecum dilated more than 10 cm.

Excessive Gas in Both Small and Large Bowel

Differential Diagnosis

■ Aerophagia: too much gas, but no air-fluid levels. Aerophagia can occur in normal patients and in those experiencing pain.
■ Paralytic ileus: large bowel, small bowel, and gastric distension with air-fluid levels. Consider prone film to distinguish colonic ileus and distal LBO; in ileus, gas will percolate up into the rectum.
■ LBO with an incompetent ileocecal valve, allowing spontaneous decompression of the distended colon backward into the small bowel.
■ SBO which is early (not enough time for evacuation of gas) or intermittent (e.g., portion of bowel episodically caught behind adhesion or in a hernia).
■ Pseudo-obstruction: inquire about associated conditions (Table 31-3).

Abnormal Pattern of Intraluminal Gas (Abnormal Bowel Wall)

■ Small bowel air-fluid levels: more than three suggest ileus or SBO.
■ Large bowel air-fluid levels: one or more beyond hepatic flexure of colon is abnormal. If dilated, consider ileus or obstruction. If nondilated, consider fluid feces from diarrhea.
■ "String of beads" pattern represents pockets of gas in primarily fluid-filled intestines forming small gas bubbles under the recesses of valvulae conniventes. This can be seen both in obstruction or ileus.
■ Thickened folds, thumb-printing, separation of bowel loops, or featureless bowel indicate inflammatory or ischemic bowel disease causing edema and enlargement of haustra or valvulae.
■ Persistent bowel pattern over time suggests aperistaltic inflamed or ischemic bowel.

Extraluminal Gas

■ Gas in portal venous system (gas within the liver, usually distal/peripheral) suggests infarcted bowel.
■ Pneumatosis (gas in bowel wall, especially nondependent) may indicate impending rupture and infarcting bowel. It is caused by gas dissecting into diseased bowel mucosa

and appears as linear collections of gas paralleling, but separate, from the bowel lumen. Rarely, benign etiologies can result in pneumatosis (corticosteroid use).

■ Pneumoperitoneum (sliver of air under diaphragm on upright radiograph or air adjacent to the liver on left lateral decubitus view, visualization of both sides of the bowel wall, or abnormally visible falciform ligament on supine or upright view) implies bowel perforation (except for patients with recent abdominal surgeries or invasive abdominal/pelvic procedures). Perforation without pneumoperitoneum can occur if there is lack of intraluminal free air.

■ Pneumobilia (gas within the liver outlining biliary system and usually close to the porta hepatis) in the setting of intestinal obstruction may be secondary to a cholecystoenteric fistula in the setting of gallstone ileus. Pneumobilia is expected and "normal" after a patient has had surgical or endoscopic manipulation of their biliary system.

■ Extraluminal, peritoneal gas can appear as amorphous collections of air outside the bowel and when focal and mottled in appearance, is suggestive of an abscess, possibly from a contained bowel perforation.

Absence of gas/air in bowel: A gasless abdomen is a nonspecific finding. This can be seen in obstruction, if most of the air has evacuated and the bowel is predominantly fluid-filled. Computed tomographic (CT) scan is necessary if obstruction is suspected in such patients.

 IMAGING WITH CONTRAST ENEMA

Indications

■ Suspected LBO.
■ Suspected distal SBO—refluxing barium through ileocecal valve to define the distal anatomy of the obstruction is faster than small bowel series.
■ Contraindicated in toxic megacolon, if pneumatosis, pneumoperitoneum, or portal venous gas are seen, and immediately following a deep biopsy (endoscopic).

Protocol

Bowel preparation is not necessary in acute obstruction. STOP immediately if there is evidence of extravasation or if patient experiences acute exacerbation of pain.

For Suspected Large Bowel Obstruction

■ Use single contrast technique under low pressure.
■ Use water-soluble contrast if there is suspicion of perforation, pseudo-obstruction, or if emergency surgery is planned; otherwise, use barium.
■ One can administer glucagon 1 mg intravenous (IV) (slow push), if necessary, to relieve spasm.
■ Only allow a trickle of contrast through the obstruction.
■ Try to reduce a sigmoid volvulus, if requested: gently administer contrast while moving patient into different positions. Monitor leading edge of contrast fluoroscopically. Abort attempt if there is a sharp increase in the size of the rectosigmoid.
■ Do not try to reduce a cecal volvulus.

For Suspected Small Bowel Obstruction

■ Perform single contrast barium enema, refluxing contrast into distal ileum.
■ Use same precautions as for evaluating LBOs (see preceding text).
■ In the setting of pneumoperitoneum, a water-soluble contrast enema will occasionally be requested to outline anatomy and identify site of perforation. In this setting, one should inform the ordering physician of the theoretic risk of pushing feces through perforation, leading to greater morbidity.
■ Use very low pressure and careful fluoroscopic monitoring.

Possible Findings

■ Cecal volvulus: beaklike narrowing at end of contrast column in ascending colon.
■ Sigmoid volvulus: "bird of prey" sign with hook-shaped narrowing at end of contrast column in sigmoid colon.
■ Diverticulitis: multiple diverticula, extravasation of contrast, and/or demonstration of an abscess with extrinsic compression of lumen.
■ Adenocarcinoma: "apple core" lesion.
■ Diverticulitis and adenocarcinoma: these can have identical appearances and can both cause mechanical obstruction. In 2–10% of cases, the two diseases occur concomitantly. Stenotic lesions more than 6 cm favor diverticulitis.
■ Adhesions: abrupt narrowing with a history of surgery.
■ Metastasis: indentation, spiculation, angulation, narrowing, displacement, and fixation of contrast-filled colon. Tumors arising from pelvic organs may invade or compress the colonic lumen. Hematogenous metastasis is usually submucosal, smooth, and sometimes ulcerated. Serosal implants from stomach or ovarian carcinoma can cause spiculation.
■ Pseudo-obstruction: no narrowing is present.

 IMAGING WITH SMALL BOWEL SERIES

Indications

■ Suspicion of SBO in setting of other indeterminate imaging findings. The procedure is safe, but slow due to long transit time. In distal SBO consider barium enema and refluxing contrast through ileocecal valve.
■ Barium should never be given by mouth in a patient with suspected LBO unless that possibility has been ruled out by contrast enema. "When in doubt, go from below."

Possible Findings

■ Malrotation: consider midgut volvulus ("corkscrew appearance"), Ladd's bands— pediatric population.
■ Double bubble sign: duodenal obstruction.
■ Triple bubble sign: jejunal obstruction with air in stomach, duodenum, and proximal jejunum.
■ Double constriction of bowel: consider hernia.
■ "Coiled spring:" consider intussusception.
■ Abrupt narrowing with history of surgery: consider adhesions.
■ Large filling defects: small bowel tumor.
■ Stricture (focal narrowing): adhesions, Crohn's disease, ischemia, radiation enteritis, or tumor.

 IMAGING WITH COMPUTED TOMOGRAPHY

Indications

■ Presumed intestinal obstruction with indeterminate radiographic findings.
■ CT can diagnose obstruction (in 95%) as well as reveal its cause in up to three fourths of patients. In addition, CT can elucidate other, extraintestinal causes for a patient's symptomatology. It is therefore often requested and performed, even in the presence of pertinent negative and absence of pertinent positive radiographic findings.

Protocol. Oral (water soluble) and IV contrast (if not contraindicated) should be administered routinely. Adequate oral contrast material is useful to prevent misidentification of a fluid-filled bowel loop for an abscess. Institutional protocols vary with regard to the optimal time interval for scanning after administration of enteric contrast. Rectal contrast can be administered immediately before CT examination if colonic obstruction is suspected.

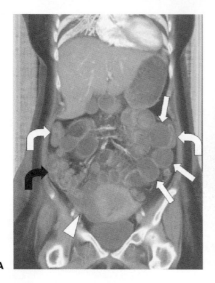
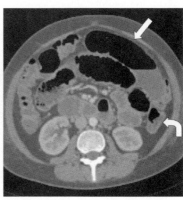

A   B

Figure 31-2. Small bowel obstruction on contrast-enhanced computed tomography (CT). **A:** Coronal volume-rendered view and **(B)** axial image demonstrate multiple dilated loops of small bowel (*straight arrows*), decompressed distal bowel (*curved arrows*), and pelvic abscess (*arrowhead*) which were responsible for the obstruction.

With the advent of multidetector CT scanning, volumetric data acquisition with isotropic voxels is commonly possible. In such cases, multiplanar images in sagittal, coronal, as well as in the traditional axial plane can be obtained. Multiplanar and three-dimensional (3D) imaging can be of great value in demonstrating a transition of caliber, given the often tortuous appearance of small bowel loops which traverse through multiple axes and obliquities. Similarly, 3D CT angiography of the mesenteric vasculature is important in situations when obstruction may be secondary to mesenteric ischemia.

Possible Findings (Fig. 31-2)

■ Interpretation of bowel distension and air-fluid levels on CT is analogous to observations made using abdominal radiographs. One aims to identify a transition point—where bowel dimensions change from dilated to nondilated caliber, signifying the presence and location of obstruction.
■ Presence and focality of stranding and inflammatory changes within mesenteric and intra-abdominal fat help determine the location and source of pathology.
■ Normal colonic wall thickness should not exceed 3 mm.
■ Presence of intraluminal soft tissue density mass can indicate underlying neoplasm, especially in cases of suspected colonic obstruction.
■ Internal hernias can appear as focally narrowed bowel, along with their associated mesentery, within a hernia sac.
■ Intussusception has a characteristic appearance on CT of collapsed proximal bowel with a rim of mesenteric fat, all within the lumen of the distal bowel (a "target" sign). Occasionally, the lead mass can be visualized (polyp, carcinoma).

IMAGING TIPS

Differentiating SBO from LBO can often be difficult radiographically. Careful examination of the geographic distribution of the bowel within the abdomen and its markings will usually separate the two. The small bowel rarely exceeds 3–5 cm when dilated, is centrally located in the abdomen, and has valvulae conniventes spanning the entire diameter of the lumen. In contrast, the large bowel usually exceeds 5 cm when dilated, is peripherally located in the abdomen, and has haustra which extend incompletely across the lumen. In addition, the valvulae conniventes are more numerous and more narrowly spaced than colonic haustra.

Ileus versus obstruction ileus can appear very similar to intestinal obstruction. Adynamic ileus is essentially a temporary reduction and/or cessation of peristalsis. The most common causes of ileus are listed in Table 31-2 and should be sought when considering this diagnosis. By definition, transit of contrast through the bowel in an ileus is delayed but not obstructed. Occasionally, ileus may present as a gasless abdomen with all bowel loops distended with fluid.

Terminology. The terms *ileus, adynamic ileus* (also known as *paralytic ileus*), *nonmechanical obstruction*, and *mechanical obstruction* can be confusing. The formal definition of ileus is intestinal obstruction, but in the United States ileus usually refers to adynamic ileus. Therefore, the terms ileus, adynamic ileus, paralytic ileus, and nonmechanical obstruction are often used interchangeably.

Rule of 3-6-9

3: More than three small bowel loops distended more than 3 cm with air-fluid levels occur 3–5 hours after initial obstruction. Thickened small bowel folds are more than 3 mm (not specific for intestinal obstruction).
6: Consider toxic megacolon when transverse colon measures more than 6 cm (i.e., $2 \times 3 = 6$) in patients with fulminant colitis, usually acute ulcerative colitis.
9: Consider impending cecal perforation when cecum distends more than 9 cm.

 ISSUES AFTER IMAGING

A partial SBO can be self-limiting, requiring only conservative measures such as NPO status, nasogastric decompression, and IV hydration/electrolyte replenishment. However, a complete SBO often requires surgical intervention. Similarly, LBOs generally require surgery.

Further Readings

Aufort S, Charra L, Lesnik A, et al. Multidetector CT of bowel obstruction: value of post-processing. *Eur J Radiol* 2005;15:2323–2329.

Brant WE, Helms CA, 2nd ed. *Fundamentals of diagnostic radiology*. Baltimore: Lippincott Williams & Wilkins, 1999:997–1023.

Donnelly LF. *Fundamentals of pediatric radiology*. Philadelphia: WB Saunders, 2001: 97–140.

Ferrucci JT. *Radiology: diagnosis, imaging, and intervention*, revised ed. Philadelphia: Lippincott Williams & Wilkins, 2003.

Horton KM, Fishman EK. The current status of multidetector row CT and three-dimensional imaging of the small bowel. *Radiol Clin North Am* 2003;41:199–212.

Maglinte DD, Kelvin FM, Rowe MG, et al. Small-bowel obstruction: optimizing radiologic investigation and non-surgical management. *Radiology* 2001;218:39–46.

Sinha R, Verma R. Multidetector row computed tomography in bowel obstruction. Part 2. Large bowel obstruction. *Clin Radiol* 2005;60:1068–1075.

Taourel P, Kessler N, Lesnik A, et al. Helical CT of large bowel obstruction. *Abdom Imaging* 2003;28:267–275.

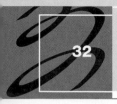

INTUSSUSCEPTION
32

Alexander M. Kowal

CLINICAL INFORMATION

Intussusception is the acquired telescoping of one portion of bowel (the intussusceptum) into another portion of bowel (the intussuscipiens).

Age at presentation. Intussusception is the most common abdominal emergency of infancy and the second most common cause of acute abdomen in children, after appendicitis. Both the incidence and etiology of intussusception are highly dependent on the age of the patient. The vast majority (75–80%) of intussusceptions occur in young children between the ages of 3 months to 2 years. The peak incidence is between 5 and 10 months with 50% younger than 1 year. Intussusceptions almost never occur before 3 months of age. After 2 years of age, the incidence declines progressively with only 5% presenting in adult patients. There is a 2–4:1 male predominance. Early diagnosis is the key to avoiding complications including bowel obstruction, necrosis, and bowel perforation.

Etiology in Children. In young children, equal to or more than 90% of intussusceptions are idiopathic with no identified pathologic lead point. These intussusceptions are virtually always ileocolic and are probably due to hypertrophied lymphoid tissue (Peyer's patches) in the distal ileum acting as a lead point. A higher incidence in the spring and autumn suggests a predisposing viral infection. After 4 years of age, the likelihood of a pathologic process causing intussusception begins to rise with the patient's age.

Differential diagnosis of pathologic lead points in children includes inverted Meckel's diverticulum, lymphoma, polyp, duplication cyst, enterogenous cyst, intramural hematoma (Henoch-Schönlein purpura), hemangioma, appendiceal inflammation, suture line from prior surgery, and inspissated meconium in the setting of cystic fibrosis.

Etiology in Adults. In adults, a specific cause or pathologic lead point is identified in equal to or more than 80% of patients with intussusception. The site of intussusception in older patients is variable. The enteroenteral type is most frequent and often related to a benign condition such as lipoma, gastrointestinal stromal tumor (GIST), adenomatous polyp, hemangioma, adhesions, lymphoid hyperplasia, or villous adenoma of the appendix. Transient, asymptomatic small bowel intussusceptions have been increasingly identified. Colonic intussusception is most often due to a malignancy such as adenocarcinoma or lymphoma but may also be due to leiomyoma, endometriosis, or a prior surgical anastomosis.

Differential diagnosis of pathologic lead points in adults also includes benign and malignant tumors, Meckel's diverticulum, aberrant pancreatic tissue, foreign body, feeding tube, chronic ulcer, prior gastroenteritis, gastroenterostomy, and trauma. In addition, intussusception can be seen without any specific lead point in adults with scleroderma, Whipple's disease, celiac disease, and fasting states.

Symptoms and Signs. In children, the classic triad of colicky intermittent abdominal pain, palpable mass, and red currant jelly stools is present in fewer than 50% of cases. Blood in the stool mixed with sloughed mucosa is a late finding, producing the characteristic "currant jelly" appearance. Infants are often irritable, may have episodes of emesis, and cry intermittently. Lethargy can accompany any one of the above symptoms. Twenty percent are painfree at presentation. Physical examination may reveal a palpable sausage-shaped mass, which can increase in size during paroxysms of pain. In adults, intussusception usually presents with nonspecific symptoms of mechanical obstruction.

 IMAGING WITH ULTRASONOGRAPHY

Indications. Ultrasonography is considered the primary imaging technique for suspected intussusception. Sensitivity is 98–100%, specificity is 88–100%, negative predictive value is 100% and the reported accuracy is 100%. The procedure is noninvasive, fast, easy, and reproducible and does not require ionizing radiation. It can detect up to 66% of pathologic lead points.

Possible Findings (Fig. 32-1)

■ An oval-shaped mass on longitudinal ultrasonography with a sonolucent rim and an echogenic center. This has been termed the *pseudokidney* appearance because it resembles the sagittal view of a kidney. The mass may also have a "sandwichlike" appearance of three parallel hypoechoic bands.
■ On transverse views, intussusception appears as a "doughnut" with a sonolucent ring and echogenic center.
■ In both views, the sonolucent rim is caused by the edematous wall of the intussuscipiens and the echogenic center corresponds to compressed mucosa and associated mesenteric fat of the intussusceptum.
■ The mass is often seen just deep to the right abdominal wall and measures between 2.5–5 cm.
■ Color Doppler is helpful to detect blood flow within the bowel wall. A lack of Doppler signal may suggest ischemia, and indicates that the chance of nonoperative reduction is decreased.
■ Trapped peritoneal fluid between serosal surfaces (<15%) is associated with decreased reduction rates and suggests ischemia.
■ False-positive examinations can occur with bowel wall thickening.

 IMAGING WITH RADIOGRAPHS

Indications. Radiography is often the first examination performed in the evaluation of abdominal pain. However, when intussusception or other abdominal pathology is strongly suspected, radiography should be avoided in favor of ultrasonography, unless perforation is suspected. Radiograph sensitivity is only 45% and a normal study does not exclude intussusception.

Protocol. In children, intussusception is best evaluated with three views: supine, prone, and left side down cross-table decubitus view. The supine view evaluates the overall gas pattern and is helpful in detecting soft tissue masses. The prone view fills the cecum with air for detecting intraluminal masses. Intussusception is effectively ruled out if the cecum and terminal ileum can be completely distended with air, but air-filled sigmoid in the right lower quadrant can be misinterpreted as cecum. Lastly, the cross-table decubitus view is used to rule out pneumoperitoneum and to fill the bowel in the right upper quadrant with air to evaluate for soft tissue masses.

Possible Findings (Fig. 32-1)

■ Appearance of intussusception is variable. Radiographs may be normal in early stages.
■ There is often an absence of air in the cecum and ascending colon.
■ A right upper quadrant soft tissue mass is seen in 78% of cases. A "target" sign (60%) representing a round soft tissue density with a concentric lucency of mesenteric fat is pathognomonic when seen in the transverse colon near the hepatic flexure. A "crescent" or "meniscus" sign (30%) is a lucency representing air outlining the apex of the intussusception.

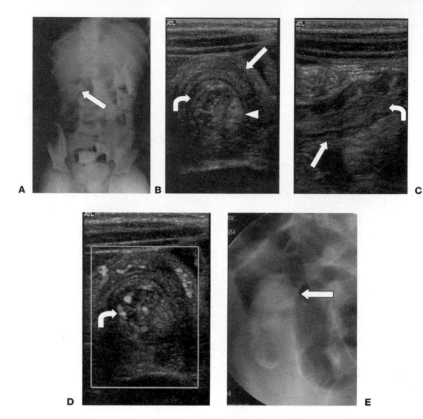

Figure 32-1. Ileocolic intussusception in 4-year-old patient who presented with crampy abdominal pain. **A:** Anteroposterior (AP) radiograph demonstrates presence of a filling defect (*arrow*) in the cecum consistent with intussusception. **B:** Transverse ultrasonography (US) view demonstrates a "target" sign with concentric rings. The outer ring corresponds to the wall of intussuscipiens (*straight arrow*) and the inner ring corresponds to the wall of intussusceptum (*curved arrow*). The mesentery of intussusceptum is pulled along and has an echogenic appearance (*arrowhead*). **C:** Longitudinal ultrasonography (US) view demonstrates sandwichlike appearance of parallel alternating hyperechoic and hypoechoic bands. The ilium or intussusceptum (*curved arrow*) is seen within the cecum or intussuscipiens (*straight arrow*). **D:** Presence of vascular flow on Doppler US in the intussusceptum (*curved arrow*) is an important predictor of successful reduction by enema. **E:** Air enema demonstrates a filling defect (*arrow*) in the cecum consistent with intussusception, which was successfully reduced during the procedure.

- Air in a dislocated appendix can be observed.
- Air fluid levels and dilatation consistent with small bowel obstruction may be seen in 42% of cases.
- Pneumoperitoneum is a relatively rare but serious complication of intussusception.

 IMAGING WITH COMPUTED TOMOGRAPHY

Indications. Computed tomography (CT)evaluation is not usually indicated in children but is useful in adults. Intussusceptions are seen on CT scans of adults who are being worked up for symptoms of mechanical bowel obstruction or nonspecific, chronic abdominal pain. CT is also helpful in evaluating lead points.

Protocol. CT of the abdomen and pelvis with both oral and intravenous contrast is preferred.

Possible Findings

- Classically appears as an intraluminal mass with a "bull's-eye" or "target" appearance on perpendicular views. The outer wall is the intussuscipiens, which contains a ring or crescent of mesenteric fat and a central soft tissue density representing the compressed intussusceptum.
- On longitudinal views, there is the appearance of a sausage-shaped mass. A rim of oral contrast may also be seen.
- There are often findings of mechanical bowel obstruction proximal to the intussusception.
- Asymptomatic, transient small bowel intussusceptions discovered incidentally on CT are common.

 ## IMAGING WITH CONTRAST ENEMA

Indications. Contrast and/or air enema is no longer considered part of the diagnostic workup of suspected intussusception but remains essential for therapeutic intervention.

Protocol. (See Chap. 57, "Intussusception Reduction.")

Possible Findings (Fig. 32-1)

- On contrast enema, intussusception appears as an intraluminal mass with contrast filling around the mass in concentric rings, producing the classic "coiled spring" appearance. The same appearance can be incidentally seen on upper gastrointestinal (GI) studies.
- On air enema, intussusception appears as an intraluminal soft tissue mass outlined by air.

 ## IMAGING WITH MAGNETIC RESONANCE

Indications. Not routinely used except with stable adult patients to help in surgical planning and evaluating pathologic lead points.

Protocol. Multiplanar HASTE (half-fourier single shot turbo spin echo).

Possible Findings

High signal will be seen within the intraluminal fluid. The bowel wall will be of low to intermediate signal.

Treatment

(See Chap. 57, "Intussusception Reduction.")

Further Readings

Applegate KE. Clinically suspected intussusception in children: evidence-based review and self-assessment module. *AJR Am J Roentgenol* 2005;185:S175–S183.

Byrne AT, Goeghegan T, Govender P, et al. The imaging of intussusception. *Clin Radiol* 2005;60:39–46.

Choi SH, Han JK, Kim SH, et al. Intussusception in adults: from stomach to rectum. *Am J Roentgenol* 2004;183:691–698.

Daneman A, Navarro O. Intussusception part 1: a review of diagnostic approaches. *Pediatr Radiol* 2003;33:79–85.

Daneman A, Navarro O. Intussusception part 2: an update on the evolution of management. *Pediatr Radiol* 2004;34:97–108.

Del Pozo G. Intussusception: still work in progress. *Pediatr Radiol* 2005;35:92–94.

Kazez A, Ozel SK, Kocakoc E, et al. Double intussusception in a child. *J Ultrasound Med* 2004;23:1659–1661.

Navarro OM, Daneman A, Chae A. Intussusception: the use of delayed, repeated reduction attempts and the management of intussusceptions due to pathologic lead points in pediatric patients. *Am J Roentgenol* 2004;182:1169–1176.

Sorantin E, Lincdbichler F. Management of intussusception. *Eur Radiol* 2004;14(Suppl 4): L146–L154.

Takeuchi K, Tsuzuki Y, Ando T, et al. The diagnosis and treatment of adult intusussception. *J Clin Gastroenterol* 2003;36(1):18–21.

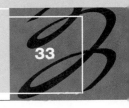

33

LIVER TRANSPLANTATION
Christopher L. Smith

$\mathcal{S}$ince the first liver transplantation was successfully performed by Thomas Starzl in 1967, orthotopic liver transplantation (OLT) has become an accepted means for the treatment of end-stage liver disease. One of the major indications for liver transplantation is cirrhosis with portal hypertension. The causes of the cirrhosis are many, including alcoholism, hepatitis, primary sclerosing cholangitis, primary biliary cirrhosis, and Wilson's disease. An emerging indication for transplantation is in treatment for hepatocellular carcinoma. In the pediatric population, the most common indications are biliary atresia and α_1-antitrypsin deficiency. In addition, a small percentage of transplantations are performed for acute hepatic failure.

PREOPERATIVE IMAGING

Indications

The preoperative evaluation of both the donor and the recipient is important.

Transplant Recipient. The objective of imaging the potential transplant recipient include evaluating the severity of the cirrhosis and associated portal hypertension, identifying conditions that may complicate the surgery or preclude transplantation, and to identifying tumor, both in the cirrhotic liver and in extrahepatic malignancy. Imaging modalities that are routinely employed in this evaluation include ultrasonography (US), computed tomography (CT), and magnetic resonance imaging (MRI). Advancements in CT and MRI have decreased the utilization of angiography.

When imaging the potential recipient, depending on the etiology of the cirrhosis, some hepatic morphologic changes can be identified on imaging which could suggest the etiology of cirrhosis. Additionally, one major role in the pretransplantation imaging is to identify vascular anomalies or pathology that may preclude transplantation. It is also important to document the patency of the hepatic vessels. One other important indication is to assess for the presence of hepatocellular carcinoma and if present, to perform accurate staging. Angiography, either computed tomography angiography (CTA), magnetic resonance angiography (MRA), or conventional angiography may be required in pediatric patients with known or suspected vascular anomalies or in the asplenia and polysplenia syndromes.

Transplant Donor. The goals of imaging the potential liver donor are to evaluate the liver parenchyma, provide data for split-liver volume assessment, and to define the liver vascular map (both intra- and extrahepatic vasculature). Both CT and MRI have been used for this evaluation. Another important objective is to evaluate the biliary tree to assess for anatomic variants. Magnetic resonance (MR) cholangiography has been reported to provide excellent definition of the biliary anatomy.

SURGICAL ANATOMY

Orthotopic Liver Transplantation. The conventional form of OLT requires suprahepatic and infrahepatic anastomoses to the native inferior vena cava (IVC). Recently, a new technique has been developed for hepatic venous anastomosis known as the *piggy-back* technique. This involves preservation of the entire retrohepatic vena cava with anastomosis of the new liver to a cuff formed from one or more of the main suprahepatic veins. Both forms involve an anastomosis of the recipient to donor portal vein, hepatic artery, and biliary tree. The arterial and biliary anastomoses are the most frequently problematic, generating most postoperative complications.

The arterial anastomosis between the donor and recipient is usually end-to-end and the site usually varies depending on the arterial anatomy and the surgeon's preference. A common recipient site of arterial anastomosis is the bifurcation of the hepatic artery into right and left branches. If this is not feasible, the next most common site is at the branch point of the gastroduodenal artery from the common hepatic artery. Less preferred, but occasionally performed, is a donor iliac arterial graft from the infrarenal aorta to the allograft.

The common bile duct is usually connected through end-to-end choledochocholedochostomy or to a loop of jejunum (Roux-en-Y choledochojejunostomy). The former option is generally preferred, as there is a higher incidence of anastomotic breakdown with the Roux-en-Y technique. Choledochojejunostomy is reserved for children, patients with sclerosing cholangitis, revisions of previous choledochocholedochostomies, and in cases where there is a large size discrepancy between donor and recipient common bile ducts.

Reduced size liver transplantation, first performed in 1984, now accounts for approximately 50% of transplantations in pediatric patients. Reduced size livers can be prepared using the entire right lobe, the entire left lobe, or the left lateral liver. The left liver provides an orientation that is most similar to native liver, facilitating correct orientation of the IVC and hilar structures. The left lateral graft technique is indicated when there is a large size disparity between donor and recipient.

Living related liver transplantation, first performed in 1989, is analogous to the reduced size left lateral segment graft: the donor left hepatic vein is anastomosed to a triangular cuff formed by the division of the native hepatic vein septae; the donor hepatic artery is connected to the recipient infrarenal aorta through interposition graft; the portal veins are connected end-to-end or side-to-side, and the biliary tree drained through Roux-en-Y hepatojejunostomy.

NORMAL POSTOPERATIVE EXAMINATION

Timing.   Routine postoperative evaluation usually consists of duplex sonography shortly after transplantation (24–48 hours) and cholangiography either through the T-tube or MRI in patients with a choledochocholedochostomy a few days after surgery and again before removal of the T-tube. Meaningful interpretation of these studies often requires knowledge of which variation of the surgical anastomoses were performed, so communication between radiologist and surgeon is important.

Ultrasonographic.   Identification of flow within the intrahepatic portal vein, hepatic vein, and hepatic artery is critical. The hepatic artery has a typical arterial pattern with pulsatile flow and low resistance forward flow in diastole. The resistive index ([peak systolic velocity–lowest diastolic velocity]/peak systolic velocity) should be greater than 0.5. The hepatic vein has a Doppler signal similar to the IVC, with a triphasic pattern. The portal vein demonstrates a continuous flow pattern, and the examiner should ascertain that the direction of flow is toward the liver (hepatopetal).

The transplanted liver is evaluated for any parenchymal abnormalities, evidence of biliary ductal dilatation, and intrahepatic or extrahepatic fluid collections. Periportal edema is considered a normal finding in the early postoperative patient (seen in 20%) and is most likely secondary to lymphedema. A small amount of fluid in the intersegmental fissure around the falciform ligament is also considered normal. A right pleural effusion is almost always present in the early postoperative period.

In patients with reduced segment transplants, it is common for the cut surface of the graft margin to appear irregular and inhomogeneous on ultrasonography. A fluid-filled Roux-en-Y loop may simulate a perihepatic fluid collection. Correlation with the surgical technique and serial exams can help to resolve these difficulties.

Magnetic Resonance Imaging. MRI with magnetic resonance (MR) cholangiography can be performed as a noninvasive evaluation of the biliary tree and hepatic vasculature. This can be performed to evaluate for biliary leaks, fluid collections, to document patency of the hepatic vasculature and MRI is especially useful in the evaluation of biliary strictures in the chronic setting.

T-tube Cholangiography. Can be performed a few days after surgery to evaluate for leakage. This most commonly occurs at the anastomotic site or at the T-tube insertion site; however, non anastomotic leaks should be searched for, as they are a much more serious complication, usually indicative of hepatic arterial thrombosis. Cholangiography is also performed before removal of the T-tube, which occurs in the uncomplicated transplant anywhere from 2 weeks to 2 months after surgery.

POSTOPERATIVE COMPLICATIONS

Acute Rejection. Rejection is the most common complication following transplantation and occurs in approximately one third of patients. Clinical findings are nonspecific, liver function tests are usually abnormal, and pathologically there is inflammatory infiltration of the allograft portal areas associated with evidence of endothelial and bile duct injury. Acute rejection can occur any time after the first 2-3 postoperative days, but it most commonly begins 1-2 weeks following surgery. Acute rejection is uncommon later than 2 months after surgery unless the patient has been inadequately immunosuppressed. There are no reliable radiologic indications of acute rejection, and the role of the radiologist is to exclude other complications. Biopsy is the only reliable method for demonstrating rejection.

Chronic Rejection. Is characterized pathologically by insidious but relentless loss of bile ducts and an obliterative arteriopathy. Chronic rejection typically occurs several months after transplantation, although the syndrome has been reported to develop as early as 3-4 weeks after surgery. Incidence of chronic rejection is estimated to be 10-15%. Again, there is little radiologic role in identifying chronic rejection, and the radiologist's role is to exclude correctable complications before biopsy is performed.

Hepatic Artery Thrombosis. Is a grave complication which often requires retransplantation. It is also the most common vascular complication, occurring in approximately 8% of adult patients and 16% of pediatric patients. Hepatic artery thrombosis usually occurs within the first few days of transplantation, but is occasionally seen as late as 2 months after surgery.

This complication is most easily identified through duplex sonography, which is able to detect up to 92% of cases of arterial thrombosis. This is usually found by failure to identify flow within the intrahepatic hepatic artery. Occasionally echogenic thrombus within the vessel lumen is seen. Lobar or peripheral areas of low echogenicity (or low attenuation on CT) within the transplanted liver are also suggestive of hepatic artery thrombosis with subsequent liver infarction. Failure to detect hepatic arterial flow by Doppler ultrasound may lead directly to surgical intervention; alternatively, in some centers arteriography is first performed for confirmation and occasionally to attempt thrombolytic therapy.

Ischemia. The donor biliary tree is particularly susceptible to ischemia following hepatic artery thrombosis as it receives its sole blood supply from the hepatic artery. Biliary ischemia can lead to nonanastomotic strictures, bile leaks, sepsis, and hepatic infarction. Nonanastomotic strictures or leaks should prompt US examination to exclude hepatic artery thrombosis: in one series, 60% of nonanastomotic strictures and 90% of nonanastomotic leaks were associated with arterial occlusion.

Hepatic artery stenosis (Fig. 33-1) is a less common complication than thrombosis and typically occurs later in the postoperative course. Stenosis usually occurs in the extrahepatic portion of the artery at the anastomotic site. Sonography demonstrates focally accelerated velocity (>2 m/second) and turbulent flow at and beyond the anastomosis. A tardus-parvus

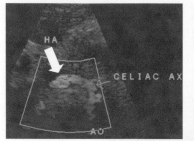
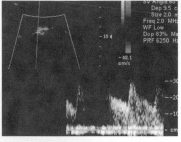

A

B

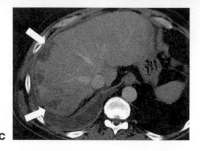

C

Figure 33-1. Hepatic artery (HA) narrowing in a patient with liver transplant. **A:** Ultrasonographic (US) image demonstrates HA (*arrow*) arising from celiac trunk. **B:** Doppler US shows marked velocity elevation compatible with stenosis. **C:** Contrast-enhanced computed tomographic (CT) image of the transplanted liver demonstrates peripheral hypodensities (*arrows*) consistent with infarcts due to HA stenosis. AO, aorta.

waveform is seen distal to the stenosis, and consists of a low systolic acceleration time and a low resistive index less than 0.5. If stenosis is suspected clinically or if a stenosis is detected on duplex examination, definitive diagnosis requires CTA, MRA, or conventional catheter arteriography. Hepatic artery stenosis can lead to thrombosis of the artery. Nonanastomotic hepatic arterial stenosis is associated with chronic rejection.

Pseudoaneurysms (Fig. 33-2) usually occur at anastomotic sites, although they can appear anywhere after biopsy. These are confirmed with ultrasonography (where turbulent flow is demonstrated within the pseudoaneurysm) or on CT where the pseudoaneurysm can be identified. One important point regarding pseudoaneurysms is to always consider the possibility of a pseudoaneurysm before performing percutaneous drainage of a fluid collection in or around the liver.

Portal vein and IVC complications are rare, occurring in 1–2% of patients. Duplex Doppler is the screening examination of choice if thrombosis or stenosis is suspected. Sonography may demonstrate a venous anastomotic stenosis directly or show indirect signs such as luminal thrombosis or slow/turbulent flow across the anastomosis.

Biliary complications constitute the second most frequent complication after acute rejection, occurring in 7–29% of patients. MRI cholangiography is the study of choice to evaluate the biliary tree, and is generally simple to perform if the T-tube is still present. Ultrasonography is useful as well, although some authors have noted that it has a decreased sensitivity for detecting biliary obstruction in transplant patients versus native livers. This is probably because more careful monitoring of liver function tests in transplant patients leads to earlier detection of obstruction and earlier requests for sonography. Ultrasonography is the first study to perform in a patient with a complicated postoperative course. If the biliary system appears abnormal, or if no abnormality is seen but biliary obstruction is suspected clinically, then cholangiography should be performed.

Biliary leakage most commonly occurs at the T-tube choledochotomy site, where it is usually self-limited. Biliary leakage at choledochocholedochostomy or

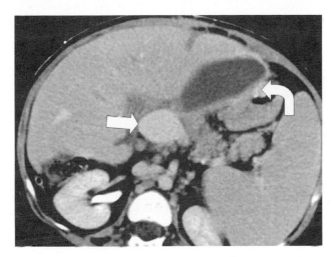

Figure 33-2. Contrast-enhanced computed tomography (CT) scan demonstrates portal vein aneurysm (*straight arrow*) and perihepatic abscess (*curved arrow*) in a patient after liver transplantation.

choledochojejunostomy sites is less frequent but has more serious complications. These have a much higher morbidity and frequently require surgical revision. As noted in the preceding text, anastomotic leaks are more common in patients with choledochojejunostomies. More proximal biliary leaks are often the result of hepatic artery stenosis or thrombosis, leading to biliary ischemia.

Bilomas are collections of bile usually in the perihepatic region. They are indistinguishable from other fluid collections on CT and ultrasonography, and therefore cholangiography or a hepatobiliary nuclear scan is the imaging modality of choice to confirm a biloma. Nuclear hepatobiliary imaging is more sensitive in detecting small leaks. Delayed images should always be obtained because slow leakage may not be apparent on early images, and abnormal collections of radiotracer can be followed to ensure that they are not in an abnormally positioned bowel loop. The fluid could also be aspirated with percutaneous catheter drainage for confirmation.

Biliary strictures appear on cholangiography, both MR and direct, as a focal narrowing with smooth walls, usually with proximal dilatation. These typically occur at anastomotic sites and can be treated with balloon angioplasty if the stricture is functionally significant. Nonanastomotic strictures are more serious in that they raise the possibility of hepatic artery thrombosis as discussed in the preceding text.

Miscellaneous Causes of Biliary Obstruction. Malpositioning of the T-tube limbs or inspissated bile occluding the T-tube or internal stent are common causes of biliary obstruction which are easily diagnosed on cholangiography. Sphincter of Oddi dysfunction is estimated to occur in up to 5% of patients following transplantation and should therefore be considered in the patient with obstruction. Endoscopic sphincterotomy is the treatment of choice. Choledocholithiasis can occur any time after transplantation and is probably associated with the increased lithogenicity of bile seen in some posttransplant patients. MRI is especially useful in this setting. Extrinsic obstruction of the common duct is usually an early complication and can be due to a biloma, hematoma, cystic duct mucocele, or other mass. MRI, CT, or ultrasonography is usually diagnostic.

Perihepatic fluid collections are a common finding in the postoperative patient, and the differential diagnosis includes abscess, hematoma, biloma, seroma, loculated ascites, and pseudoaneurysm. The significance of a perihepatic collection depends largely on the clinical status of the patient. Percutaneous aspiration and drainage under CT or ultrasonographic guidance is diagnostic; however, always confirm with Doppler ultrasound or contrast enhanced CT or MRI that the fluid collection is not a pseudoaneurysm.

Infection.   All liver transplant patients are immunosuppressed, and it is not surprising that there is a high incidence of postoperative infection (Fig. 33-2). Common organisms are gram-negative enteric bacteria, *Staphylococcus*, cytomegalovirus (CMV), and Epstein-Barr virus (EBV). Most infections occur within 3 months of surgery. Ten percent of patients develop an abdominal abscess; 80% of these are intrahepatic. Chest x-ray and abdominal CT are indicated in the febrile posttransplant patient.

    Hemobilia is most often the result of liver biopsy or percutaneous cholangiography. It is usually self-limited.

Other Complications.   Extrahepatic complications include right adrenal hemorrhage secondary to clamping of the adrenal vein during IVC anastomosis, pancreatitis, cyclosporin-induced lymphoma or lymphoproliferative disorder, recurrent primary hepatic tumor, intracranial hemorrhage, cerebral edema, bowel perforation, and splenic infarction.

Further Readings

Dodson TF. Surgical anatomy of hepatic transplantation. *Surg Clin North Am* 1993;73: 645–659.

Eghtesad B, Kadry Z, Fung J. Technical considerations in liver transplantation: what a hepatologist needs to know (and every surgeon should practice). *Liver Transpl* 2005;11(8):861–871.

Hoeffel C, Azizi L, Lewin M, et al. Normal and pathological features of the postoperative biliary tract at 3D MR cholangiopancreatography and MR imaging. *Radiographics* 2006;26:1603–1620.

Olmusa O, Federle MP. Abdominal imaging and intervention in liver transplantation. *Liver Transpl* 2006;12:184–193.

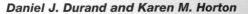
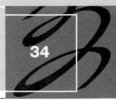

NEPHROLITHIASIS

Daniel J. Durand and Karen M. Horton

34

*N*ephrolithiasis is the most common cause of urinary tract obstruction. Approximately 90% of calculi are radiopaque on radiographs whereas almost all stones are radiopaque on computed tomography (CT). The only exceptions are radiolucent stones that can form in patients on protease inhibitors such as Indinavir. Renal stones are commonly classified according to their predominant chemical composition (Table 34-1). In addition to obstruction, renal calculi can also cause stricture formation, chronic renal infection, or loss of renal function.

CLINICAL INFORMATION

The major etiologies of nephrolithiasis are listed in Table 34-2.

Symptoms and signs of passing a ureteral stone include pain and hematuria, although stone passage is occasionally asymptomatic. The pain usually begins in the flank and gradually increases over minutes to hours until it is so severe that narcotics may be required for pain control. Classically, the pain fluctuates and is known as *renal colic*. Downward migration of the pain toward the groin indicates passage of the stone into the distal third of the ureter. Hematuria is present in approximately 85% of cases.

Differential diagnosis of renal colic includes urinary tract infection, appendicitis, diverticulitis, gynecologic conditions, lumbar disc disease, and abdominal aortic aneurysm (with or without dissection).

IMAGING OVERVIEW

Radiologic imaging has always played a central role in the evaluation of suspected nephrolithiasis. Although several imaging modalities are potentially useful in detecting stones or secondary signs of obstruction such as hydronephrosis, noncontrast CT (NCCT) has become the test of choice over the last decade due to its speed and accuracy. Nevertheless, other modalities such as ultrasonography may be of use in situations when there are concerns over radiation exposure or cost.

IMAGING WITH RADIOGRAPHS

Indications. Because most renal stones are radiopaque, the workup often begins with a plain abdominal radiograph. The stone may be difficult to visualize, however, due to overlying bowel gas, fecal material, and phleboliths. Recent studies indicate that abdominal radiographs have a sensitivity and specificity of 53–59% and 71–74%, respectively.

Protocol. Typically, a kidney, ureter, and bladder (KUB) is obtained. Oblique views can sometimes help to determine if a suspicious calcification is in the kidney or ureter. On the oblique view, a potential stone should "move" with the kidney and the expected course of the ureter.

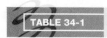

TABLE 34-1   Types of Renal Stones

Type	Percentage of total cases	Radiograph radi-opacity	Comments
Calcium salts (oxalate, phosphate)	75–85	+++	Male predominance
Struvite ($MgNH_4PO_4$)	10–15	++	Associated with urease-producing organisms and staghorn calculi; female predominance
Uric acid	5–8	0	Approximately half have gout
Cystine	1	+	Mildly radiopaque due to sulfur content

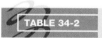

TABLE 34-2   Causes of Urolithiasis

Etiology	Approximate percentage of total cases
Idiopathic hypercalcuria (usually familial)	
Idiopathic with normocalcuria	45
Hyperuricosuria (excessive purine intake)	20
Hypercalcemic disorders	15
Primary hyperparathyroidism	—
Immobilization	4
Sarcoidosis	—
Cushing's syndrome	—
Hypervitaminosis D	—
Milk-alkali syndrome	—
Secondary urolithiasis	—
Infection (struvite stones)	—
Urinary obstruction (e.g., bladder outflow)	10–15
Medullary sponge kidney	—
Urinary diversion procedure	—
Indwelling catheter	—
Intestinal hyperoxaluria (oxalate overabsorption)	<1
Drug-related (e.g., Indinavir)	—
Uric acid lithiasis	—
Gout	2–4
Idiopathic (but usually familial)	2–4
Myeloproliferative disease	—
Renal tubular acidosis (type I, distal)	Rare

Possible Findings

A radiopaque calculus may be seen in the kidney or along the course of the ureter on radiography. It can be difficult or even impossible to distinguish calculi from other abdominal calcifications, including phleboliths, calcified mesenteric lymph nodes, gallstones, and costal cartilage calcifications. The inherent limitations of radiography often necessitate a follow-up CT, which is why most contemporary practitioners proceed directly to CT.

 ## IMAGING WITH NONCONTRAST COMPUTED TOMOGRAPHY

Indications. NCCT of the abdomen and pelvis is now the modality of choice for investigation of suspected nephrolithiasis. Recent studies indicate that CT is 96–100% sensitive and 95.5–100% specific in detecting urinary stones. NCCT also eliminates concerns related to renal toxicity and contrast allergies. It is also far more rapid than intravenous urogram (IVU) and is far more sensitive in detecting secondary effects of calculi (e.g., hydronephrosis) and noncalculus causes of flank pain and obstruction (e.g., pelvic masses, appendicitis). Some notable disadvantages of CT are its high cost, radiation exposure, and inability to visualize renal enhancement.

Protocol. Images are typically obtained without contrast from the top of the kidneys through the bladder base using a conventional helical CT scanner. Slices are typically 2–3 mm and tube currents run from 150–200 mAs depending on the generation of scanner used. In some patients obtaining additional scans may be helpful. For example, when a calculus is observed at the ureterovesicular junction (UVJ), prone imaging can be added to determine if the calculus is free floating within the bladder or impacted in the distal ureter. Also, it may be difficult to determine if a pelvic calcification is actually within the ureter or outside the ureter. In these cases, it is helpful to administer intravenous (IV) contrast and scan during the excretory phase, once the ureters are opacified. In situations where NCCT does not detect the cause of the patient's symptoms, it may be useful to perform a second scan with oral and IV contrast, because this greatly improves the sensitivity for detecting other diagnoses that can cause hematuria and flank pain. It is therefore advisable to review initial noncontrast images before releasing the patient from the scanning room.

Possible Findings (Fig. 34-1)

- A calculus appears as a hyperdense focus of bone density within the kidney or ureter. Calculi less than 1 mm may not be detected on NCCT due to volume averaging. It is important to be able to distinguish distal calculi from pelvic phleboliths. Most calculi have a "rim" of circumferential soft tissue thickening, which represents the obstructed ureter. This "rim" is present in 50–77% of calculi and absent in more than 90% of extraurinary calcifications. Following the ureter from the site of obstruction back to the renal pelvis is also useful and multiplanar reconstruction can be especially helpful when doing so.
- **Hydronephrosis and hydroureter.** On CT, hydronephrosis appears as dilation of the renal pelvis with clubbing of the calyces in the upper and lower poles. It is often associated with obliteration of renal sinus fat, asymmetric perinephric stranding, and enlargement and hypoattenuation of the entire kidney. Hydroureter appears as a dilated ureter.

 ## IMAGING WITH ULTRASONOGRAPHY

Indications. Ultrasonography is readily available, inexpensive, and can be especially useful when seeking to minimize radiation exposure to pregnant women and children. Ultrasonography is best suited for detecting hydronephrosis, although this is sometimes absent early in obstruction. Furthermore, a substantial proportion of pregnant women have physiologic hydronephrosis secondary to the mass effect of the gravid uterus compressing the ureters.

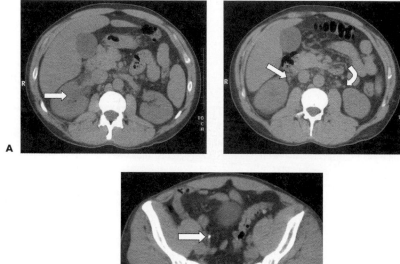

A

B

C

Figure 34-1. A: Computed tomography (CT) scan demonstrates minimal hydronephrosis of the right kidney (*arrow*). **B:** The right ureter (*straight arrow*) is minimally dilated in comparison the left (*curved arrow*). **C:** There is a tiny calculus (*arrow*) in the right ureter accounting for the hydronephrosis and hydroureter.

Ultrasonography is highly sensitive (96–100%) at detecting renal calculi greater than 5 mm, but less sensitive in detecting smaller stones. Owing to overlying bowel gas, ultrasonography can detect just 37% of ureteral calculi, although its sensitivity nearly doubles when hydronephrosis is included as a positive sign. Ultrasonography is even less effective in obese patients.

Protocol.   In assessing for hydronephrosis, be sure the bladder is empty. Try to visualize both the ureteropelvic junction (UPJ) and the UVJ to look for dilatation and impacted stones.

Possible Findings (Fig. 34-2)

- A calculus appears as a strongly echogenic focus accompanied by strong acoustic shadowing. Calculi as small as 3–5 mm may be detected by ultrasonography. Air within the renal collecting system or parenchyma can also appear echogenic but typically demonstrates "dirty" shadowing.
- Hydronephrosis and hydroureter. If hydronephrosis is present, try to visualize the proximal ureter, if possible. Also, consider that the hydronephrosis could be chronic—observe if the renal parenchyma is atrophied due to chronic renal failure.

IMAGING WITH INTRAVENOUS UROGRAM

Indications.   Although no longer a first-line imaging study for the detection of nephrolithiasis, in cases where CT is not available, too costly or nondiagnostic in the context of extremely high suspicion, an IVU may be of use. IVU has the added advantage of providing physiologic information on the functional status of the kidneys. As a secondary

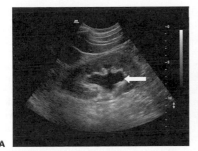
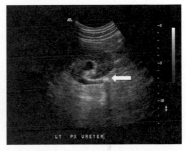

A   B

Figure 34-2. A: Ultrasonography of the kidney demonstrates moderate hydronephrosis (*arrow*), suspicious for obstruction. **B:** Examination of the proximal ureter shows an echogenic focus with shadowing (*arrow*), compatible with a calculus, responsible for the obstruction.

benefit, the diuretic effect of IV contrast may facilitate the passage of an obstructing ureteral stone, if one is present.

Protocol. IV contrast should be injected over 60–90 seconds and a film of the kidneys taken immediately. The diagnosis of ureteral obstruction can often be suspected from this first film. A series of timed films are then obtained. If obstruction is present, delayed films are often necessary to visualize the level of obstruction.

Possible Findings

■ Delayed appearance of nephrogram compared to the asymptomatic side. This finding may only be evident on the early films of the study.
■ Intensifying nephrogram over the hour following contrast injection. Normally, peak nephrogram opacity occurs a few minutes following contrast injection.
■ Delayed appearance of contrast and poor contrast concentration in the ipsilateral calyces and renal pelvis. Patients with renal colic are often aggressively hydrated, and this may contribute to the dilution of contrast in the collecting system (compare with the asymptomatic side).
■ Persistent column of contrast within the collecting system and ureter, ending at the level of the obstruction. This finding can be confirmed on a follow-up film after having the patient sit or stand up. Renal stones commonly lodge in one of three locations of relative narrowing: the UPJ, the lower ureter as it crosses over the pelvic brim, and the UVJ.
■ Filling defect(s) due to stone(s), not all of which may be causing acute obstruction. The classic differential diagnosis of filling defects in the urinary system should be kept in mind: blood clot, sloughed renal papilla, transitional cell carcinoma, and fungus ball.
■ Hydronephrosis and hydroureter may be mild or absent in the first 48 hours of obstruction. Mild collecting system dilatation may also be present following a recently passed stone, but a follow-up film (after the patient has been sitting upright) will demonstrate drainage of contrast, differentiating this case from true obstruction. If hydronephrosis is present, one should also consider if it represents chronic obstruction; this possibility can be evaluated by looking for thinning of the renal parenchyma due to chronic loss of renal function.
■ Calyceal rupture is a complication of acute obstruction caused by high intraluminal pressure. Extravasated contrast tracks along fascial planes paralleling the urinary tract, giving the IVU a "streaky" appearance.

 FUTURE DIRECTION IN IMAGING

Computed Tomography Advancements.   As the resolution of contemporary CT scanners increases and slices become incrementally thinner, the sensitivity and specificity of NCCT for nephrolithiasis will likely approach 100% as volume-averaging artifacts are gradually overcome. NCCT will likely remain the dominant modality for diagnosing nephrolithiasis for the foreseeable future.

Radiation Considerations.   The primary limitation of NCCT is the use of ionizing radiation, which is of particular concern in children, young adults, and pregnant women. The skin dose for NCCT is 3–5 rad, far more than the 0.25–0.30 rad of IVU and the 0 rad of ultrasonography. Accordingly, the first test given to a pregnant woman, child, or young adult should be an abdominopelvic ultrasonography which can be followed, when necessary, by a limited IVU. For example, a limited IVU might consist of a scout image followed by a coned anteroposterior (AP) view of the kidneys 2 minutes after injection, a full abdominal view at 10 minutes and a delayed image at 25 minutes. If NCCT cannot be avoided, some authors have suggested that tube currents as low as 100 mA can be used with little decrement in accuracy.

Magnetic Resonance Imaging.   Although magnetic resonance imaging (MRI) has the inherent advantage of not exposing the patient to ionizing radiation, it is currently slower, more costly, and less well characterized than CT for detecting stones. For the most part, the use of magnetic resonance (MR) in this application is limited to centers of research. Generally speaking, there are two techniques in development that use T1- and T2-weighted images, respectively. The T2-weighted techniques are more rapid but less sensitive whereas the T1-weighted techniques use gadolinium-based contrast agents to image the ureters and are more sensitive but require much longer acquisition times.

 TREATMENT AND POSTIMAGING ISSUES

Radiographic information regarding the size of the stone has an important influence on treatment, as more than 90% of stones less than 4 mm in diameter will pass spontaneously whereas those larger than 8 mm usually require intervention. The first-line treatment for nephrolithiasis is extracorporeal shock-wave lithotripsy (ESWL), which is approximately 90% successful at breaking stones into smaller fragments that can be passed sponta-neously. Stones greater than 24 mm in size and staghorn calculi often fail ESWL and necessitate other strategies. The radiologist is essential in this instance, as the location and shape of the stone often determine the mode of treatment. Open surgery is undertaken only as a last resort when less invasive strategies such as endoscopic interventions have failed.

If urinary obstruction is associated with symptoms and signs of urinary tract infection, percutaneous drainage may be necessary to prevent fulminant infection of a closed space (see Chap. 58, "Nephrostomy"). Percutaneous nephrostomy tracts are usually large enough to allow the passage of endoscopic equipment for stone removal.

Patients undergoing conservative management should have their urine sieved in order to detect the passage of stones and collect them for chemical analysis, which is necessary for proper medical treatment of nephrolithiasis. Most patients who form a single calcium stone will eventually develop more. On average, such patients form a stone every 2–3 years.

Further Readings
Asplin JR, Coe FL, Favus MJ. Nephrolithiasis. In: Kasper DL, Braunwald E, Fauci AS, et al. eds. *Harrison's principles of internal medicine*, 16th ed. New York: McGraw-Hill, 2005;1710–1713. (Newer editions exist).

Fowler KA, Locken JA, Duchesne JH, et al. US for detecting renal calculi with nonenhanced CT as a reference standard. *Radiology* 2002;222:109–113.

Heneghan JP, McGuire KA, Leder RA, et al. Helical CT for nephrolithiasis and ureterolithi-asis: comparison of conventional and reduced radiation-dose techniques. *Radiology* 2003;229:575–580.

Sheafor DH, Hertzberg BS, Freed KS, et al. Nonenhanced helical CT and US in the emergency evaluation of patients with renal colic: prospective comparison. *Radiology* 2000;217:792–797.

Springhart WP, Preminger GM. Advanced imaging in stone management. *Curr Opin Urol* 2004;14:95–98.

Tamm EP. Evaluation of the patient with flank pain and possible ureteral calculus. *Radiology* 2003;228:319–329.

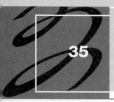

35   RENAL FAILURE
Brad P. Barnett and Satomi Kawamoto

CLINICAL INFORMATION

Radiologic evaluation in the setting of renal failure includes determining the number, size, position, and degree of perfusion of the kidneys, and whether urinary obstruction is present. Obstructive uropathy is a surgically correctable cause of acute renal failure (ARF). Imaging is also useful in detecting underlying vascular or embolic causes of renal failure.

The size of the kidneys and the thickness of the parenchyma should be noted.

- Normal adult kidney size is 9–12 cm in length.
- Normal parenchymal thickness is 2–2.5 cm.
- Enlarged kidneys with thick parenchyma are usually indicative of an acute disorder, whereas small kidneys with thin parenchyma are often present in chronic renal disease. Causes of ARF are classically placed in one of three categories
- **Prerenal etiologies** account for approximately 70% of all ARF cases and should be diagnosed by nonradiologic methods (↑ blood urea nitrogen [BUN] and creatinine with inherently normal renal function). Hypoperfusion secondary to volume depletion, sepsis, cardiac failure, liver failure, burns, bilateral renal artery stenosis, or pharmacologic agents (such as cyclooxygenase [COX] inhibitors or angiotensin-converting enzyme [ACE] inhibitors) are the most common causes of prerenal failure.
- **Renal etiologies** result from damage to the kidney parenchyma itself. Acute tubular necrosis is the most common type of intrinsic renal disease and is found in cases of prolonged hypotension, secondary to gram-negative sepsis, trauma, hemorrhage, or direct toxins (e.g., mercuric chloride). Other causes include large vessel disease (thrombosis, emboli, dissection), small vessel disease (vasculitis, thrombotic thrombocytopenic purpura [TTP], and disseminated intravascular coagulation [DIC]), interstitial nephritis (urate, myeloma, drugs), and cortical necrosis. Glomerulonephritis is a relatively uncommon intrinsic renal disease, which may occasionally cause ARF but more commonly presents in the context of chronic renal failure (CRF).
- **Postrenal failure** is secondary to obstruction of urine outflow from the kidneys. To cause renal failure, obstruction must be bilateral unless the contralateral kidney is absent or diseased. The most common sources of obstruction include stricture, prostatic hyperplasia, and bladder neck obstruction. Postrenal failure is a relatively uncommon cause of ARF, accounting for less than 5% of cases.

Causes of CRF are commonly classified according to underlying disease. The major causes of CRF in decreasing prevalence are diabetes mellitus, hypertension, and glomerulonephritis. Disease progression can be characterized by three stages: (1) diminished renal reserve, (2) renal insufficiency (azotemia), and (3) uremia.

IMAGING WITH RADIOGRAPHS

Indications. Radiographs of the abdomen are not typically helpful for evaluation of renal failure. However, incidental findings suggestive of ARF can be seen on abdominal films acquired for other reasons.

Protocol. Supine position. Include kidneys and area of ureters and bladder.

Possible Findings

- Abnormal renal size, shape, and position.
- Radiopaque calculi in kidneys, ureters, or bladder.
- Abnormal gas collections in urosepsis.
- Calcifications of vascular structures, lymph nodes, cysts, or tumors.
- Abnormal bones in renal osteodystrophy.

 IMAGING WITH ULTRASONOGRAPHY

Indications. Because of lack of ionizing radiation and low cost, ultrasonography (US) should be the first imaging modality employed in every new case of renal failure. US is considered the method of choice for differentiating the postrenal and renal causes of ARF after prerenal failure has been excluded clinically.

Protocol. Patients should be well hydrated and the bladder should be empty because a distended bladder can cause upper tract dilatation in a normal patient, giving a false impression of obstruction. Kidneys are imaged with at least a 3.5 MHz transducer (preferably, 5.0 MHz for children) Color Doppler is used to evaluate renal perfusion, renal vasculature, and ureteral bladder jets.

Possible Findings (Fig. 35-1)

- Abnormal number or position. Absent kidney: renal agenesis, previous nephrectomy. Ectopic kidney: pelvic, intrathoracic (rare), crossed fused.
- Abnormal renal size. Normal adult kidney size is 9–12 cm in length. Normal or large-sized kidneys generally indicate ARF and small kidneys generally indicate CRF. (Exception: adult or infantile polycystic kidney disease and bilateral hydronephrosis.)

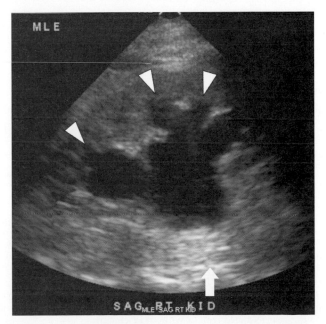

Figure 35-1. Sagittal ultrasonographic (US) image of the right kidney demonstrates dilatation of the renal pelvis (*arrow*) and renal calyces (*arrowheads*) in a patient who presented with renal failure. Subsequent evaluation demonstrated cervical cancer that caused ureteral obstruction.

- Dilatation of upper urinary tract (calyces, renal pelvis, ureters)/hydronephrosis, indicating obstructive uropathy. The false positive rate is 8–26%.
- False positives (i.e., nonobstructive dilatation of the pelvocalyceal system) include the following
  - Reflux nephropathy.
  - Congenital megacalyces.
  - Congenital megaloureters and prune belly syndrome.
  - Parapelvic cysts, calyceal cysts, and polycystic kidney disease may also lead to confusion.
- False negatives can occur in four circumstances, as follows:
  - Acute or early obstruction, when dilatation of the collecting system may be minimal to absent.
  - Staghorn calculi, which may obscure visualization of pelvocalyceal dilatation due to dense echoes and acoustic shadowing.
  - ARF superimposed on chronic obstruction, where urine output is so low that pelvocalyceal or ureteral dilatation cannot occur.
  - Encasement of the pelvocalyceal system or ureter by a retroperitoneal mass or fibrosis so that these structures are not distensible even in the presence of obstruction.
- Increased cortical echogenicity ($\geq$ adjacent liver) is seen in renal parenchymal disease. However, the false positive rate is 72% and the false negative is 63%.
- Decreased cortical echogenicity can be seen in lymphoma, acute pyelonephritis, and acute or subacute renal vein thrombosis.
- Increased medullary echogenicity can be seen in gouty nephropathy, medullary nephrocalcinosis, renal tubular acidosis, and medullary sponge kidney.
- Abnormal Doppler waveform in the main renal artery or vein
  - In renal artery stenosis: (1) peak systolic velocity greater than 180 cm/second and (2) ratio of renal artery peak systolic velocity to aortic peak systolic velocity greater than 3.5 for greater than 60% stenosis (sensitivity 84–98%, specificity 90–98%).
  - In renal vein thrombosis: absence of a venous waveform, or complete or partial filling defect in the renal vein.
- Renal calculi, which appear as echogenic foci with acoustic shadowing.
- Incidental mass.

IMAGING WITH COMPUTED TOMOGRAPHY

Indications. Computed tomography (CT) should be employed if US is inconclusive. CT is particularly useful in localizing small or ectopic kidneys, in detecting obstructions and their causes, in evaluating retroperitoneal pathology, and detecting nephrocalcinosis and urolithiasis.

Protocol. Noncontrast CT is required to evaluate nephrocalcinosis or urolithiasis. Intravenous (IV) contrast is not required in most cases and may be contraindicated in severe renal failure (especially diabetic nephropathy and multiple myeloma–associated nephropathy).

For patients with borderline renal function in which contrast is necessary, N-acetylcysteine (NAC) may be given orally on the day before and on the day of contrast administration unless acute etiologies are suspected and the administration of NAC would delay therapeutic intervention.

Possible Findings (Fig. 35-2)

- Kidney size, position, and configuration, and degree of cortical atrophy can be evaluated.
- Obstruction can be confirmed or excluded in many cases and the level of ureteral obstruction can be determined with or without IV contrast.
- Small or "nonopaque" calculi can be detected. Indinavir (Crixivan) may appear lucent on CT scans. Very rare pure matrix stones of mucoprotein and fibrin may be undetectable on CT.

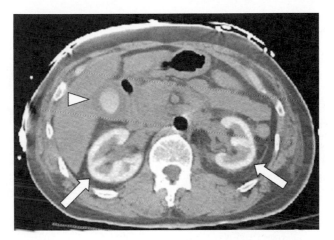

Figure 35-2. Contract-induced acute tubular necrosis. Noncontrast computed tomography (CT) scan obtained in a patient with acute renal failure after cardiac catheterization shows persistent bilateral renal nephrograms (*arrows*) and vicarious contrast excretion into the gallbladder (*arrowhead*). No contrast is seen elsewhere.

- Delayed nephrogram if IV contrast was given.
- Renal vein thrombosis sensitivity is approximately 100% with dynamic CT.
- Renal arterial stenosis or dissection requires IV contrast and may require multiplanar or 3D reconstruction. Differential perfusion of the kidneys is an indirect finding.
- Wedge-shaped perfusion defects compatible with embolic disease.

 IMAGING WITH NUCLEAR MEDICINE

Indications. Radionucleotide scanning provides a good means of assessing global function and renal reserve, and is helpful in differentiating reversible causes of renal failure such as acute tubular necrosis from other conditions with a poorer prognosis like cortical necrosis. Unfortunately, the accuracy of nuclear medicine in determining global renal function decreases as renal function deteriorates due to predominance of background activity.

Protocol. ^{99m}Technetium (^{99m}Tc)-diethylene triamine pentaacetic acid (DTPA) (glomerular filtration) and ^{99m}Tc-mercaptoacetyltriglycine (MAG3) (tubular secretion) are the two most commonly employed agents. Typical study includes the following:

- Bolus injection.
- Flow imaging with 1 second/frame for 60 seconds.
- Delayed imaging with 1 minute/frame for 30 minutes.
- If persistent collecting system activity is present at 30 minutes, diuretic scan should be performed by administering furosemide (Lasix) 0.5 mg/kg IV. Perform additional imaging with 1 minute/frame for 30 minutes.
- ACE inhibitor scan requires a baseline study for comparison, which is typically performed with low dose of ^{99m}Tc-DTPA. Following 4–6 hours to allow for tracer washout, another renal scan is performed 1 hour after oral administration of captopril, 50 mg. Before the test, withhold diuretics for 48 hours and ACE inhibitors for at least 1 week.

Possible Findings

Normal
- Renal activity should be seen within 6 seconds after aortic peak in normal kidneys.

■ Peak cortical activity should occur at 3–5 minutes.
■ Collecting system activity should appear at 5 minutes.

Obstruction

■ More than 20 minutes renal parenchymal clearance. Tracer accumulation in dilated nonobstructed collecting system may create a false positive requiring diuretic administration.
■ Lack of response to Lasix within 15 minutes with persistent parenchymal and or collecting system activity. Lasix may not work in patients with severe renal failure resulting in a false-positive study.
■ Nonvisualization of ureter in severe obstruction.

Renovascular Hypertension

■ Unilateral renal artery stenosis results in the following:
  • Decreased flow.
  • Prolonged cortical transit time.
  • Prolonged washout.
  • Bilateral renal artery stenosis is a common cause of false negative study.

 ## IMAGING WITH MAGNETIC RESONANCE

Indication.   Magnetic resonance imaging (MRI) is a useful alternative to CT in patients in whom the use of iodinated contrast material is contraindicated. The indications and findings are similar to those of CT, although magnetic resonance angiography (MRA) to assess for renal artery stenosis is the most common indication. Further, diffusion-weighted (DW) MRI may provide information as to degree of kidney dysfunction, and may assist in the differentiation of various renal abnormalities.

Protocol.   A renal MRI study should include a T1- and T2-weighted image in at least one plane. Fast gradient echo images allow for acquisition of images in time-efficient manner. Gd can be delivered as a bolus with dynamic image acquisition. This approach permits evaluation of the enhancement properties of a focal renal lesion or estimation of the degree of functional impairment associated with hydronephrosis or parenchymal abnormalities.

 ## NOTE OF CAUTION

Nephrogenic systemic fibrosis/nephrogenic fibrosing dermopathy (NSF/NFD) is a newly described complication of Gd in patients with renal failure.

NSF/NFD is seen in patients who have noticeably advanced renal failure. The disease causes fibrosis of the skin and connective tissues throughout the body. Patients develop skin thickening that may prevent bending and extending joints, resulting in decreased mobility of joints. In addition, patients may experience fibrosis that has spread to other parts of the body such as the diaphragm, muscles in the thigh and lower abdomen, and the interior areas of lung vessels. The clinical course of NSF/NFD is progressive and may be fatal.

Before Gd is administered to patients with renal failure, your department's policy regarding NSF/NFD should be consulted.

 ## ANGIOGRAPHY

Indication.   Renovascular disease is an important cause of CRF. Approximately 10% of dialysis patients have renovascular disease as their primary diagnosis. Correction of renovascular disease by angioplasty or other means can significantly improve renal function.

Over recent years, contrast-enhanced MRA and CT angiography have rapidly developed into an acceptable alternative to traditional angiography. Conventional angiography is typically performed if other imaging is inconclusive, or if a stenosis has been detected in a viable kidney and therapeutic angioplasty/stenting is requested.

 IMAGE-GUIDED RENAL BIOPSY

Indication.   To provide definitive diagnosis in renal parenchymal disease and in patients with unexplained ARF image guided renal biopsy is indicated. Small kidneys with parenchymal thickness of 1 cm or less are not usually biopsied due to nonspecific histologic findings and increased associated complication rate.

Protocol.   Real-time US guidance is most commonly employed, although CT may also be used. The patient is instructed to hold breath on inspiration for each needle advance. Core biopsy specimens are usually taken from the lower pole of the kidney just deep to the capsule, thereby obtaining cortex and not medulla.

Further Readings

Davidson AJ, Hartman DS. *Radiology of the kidney and urinary tract*, 3rd ed. Philadelphia: WB Saunders, 1999.

Grainger RG, Allison DJ. *Diagnostic radiology*, 4th ed. New York: Churchill Livingstone, 2001·1671–1679.

Hagen-Ansert SL. *Textbook of diagnostic ultrasonography*, 5th ed. St. Louis: Mosby, 2001:274–289.

Ota H, Takase K, Rikimaru H, et al. Quantitative vascular measurements in arterial occlusive disease. *Radiographics* 2005;25:1141–1158.

Kawashima A, Sandler CM, Ernst RD, et al. CT evaluation of renovascular disease. *Radiographics* 2000;20(5):1321–1340.

Kawashima A, Vrtiska TJ, LeRoy AJ, et al. CT Urography. *Radiographics* 2004;24(Suppl 1): S35–S54.

Kim SH. *Uroradiology illustrated*. Philadelphia: WB Saunders, 2003.

Liu R, Deepu N, Joachim I, et al. N-Acetlycysteine for the prevention of contrast-induced nephropathy. *J Gen Intern Med* 2005;20:193–200.

Resnick MI, Rifkin MD. *Ultrasonography of the urinary tract*, 3rd ed. St. Louis: Mosby, Elsevier Science, 2004.

Rumack CM, Wilson SR, Charboneau JW. *Diagnostic ultrasound*, 3rd ed. St. Louis: Mosby, Elesevier Science, 2005.

Sandler CM, Newhouse JH, Amis ES, et al. *Textbook of uroradiology*, 3rd ed. Williams & Wilkins: Baltimore, 2001.

Williamson MR, Smith A. *Fundamentals of uroradiology*. Philadelphia: WB Saunders, 1999.

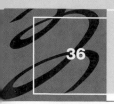

36

RENAL TRANSPLANTATION
Benjamin Tubb

PREOPERATIVE EVALUATION OF RENAL DONORS

Imaging of renovascular and ureteral anatomy in prospective renal donors is valuable for surgical planning, especially as living donor nephrectomies are increasingly performed laparoscopically. Traditional catheter angiography has largely been replaced by computed tomographic (CT) angiography and magnetic resonance (MR) angiography for preoperative donor evaluation. Radiologists must assess for variant anatomy such as accessory renal arteries, prehilar renal artery branching, and renal venous variants such as retroaortic or circumaortic left renal vein and large connections to lumbar veins which might necessitate open surgical approach rather than laparoscopic. Cross-sectional imaging allows identification of duplicated collecting systems and parenchymal abnormalities (masses, calculi, abnormally located kidney, or cysts suggesting possible polycystic kidney disease) that might alter or preclude graft harvesting. CT and MR can both be used for evaluation of prospective donors, although MR is less sensitive for small calculi.

SURGICAL TECHNIQUE

Transplant kidneys are usually placed in extraperitoneal location within the iliac fossa, with end-to-side vascular anastomosis to the external iliac vessels. The common method of urinary drainage is ureteroneocystostomy, with transplant ureter implanted into the wall of the bladder. Variations include intraperitoneal graft placement, anastomosis to internal iliac artery, and connection of transplant collecting system to the recipient ureter or interposed bowel segment. Operative notes should be reviewed to clarify transplant anatomy.

COMMON POSTOPERATIVE FINDINGS

Doppler ultrasound examinations of renal allografts are routinely performed in the immediate postoperative period to evaluate blood flow in the transplant organs and to exclude early complications. Mild hydronephrosis is often seen, possibly due to denervation of the collecting system during transplantation and edema at the ureteral anastomosis. Small perinephric fluid collections are often present after surgery, usually representing postoperative seromas or small hematomas. Doppler examination of intrarenal vessels should demonstrate antegrade diastolic flow with low resistance waveform, with resistive index (RI) less than 0.70. However, cadaveric allografts can have transient edema related to ischemia (some degree of ischemia is inevitable during transport), which can cause high resistance flow in intrarenal arteries during the immediate postoperative period.

RENAL TRANSPLANT COMPLICATIONS

Acute tubular necrosis (ATN) occurs postoperatively in 30–50% of cadaveric transplants due to ischemia during transport and transplantation. Most will return to normal function in 2 weeks. ATN is rare in living donor transplants. Recovery usually occurs, often heralded by slow rise in urine output followed by large diuresis. ATN causes elevated creatinine and oliguria. These are very nonspecific findings, and imaging studies are often performed to exclude other causes of decreased transplant function.

Perinephric collections can cause compression of transplant vasculature or ureter and may present with fever, tenderness, worsening renal function, oliguria, or hypertension. Causes include the following:

- **Seroma.** Virtually a normal postoperative finding, often appearing as crescentic collection of simple fluid along border of the transplanted kidney. Only problematic if compressing adjacent structures or enlarging.
- **Hematoma.** May indicate bleeding from vascular anastomoses. Usually occurs in first few days postoperatively. Small hematomata usually resolve spontaneously. May also occur after biopsy of transplanted kidney.
- **Abscess.** Increased risk due to immunosuppression. Usually seen a few days after surgery. Any form of perinephric collection can become infected and lead to abscess formation, necessitating drainage.
- **Urinoma.** Due to leakage at ureteral anastomosis, collecting system rupture from obstruction, or rarely calyceal leakage from segmental infarction in transplant organ (e.g., accessory renal artery was not identified or anastomosed). Usually occurs within days to weeks after surgery. Often located between transplant and bladder; can occur in unusual locations such as scrotum/labia or thigh. May rapidly increase in size. Aspirated fluid demonstrates higher creatinine than other collections. Treated with nephrostomy tube placement, ureteral stenting, and/or surgical repair.
- **Lymphocele.** Secondary to disruption of native lymphatic channels in the operative bed or leakage from lymphatics of the allograft. Lymphoceles usually present 4–12 weeks after surgery but can occur years later. They usually occur medial to transplant around iliac vessels and may appear septated. These are the most common collection to cause transplant hydronephrosis; can even cause leg swelling from pressure on iliac vein. They commonly recur after drainage and may require sclerotherapy or marsupialization.

Urinary obstruction occurs in 2% of transplantations, usually within the first 6 months postoperatively. Obstruction may not be evident until nephroureteral stent is removed. The most common cause is stenosis of distal ureter at site of implantation in bladder, related to ischemia or rejection. Other causes include obstructing material such as calculi, blood clots, fungus balls, or papillary necrosis. Extrinsic compression of ureter by perinephric collections can also cause hydronephrosis. Importantly, the transplanted kidney is denervated, so patients will not experience colicky pain due to obstruction. The only indication of obstruction may be elevated serum creatinine and/or oliguria. Diagnosis of urinary obstruction can be complicated in transplanted kidneys. Incompetence of the ureteral anastomosis to the bladder may cause mild to moderate collecting system dilatation when the patient's bladder is full. It is important to reevaluate after bladder is empty. Denervation of the transplant collecting system decreases its tone, so mild dilatation may be a stable postoperative finding. Moreover, prior episodes of obstruction may yield persistently dilated collecting system, despite resolution of the obstruction. Alternatively, fibrosis related to rejection may prevent hydronephrosis in some cases of obstruction. For these reasons, assays such as Whitaker test (invasive test with direct measurement of pressure gradient from renal pelvis to bladder during fluid instillation in renal pelvis) or functional assays such as nuclear medicine examinations are used to diagnose true urinary obstruction with consequent delayed renal function.

Vascular complications occur in approximately 2% of transplant recipients. These include renal artery stenosis or thrombosis, renal infarction, renal vein thrombosis, and postbiopsy complications such as arteriovenous (AV) fistula or pseudoaneurysm formation.

- Renal artery stenosis usually manifests in the first year and occurs most commonly at anastomosis (related to surgical technique or fibrosis), but can occur distally in transplant renal artery (due to rejection occurring in vessel wall, extrinsic compression by perinephric collections, or mechanical kinking or twisting of vessels related to transplant position) or proximal to the anastomosis (native vessel atherosclerotic disease). Renal artery stenosis may present with severe/persistent hypertension, refractory to medical therapy, and decreased renal function.

- Renal artery thrombosis may be due to hyperacute rejection (usually evident at surgery), occlusion or kinking at anastomosis, or renal artery dissection. Acute transplant infarction can present with anuria and swelling and tenderness over the kidney. Despite denervation of the transplant, any cause of inflammation in the transplanted kidney can irritate adjacent structures in the pelvis and cause pain.
- Vasculitis usually affects smaller renal vessels and leads to small segmental infarcts.
- Renal vein thrombosis is a rare postoperative complication and a surgical emergency requiring immediate intervention (venous collaterals are absent in transplant organ). This usually occurs in the first week postoperatively and classically presents with abruptly decreased renal function and swelling and tenderness over the graft.
- AV fistula or pseudoaneurysm formation affecting small vessels in the renal parenchyma are occasional complications of renal biopsy; these are usually managed conservatively when they are small. Gross hematuria occurs in 5–7% of patients following biopsy and usually resolves spontaneously.

Infections occur in 80% of transplant recipients during the first year after surgery. In the first several weeks, these infections are similar to those of other surgical procedures: pneumonia, wound infection, urinary tract infection, and infected perinephric fluid collections leading to abscess formation. Pyelonephritis can mimic acute rejection. Opportunistic infections related to immunosuppression characteristically occur 1–6 months postoperatively.

Immune Rejection

- **Hyperacute**. Due to preformed antibodies. Blue boggy kidney may be seen intraoperatively immediately after anastomosis is performed.
- **Accelerated acute**. Seen in recipients of living related donor kidneys who have received prior blood transfusion from donor. Decreased function occurs within 5 days postoperatively.
- **Acute**. Due to cell-mediated and/or humoral attack on foreign antigens. Seen from 1 week to several months after transplantation, presenting with oliguria, weight gain, hypertension, and elevated creatinine. May present with enlargement and tenderness of the graft related to infiltration by immune cells, and patient may be febrile with elevated erythrocyte sedimentation rate (ESR). This is a progressive inflammatory process that can be treated with high-dose steroid therapy. There has been a decreased incidence of acute rejection during the last 2 decades with new medication regimens.
- **Chronic**. Due to humoral and cellular factors causing characteristic vascular changes in the graft, as seen on biopsy. Gradual decreased renal function with proteinuria and hypertension. Kidney demonstrates vascular changes, fibrosis, tubular atrophy, and glomerulosclerosis. No effective therapy at present. Chronic rejection now represents the leading cause of transplantation failure.

Calcineurin inhibitor toxicity occurs after 1 month after transplantation. Calcineurin inhibitors are a class of commonly used immunosuppressive medications including cyclosporine and tacrolimus. Patients are usually asymptomatic with rising creatinine. Blood levels of the medication should be drawn, and if levels are high the drug is decreased or withheld and creatinine is followed. If creatinine drops, it is assumed that drug toxicity was the reason for the renal failure. Classically this occurred with high levels of cyclosporine; less frequent with new medication regimens.

IMAGING WITH ULTRASONOGRAPHY

Indications.   Emergently in postoperative period to assess transplant vasculature and exclude significant perinephric fluid collections if kidney is anuric or severely oliguric. Other indications include oliguria, hypertension, or rising creatinine at any point, to assess kidney for rejection or surgical complication, and in case of sepsis to evaluate for perinephric abscess.

Protocol.   Transverse and longitudinal images of transplanted kidney, attempting to follow ureter as far as possible, including images of bladder and attempt to identify ureteral anastomosis. Color Doppler to assess vasculature, including waveforms and quantitative measures of main renal artery systolic and diastolic velocities (avoid applying excess pressure from transducer during these measurements). Importantly, bladder should be fully drained at start of examination, as noted earlier in discussion of urinary obstruction.

Possible Findings (Figs. 36-1 through 36-3)

- Hydronephrosis may indicate obstruction at the ureteral anastomosis from edema (early postoperatively this is usually temporary), stricture (occurs later), blood clot, calculus, or extrinsic compression by perinephric fluid collection. Remember that pelvicalyceal system of renal transplant normally appears prominent because it is closer to the transducer than the native kidney. It is important to confirm that the bladder is empty when evaluating hydronephrosis, because the ureteral anastomosis is frequently incompetent.
- Perinephric fluid collections include abscess, lymphocele, hematoma, and urinoma, all of which appear as anechoic or hypoechoic collections, possibly compressing the ureter and causing obstruction. Abscesses and hematomas may have septations and debris. Small seromas are common postoperatively. It is important to consider whether perinephric fluid collections appear to be distended and under pressure, as these are the collections which may cause ureteral obstruction.
- Enlarged kidney. It is helpful to have a baseline study to assess for change. This is a nonspecific finding which can be prominent in acute rejection but can also be seen in cases of ATN and renal vein thrombosis.
- Elevated RI in intrarenal arteries, RI is defined as $(S - D)/S$, where S is systolic Doppler frequency shift and D is diastolic shift. Normal RI value in intrarenal arteries is approximately 0.7. Cases of acute rejection often demonstrate progressive increase in RI of intrarenal arteries. However this is a nonspecific finding, and ATN (common in immediate postoperative period) can cause a transient increase in intrarenal resistive indices. Other causes of elevated RI include drug toxicity, renal vein thrombosis, and increased pressure on the transplant kidney from any source, including subcapsular or perinephric collections or artifact from excessive pressure on transducer during examination.
- Vascular problems. Pseudoaneurysm may look like a simple or complex renal cyst on grayscale images; color Doppler allows visualization of turbulent flow. If the pseudoaneurysm is enlarging, larger than 2 cm, or extrarenal (risk of rupture), surgical

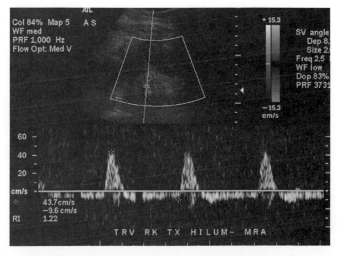

Figure 36-1. Renal vein occlusion in a patient after liver transplantation. Doppler ultrasonography (US) demonstrates reversal of diastolic flow in main renal artery at the hilum.

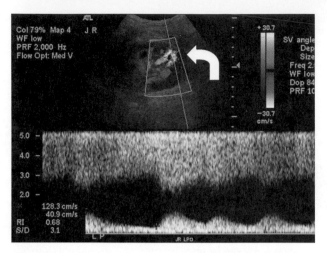

Figure 36-2. Arteriovenous fistula (*arrow*) in transplanted kidney following a biopsy. Doppler ultrasonography (US) demonstrates markedly abnormal waveform with increased diastolic flow.

treatment is necessary. AV fistula causes arterial-type pulsations in an enlarged draining vein. Renal artery stenosis may cause a high velocity jet through the stenotic area with distal turbulence. Importantly, intrarenal arterial waveforms may show a slow or blunted systolic upstroke (tardus et parvus waveform) distal to the stenosis, and often this is the only evidence of a stenosis proximally in the main renal artery (which may not be well visualized itself). If the entire main renal artery is visualized and no areas of stenosis are seen, arteriography is not needed. If there is suspicion for stenosis but the main renal artery is not well visualized, then arteriography may be indicated. Renal vein thrombosis is a rare but important condition characterized by absence of venous flow in the kidney with high-resistance arterial flow, classically demonstrating reversal of diastolic flow

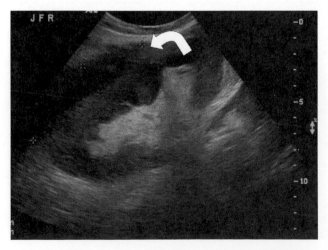

Figure 36-3. Subcapsular hematoma (*arrow*) on ultrasonography (US) deforming the transplanted kidney.

(to-and-fro flow in renal arteries). Renal vein thrombosis is an urgent finding and should be communicated to referring clinicians immediately. Renal artery thrombosis results in absence of arterial and venous flow in the kidney during the early postoperative period.

IMAGING WITH COMPUTED TOMOGRAPHY AND MAGNETIC RESONANCE

Indications. CT and magnetic resonance imaging (MRI) are increasingly used in evaluation of renal transplant complications, providing comprehensive anatomic information and—when contrast agents are administered—angiographic and limited functional evaluation. Ultrasonography remains the initial examination in most cases but may be limited in obese patients and provides limited characterization of perinephric collections and masses. CT and MR angiography have largely replaced catheter angiography in the detailed evaluation of transplant vasculature when ultrasonographic examination is technically limited.

Contrast Agent Considerations. Unenhanced CT and MRI examinations pose minimal risk and can serve to characterize size/distribution of perinephric collections. However, in order to characterize the transplant vasculature and function, intravascular contrast agents are required. Iodinated CT contrast agents increase risk of contrast-induced nephropathy and are generally avoided in patients with decreased transplant function. When administered to patients with good transplant function, low osmolality CT contrast agents should be used at the lowest dose possible and accompanied by efforts to keep the patient well hydrated. Diabetic patients should stop taking metformin before and following examination until renal function is reevaluated. The decision regarding administration of iodinated CT contrast should be made together with referring clinicians. Gadolinium-containing MR contrast agents pose lower risk of contrast-induced nephropathy but should also be used at lowest reasonable dose.

Protocol. CT examination protocols for transplant kidneys are similar to renal protocol examinations of native kidneys. Unenhanced images are obtained, followed by contrast administration (if necessary) with imaging in early arterial phase (for angiographic evaluation), venous or corticomedullary phase (for renal parenchymal evaluation), and delayed excretory or pyelographic phase (for collecting system evaluation). MR examination protocols include fat-suppressed T2-weighted images and T1-weighted pre- and postcontrast images obtained in multiple phases as mentioned earlier, including early arterial phase acquisition suitable for MR angiography. Note that similar to ultrasonographic examinations, CT and MR examinations should be performed with the bladder emptied immediately before study and Foley or suprapubic catheter then clamped to allow visualization of contrast accumulation in the bladder during the examination (and unclamped following examination).

Possible Findings

These are similar to ultrasonographic findings listed earlier. CT and MRI provide accurate characterization of hydronephrosis and the size and extent of perinephric fluid collections and may demonstrate inflammatory changes suggesting infection. Contrast-enhanced examinations allow evaluation of the timing and uniformity of cortical and corticomedullary enhancement in the transplant kidney. Delayed images show contrast progress through the transplant collecting system to the bladder and potential leaks. CT and MR angiography directly evaluate the transplant vasculature and related complications as listed earlier. Importantly, CT and MRI provide additional information about the patient's native kidneys, which can be complicated by hydronephrosis, infection, or malignancy.

IMAGING WITH NUCLEAR MEDICINE

Indications. Nuclear medicine provides a functional, rather than anatomic, evaluation of the renal transplant. Renal scintigraphy was previously used to follow allograft function over time and might help to differentiate ATN from acute rejection. Now scintigraphy is more often performed with diuretic administration to distinguish obstructive hydronephrosis from nonobstructive dilatation of the renal collecting system related to denervation/reflux.

Protocol. Radiotracer is usually ^{99m}Technetium (^{99m}Tc)mercaptoacetyltriglycine (MAG3) rather than ^{99m}Tc diethylenetriamine pentaacetate (DTPA), as MAG3 is cleared by tubular secretion and has high extraction efficiency even in kidneys with poor function. The camera is positioned anteriorly over the pelvis including visualization of urinary bladder. Initial flow images are obtained to evaluate allograft perfusion, followed by functional images over 30 minutes or more. If evaluating for obstruction, a diuretic such as furosemide is given intravenously, dosed according to patient size and creatinine level, and further dynamic images are obtained. When the urine collection bag is present during the immediate postoperative period, include bag in images to evaluate excretion because the collecting system itself may not be well visualized when nephroureteral stent and Foley catheter are present. The bag should be emptied before study. Alternatively, the bladder can be drained at start of examination and the Foley catheter temporarily clamped during examination to allow visualization of radiotracer accumulation in bladder.

Possible Findings

- Reduced renal blood flow. Activity within allograft is usually visualized within 3–6 seconds of peak activity in adjacent iliac artery. The peak activity in allograft kidney should match or exceed the iliac artery. If these conditions are not met, there is reduced renal blood flow. This may be appreciated in the initial dynamic flow images, or it may be better appreciated as decreased slope of radiotracer uptake in first minutes of the time–activity curve obtained from the functional images. Reduced perfusion is most prominently seen in acute rejection and less frequently in cases of drug toxicity. Conversely, perfusion is usually near normal or minimally reduced in ATN. Note that acute rejection and ATN are also differentiated by their usual time courses, with ATN occurring in immediate postoperative period and then resolving, whereas acute rejection usually begins from 1 week to months postoperatively and progressively worsens without treatment. Also note that reduced perfusion is nonspecific; other possible causes include infection and vascular complications such as renal vein thrombosis.
- Poor initial parenchymal uptake with progressive parenchymal accumulation. After 2–3 minutes, renal activity should appear at least two to three times more intense than liver or spleen, and renal activity should peak at 3–4 minutes after injection. When radiotracer used is DTPA (excreted through glomerular filtration), cases of ATN typically show early (<3 minutes) peak activity with rapid washout of tracer, reflecting vascular delivery and washout of tracer without functional uptake. Cases of acute rejection typically show poor initial perfusion and then progressive accumulation of DTPA in the renal parenchyma. When radiotracer used is MAG3 (cleared by tubular secretion with high extraction efficiency), both ATN and acute rejection typically show progressive accumulation of radiotracer in renal parenchyma. Differentiation is based on initial flow images and time course postoperatively (as described in preceding paragraph). Note that considerable overlap exists between the appearance of ATN, acute rejection, and drug toxicity; baseline scan at 24–48 hours postoperatively and sequential examinations are helpful in distinguishing these causes of decreased allograft function.
- Delayed or poor visualization of collecting system. Activity in collecting system should be visualized by approximately 4 minutes. Delay is typical in ATN, rejection, and drug toxicity. Delayed collecting system activity may also be seen in severe obstruction.
- Progressive accumulation of radiotracer in collecting system is seen with obstruction (true anatomic obstruction) or hydronephrosis due to denervation/reflux (sometimes called *functional obstruction*). After diuretic administration, activity should gradually clear from renal collecting system to bladder in cases of hydronephrosis due to denervation/reflux, versus absent or poor clearance in cases of true anatomic obstruction.
- Extrarenal activity. If radiotracer activity is seen outside the normal confines of the collecting system, suspect a leak. To confirm this, assess whether moving the patient

causes the collection to move, obtain oblique or lateral views, obtain delayed views to see if collection intensifies, or have the patient void to assess if activity is from the bladder.

Further Readings

Akbar SA, Jafri SZ, Amendola MA, et al. Complications of renal transplantation. *Radiographics* 2005;25(5):1335–1356.

Alonso-Torres A, Fernandez-Cuadrado J, Pinilla I, et al. Multidetector CT in the evaluation of potential living donors for liver transplantation. *Radiographics* 2005;25(4):1017–1030.

Friedewald SM, Molmenti EP, Friedewald JJ, et al. Vascular and nonvascular complications of renal transplants: sonographic evaluation and correlation with other imaging modalities, surgery, and pathology. *J Clin Ultrasound* 2005;33(3):127–139.

Hohenwalter MD, Skowlund CJ, Erickson SJ, et al. Renal transplant evaluation with MR angiography and MR imaging. *Radiographics* 2001;21(6):1505–1517.

Sebastia C, Quiroga S, Boye R, et al. Helical CT in renal transplantation: normal findings and early and late complications. *Radiographics* 2001;21(5):1103–1117.

Ziessman HA, O'Malley JP, Thrall JH. *Nuclear medicine: the requisites.* Philadelphia: Mosby, Elsevier Science, 2006.

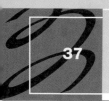

RETROPERITONEAL HEMORRHAGE

37

Mandeep Dagli

*R*etroperitoneal hemorrhage is most commonly seen following blunt or penetrating trauma (often in association with pelvic fracture), but it can also occur with anticoagulation medication, ruptured abdominal aortic aneurysm, renal tumors, or bleeding diathesis. Rarely, it may be spontaneous. It is associated with a high mortality rate when due to trauma.

 CLINICAL INFORMATION

Anatomy of the Retroperitoneum

An understanding of basic retroperitoneal anatomy is essential to both the interpretation of imaging findings and management of retroperitoneal hemorrhage. The retroperitoneum consists of three main compartments: the anterior pararenal space, the perirenal space (PRS), and the posterior pararenal space which are defined by three fascial planes: the anterior renal fascia, the posterior renal fascia, and the lateroconal fascia, respectively.

In general, hemorrhage will be confined to the compartment of origin, thereby limiting the differential diagnosis (Fig. 37-1).

- **Anterior pararenal space:** ascending and descending colon, pancreas, second and third portions of the duodenum.
- **Perirenal space (PRS):** kidney, adrenal gland, proximal ureter, renal vessels and lymphatics.
- **Posterior pararenal space:** mainly fat.

In cases of substantial hemorrhage, blood can spread between compartments through perinephric bridging septa. Superiorly, the PRS is open to the bare area of the liver. Inferiorly, the PRSs communicate at the level of lower lumbar spine. The blood can also extend across the midline through thin communication that is present anterior to aorta and inferior vena cava (IVC) at the level of lower lumbar spine.

Symptoms and Signs

History of trauma (especially pelvic fracture), back/flank pain, falling hematocrit, hypotension (the retroperitoneum can hold up to 4 L of blood), hematuria, Grey-Turner sign (bluish discoloration of flanks).

Etiology

- Iatrogenic anticoagulation, catheterization, recent percutaneous abdominal intervention.
- Arterial: aneurysms.
- Neoplasm: renal cell carcinoma, renal adrenal myelolipoma (AML), adrenal carcinoma, and AML
- Trauma: penetrating and blunt trauma which can result in organ, bony, or vascular injury. Life-threatening hemorrhage in pelvic fractures may be secondary to fractured bone, venous plexus, major pelvic veins, or iliac arterial branches.
- Inflammation: pancreatitis or infection leading to vascular injury.

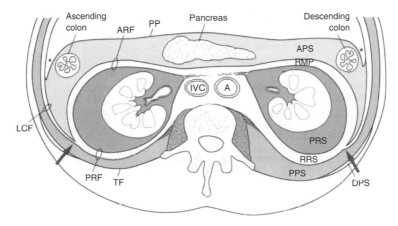

Figure 37-1. Retroperitoneal and interfascial planes. Drawing at level of renal hila shows that renal and lateroconal fasciae are laminated planes composed of apposed layers of embryonic mesentery. Thickness of interfascial planes is exaggerated to illustrate their potentially expansile nature. Note that perirenal spaces (PRSs) are closed medially. Retromesenteric space is continuous across midline. Retromesenterio anterior interfascial space (RMP), retrorenal posterior interfascial space (RRS), and lateroconal fascia communicate at fascial trifurcation (*arrows*). ARF, anterior renal fascia; PP, parietal peritoneum; APS, anterior pararenal space; *asterisk*, posterior peritoneal recess; IVC, inferior vena cava; A, aorta; LCF, lateroconal fascia; PRF, posterior renal fascia; TF, transversalis fascia; PPS, posterior pararenal space; DPS, dorsal pleural sinus. (Adapted from Ishikawa K, Tohira H, Mizushima Y, et al. Traumatic retroperitoneal hematoma spreads through the interfascial planes. *J Trauma* 2005;59:595–608.)

 IMAGING WITH RADIOGRAPHS

Indications. Not sensitive for diagnosis of retroperitoneal hematoma, although may be obtained for other reasons.

Possible Findings

- Pelvic fractures are commonly associated with hemorrhage.
- Diffuse enlargement or bulging psoas shadow if hematoma involves the psoas.
- Obliteration of the upper psoas shadow or an abnormal renal outline if perirenal hematoma is present.

 IMAGING WITH COMPUTED TOMOGRAPHY

Indications. Computed tomography (CT) is the modality of choice for evaluating retroperitoneal hemorrhage in both traumatic and nontraumatic situations. In trauma, CT provides rapid and comprehensive evaluation of injury extent. Generally, a CT is not obtained when patients are unstable.

Protocol. Retroperitoneal hematoma can be readily detected on noncontrast CT; however, intravenous (IV) contrast may be helpful for identification of potential causes. Following trauma, IV contrast is essential to detect active contrast extravasation as well as solid organ injury.

Possible Findings (Fig. 37-2 and 37-3)

- Acute blood is represented by high-density fluid (60–80 HU), which is denser than muscle (Fig. 37-1).

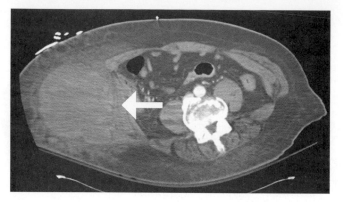

Figure 37-2. Right flank hematoma (*arrow*) on contrast-enhanced computed tomography (CT) scan.

- Chronic bleeding is usually of lower density (20–40 HU), ranging from simple to complex fluid, usually less dense than muscle.
- Active bleeding has very high density (80–370 HU), secondary to contrast extravasation, and usually has a linear or globular appearance.
- Swirled appearance is common to hematomas due to multiple episodes of bleeding.
- Psoas thickening due to hematoma (Fig. 37-1).
- Remember to evaluate for distribution of hemorrhage, likely origin, evidence of vascular or traumatic injury, and mass effect.

Issues After Diagnosis

Retroperitoneal hemorrhage due to coagulation disorders requires correction of the underlying coagulopathy. Transarterial embolization can be performed when there is evidence of active retroperitoneal hemorrhage. It may also be used in situations of pelvic trauma

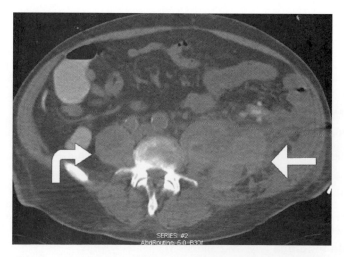

Figure 37-3. Left psoas hematoma (*straight arrow*) on computed tomography (CT) scan. Compare to normal left side (*curved arrow*).

with hemorrhage uncontrollable by fracture stabilization and C-clamp compression. In the setting of trauma, the zonal concept of management divides the retroperitoneum into three zones. Zone I hemorrhage (middle retroperitoneum) warrants surgical exploration because of the high likelihood of great vessel injury. Zone II hemorrhage (perinephric) may be treated by observation except in the setting of instability or an expanding hematoma. Zone III hemorrhage (pelvic) warrants pelvic stabilization with or without embolization in the setting of blunt trauma and exploration in the setting of penetrating trauma (because of the high likelihood of iliac vessel injury). Although widely used, the zonal concept of management is controversial because hemorrhage is not always clearly classified.

Further Readings

Aizenstein RI, Wilbur AC, O'Neil HK. Interfascial and perinephric pathways in the spread of retroperitoneal disease: refined concepts based on CT observations. *Am J Roentgenol* 1997;168:639–643.

Dondelinger RF, Trotteur G, Ghaye B, et al. Traumatic injuries: radiological hemostatic intervention at admission. *Eur Radiol* 2002;12:979–993.

Federle MP, Jeffrey RB, Dresser TS, et al. *Diagnostic imaging: abdomen*, 1st ed. Utah: Amirsys, 2004.

Feliciano DV. Management of traumatic retroperitoneal hematoma. *Ann Surg* 1990;211: 109–123.

Gore RM, Balfe DM, Aizenstein RI, et al. The great escape: interfascial decompression planes of the retroperitoneum. *Am J Roentgenol* 2000;175:363–370.

Ishikawa K, Tohira H, Mizushima Y, et al. Traumatic retroperitoneal hematoma spreads through the interfascial planes. *J Trauma* 2005;59:595–608.

Korobkin M, Silverman PM, Quint LE, et al. CT of the extraperitoneal space: normal anatomy and fluid collections. *Am J Roentgenol* 1992;159:933–941.

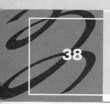

NECROTIZING ENTEROCOLITIS
Douglas E. Ramsey

CLINICAL INFORMATION

Necrotizing enterocolitis (NEC) is one of the most common surgical emergencies in neonates. A high index of suspicion and early diagnosis are critical to improving the chance of survival. Although radiologic findings may be nonspecific, prompt communication with clinicians is crucial when necrotizing enterocolitis is considered in a differential diagnosis.

Pathogenesis and Epidemiology.   The precise mechanism underlying NEC is not well understood. A leading explanation postulates that intestinal ischemia allows bacterial overgrowth, which may ultimately cause bowel perforation. Conditions which may cause ischemia, such as perinatal hypoxia, congenital heart disease, and hypotension, intestinal allows bacterial overgrowth, which cause bowel perforation are all risk factors for NEC. Introduction of milk or formula then provides a medium for bacterial overgrowth and infiltration of the bowel. Several risk factors have been statistically associated with necrotizing enterocolitis, including advanced maternal age, premature rupture of membranes, preterm delivery, low birth weight ($<2,000$ g), and maternal cocaine exposure.

Most infants diagnosed with necrotizing enterocolitis are small for gestational age and/or preterm, however full-term neonates may also be affected if they develop intestinal ischemia. Prevalence of NEC is as high as 4% in children with birth weights less than 2,000 g, affecting both sexes equally. NEC accounts for approximately 2% of neonatal intensive care unit (NICU) admissions.

Signs and Symptoms.   Feeding intolerance and abdominal distension may be the first signs of NEC, especially in full-term infants. Most patients with NEC have guaiac-positive stool or frank hematochezia. Peritonitis, including abdominal tenderness, is a typically later sign that may suggest perforation. Signs of generalized sepsis, including worsening metabolic acidosis, apnea, lethargy, and hypotension are seen in fulminant cases. Patients may have fever, leukocytosis, or even manifest disseminated intravascular coagulation, with thrombocytopenia. Blood and stool cultures may reveal any of a variety of organisms, all of which could precipitate NEC.

IMAGING WITH RADIOGRAPHS

Indications.   NEC is a clinical diagnosis that is supported by radiologic findings. Abdominal radiographs remain the modality of choice for the diagnosis of NEC. Water-soluble contrast enemas have been shown to reduce unnecessary surgery, but they are seldom performed for NEC, as a positive study will typically show only edema and nonspecific mucosal abnormalities. Although computed tomography (CT) could be used to detect questionable pneumatosis or free air, it is not commonly used. When radiographic findings are equivocal in light of toxic clinical presentation, treatment should precede radiologic evidence.

Protocol.   Whenever NEC is suspected, a supine view may be insufficient to find free intraabdominal air. A left decubitus or cross-table lateral view is essential to reliably detect pneumoperitoneum, which is an indication for surgery.

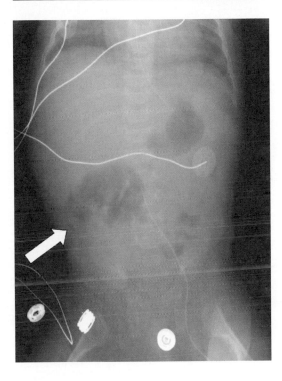

Figure 38-1. Anteroposterior (AP) view of the abdomen, obtained in a premature neonate demonstrates pneumatosis involving the hepatic flexure (*arrow*), consistent with necrotizing enterocolitis.

Possible Findings (Fig. 38-1)

- In early stages of NEC, abdominal radiographs may be normal, or only demonstrate minimal distention of bowel with air.
- Pneumatosis intestinalis in a premature neonate (Fig. 38-1) is essentially pathognomonic for NEC and should be communicated to the referring clinician immediately.
- In challenging cases where pneumatosis is in question, follow-up examinations should be obtained every 6 to 8 hours. Whereas pneumatosis is unlikely to move, gas bubbles in stool will migrate over time.
- Portal venous gas is an ominous finding that is associated with a poor outcome.
- A less sensitive radiographic finding is the "persistent loop" sign, where a dilated bowel loop retains the same appearance over at least 24 hours.
- Development of ascites may also indicate impending bowel perforation.
- Asymmetric distension of bowel with air is also suggestive of NEC.

Treatment and Outcomes

Depending on the clinical presentation, NEC can be managed medically or surgically. Clinically benign patients who manifest radiologic or isolated clinical data suggestive of NEC are often treated with intravenous antibiotics, hydration, and close monitoring. Oral feedings are stopped, and the bowel should be decompressed. Patients who present with severe peritonitis, pneumoperitoneum, or portal venous gas are usually referred for emergent laparotomy and bowel resection. Despite improved medical and surgical management of NEC, survival rates have not changed. Improving viability of increasingly premature infants has increased the prevalence and complexity of NEC. Survival rates are correlated with birth weight; infants weighing less than 1,000 g have a 43% survival rate, whereas survival increases to 80% for babies weighing more than 2,500 g. Bowel strictures and intestinal malabsorption are chronic complications of NEC.

Further Readings

Buonomo C. The radiology of necrotizing enterocolitis. *Radiol Clin N Am* 1999;37:1187–1198.

Johnson KB, Oski FA, eds. *Oski's essential pediatrics*. Philadelphia: Lippincott-Raven, 1997:421–425.

Neu J. Neonatal necrotizing enterocolitis: an update. *Acta Paediatr* 2005;94(Suppl 449):100–105.

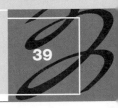
MALROTATION AND MIDGUT VOLVULUS
Sarah Mezban

CLINICAL INFORMATION

Malrotation results when the normal embryologic sequence of bowel development and fixation is interrupted. Malrotation predisposes to two problems: midgut volvulus and small bowel obstruction. Because of the potential for midgut volvulus and infarction of the entire small bowel, malrotation with midgut volvulus is a life-threatening surgical emergency in the newborn.

Embryology. Normal rotation of the proximal duodenojejunal loop and the distal cecocolic loop takes place around the superior mesenteric artery (SMA) as the axis, and is usually divided into three stages:

■ **Stage I.** Physiologic herniation of the gut through the umbilicus at sixth week of gestation is accompanied by a 180-degree counterclockwise rotation of the developing intestine around the SMA. The midgut lengthens along the SMA, and as rotation continues, a very broad pedicle is formed at the base of the mesentery.
■ **Stage II.** At the 10th week of gestation the bowel returns to the abdominal cavity. As it returns, the duodenojejunal loop rotates an additional 90 degrees to end at the anatomic left of the SMA. The cecocolic loop turns 180 degrees more as it reenters the abdominal cavity. This turn places it to the anatomic right of the SMA.
■ **Stage III.** Occurs from 11 weeks' gestation until term. It involves the descent of the cecum to the right lower quadrant and fixation of the mesenteries. Normal small bowel mesentery has a broad attachment stretching diagonally from the duodenojejunal junction (DJJ) (in the left upper quadrant) to the cecum (in the right lower quadrant). The point of attachment at the DJJ is referred to as the *ligament of Treitz*.

Pathophysiology. The cause of intestinal malrotation is disruption in the normal embryological development of the bowel at any stage.

Nonrotation

■ Arrest in development at stage I results in nonrotation. Subsequently, the DJJ does not lie inferior and to the left of the SMA, and the cecum does not lie in the right lower quadrant. The mesentery in turn forms a narrow base which is prone to clockwise twisting, leading to midgut volvulus. The width of the base of the mesentery is different in each patient, and not every patient develops midgut volvulus.

Incomplete Rotation

■ Stage II arrest results in incomplete rotation and is most likely to result in duodenal obstruction. Typically, peritoneal bands running from the misplaced cecum to the mesentery compress the third portion of the duodenum.

Incomplete Fixation

■ Malrotation is most often associated with malfixation. Potential hernial pouches form when the mesentery of the right and left colon and the duodenum do not become fixed retroperitoneally.

Frequency.   Malrotation frequency is unknown since many asymptomatic patients may never present; it is estimated to occur in 1 in 500 live births.

Age.   In 60% of patients, malrotation presents by age 1 month. Another 20–30% of patients present at age 1–12 months. Malrotation may remain clinically "silent" for some time and can present at any age.

Clinical Presentation.   The typical history of a patient with intestinal malrotation depends on age at presentation and degree of obstruction.

- Malrotation with midgut volvulus classically presents in the neonate with bilious vomiting and symptoms of proximal intestinal obstruction.
- Older children may show failure to thrive, chronic recurrent abdominal pain, malabsorption, or other vague presentations.
- Nonrotation of the intestine may be asymptomatic; therefore it is an incidental finding on upper gastrointestinal series (UGI) performed for other reasons.
- Peritoneal bands (Ladd's bands) leading to compression or kinking of the duodenum can present at infancy with forceful vomiting, which may or may not be bile stained, depending on the location of the obstruction with respect to the entrance of the common bile duct. This can also have a more chronic presentation.
- Internal herniation usually has more chronic presentation with recurrent abdominal pain, which may progress from intermittent to constant.

 IMAGING

Preferred Examination.   The diagnostic test of choice in a child with possible malrotation with or without midgut volvulus is a UGI series and should be performed unless delaying surgery will compromise outcome, as in the case of an unstable or moribund child.

Imaging with Radiographs

Indication.   In malrotation without midgut volvulus, radiographs have limited use for defining obstruction because infants may have a gasless abdomen or one that is almost normal. On the other hand, radiographs are rarely normal in malrotation with midgut volvulus.

Protocol.   Routine supine and erect film of the abdomen.

Possible Findings

- In simple malrotation, radiographs may appear normal (normal abdominal film does not exclude malrotation).
- In midgut volvulus, the classic radiographic finding is a partial duodenal obstruction (dilation of both the stomach and proximal duodenum, with a small amount of distal bowel gas).
- Complete obstruction of the duodenum may also be found.
- Less frequent but more ominous signs are a gasless abdomen, ileus, or distal small bowel obstruction with multiple dilated loops and air–fluid levels.

Imaging with Upper Gastroesophageal Series

Indication.   The UGI series provides a high degree of confidence in the diagnosis of malrotation and midgut volvulus. The sensitivity of the UGI series is 85–95% with a higher specificity (false positives are rare). Contrast studies may not be possible in patients who are actively vomiting or are unstable and need immediate surgical exploration.

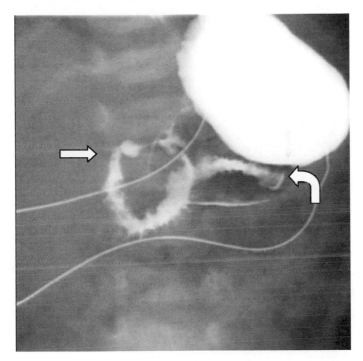

Figure 39-1. Normal rotation on upper gastrointestinal (UGI). Ligament of Treiz (*curved arrow*) is to the left of the spine and at the same level as duodenal bulb (*straight arrow*). Image courtesy of Renee Flax-Goldeberg, MD, Johns Hopkins Hospital.

Protocol. Performed with barium administered either by bottle or through a nasogastric tube. Water-soluble agents should be used if the study is being performed before imminent surgery. It is important to identify the location of the DJJ on the first pass of oral contrast before the more distal small bowel opacifies and obscures the DJJ.

Possible Findings (Figs. 39-1 and 39-2)

- Normal rotation
  - After the C loop, the duodenum crosses the midline, with the DJJ seen to the left of the spine higher than or at the level of the duodenal bulb.
- Malrotation
  - DJJ displaced downward and to the right on the frontal view.
  - An abnormal course of the duodenum on lateral view.
  - An abnormal position of the jejunum (lying on right side of abdomen) should alert one to the possibility of a malrotation but should not be relied upon to either make or exclude the diagnosis.
- Malrotation with midgut volvulus
  - A dilated, fluid-filled duodenum.
  - A proximal small bowel obstruction.
  - A "corkscrew" pattern (proximal jejunum spiraling downward in right or mid upper abdomen in midgut volvulus, which is rare).
  - Mural edema, thick folds.

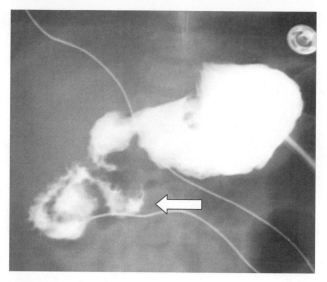

Figure 39-2. Malrotation on upper gastrointestinal (UGI) with abnormal duodenal course (*arrow*). Image courtesy of Renee Flax-Goldeberg, MD, Johns Hopkins Hospital.

Imaging with Ultrasonography

Ultrasonography may suggest the diagnosis of malrotation; however, sensitivity and specificity are low compared to the UGI series; therefore, a UGI examination is mandatory to confirm the diagnosis if suspected on ultrasonography.

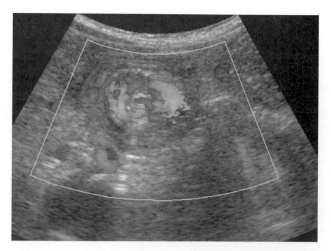

Figure 39-3. Midgut volvulus, with Doppler ultrasound (US) showing "the whirlpool sign" of vessels twisting around superior mesenteric artery in midgut volvulus. (Source: Epelman E. The whirlpool sign. *Radiology* 2006;240:910–911.)

Possible Findings (Fig. 39-3)

■ When the superior mesenteric vein (SMV) lies to the left of or posterior to the SMA this suggests malrotation.

■ Normal vascular positioning (SMV slightly ventral and to the right of SMA) can be seen in approximately 30% of patients with malrotation.

■ Color Doppler demonstrates mesentery and Doppler flow within the SMV wrapping around the SMA (in a clockwise direction) "whirlpool sign," indicating malrotation with volvulus.

■ A dilated, fluid-filled duodenum frequently is seen in patients with obstruction without volvulus.

Further Readings

Herba A. *Intestinal volvulus*. www.emedicine.com. Feb. 2004.

Millar AJ, Rode H, Cywes S. Malrotation and volvulus in infancy and childhood. *Semin Pediatr Surg* 2003;12(4):229–236.

Parish A. *Intestinal malrotation*. www.emedicine.com. Dec. 2002.

Strouse PJ. Clinics in diagnostic imaging midgut malrotation with volvulus. *Singapore Med J* 2002;43(6):325–328.

Zerin JM, DiPietro MA. Superior mesenteric vascular anatomy at US in patients with surgically proved malrotation of the midgut. *Radiology* 1992;183(3):693–694.

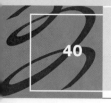

40

HYPERTROPHIC PYLORIC STENOSIS
Jennifer E. Swart

 ## CLINICAL INFORMATION

Mechanism and Epidemiology.   Hypertrophic pyloric stenosis is an idiopathic hypertrophy, or thickening, of the circular muscle bundles of the stomach pylorus. This hypertrophy is progressive, resulting in gradual development of gastric outlet obstruction. The etiology of the condition remains unknown, although postulated mechanisms include abnormal myenteric plexus nerve cells of the pylorus as well as excessive spasm or overactivity of the pylorus leading to eventual muscular hypertrophy.

The age at presentation is typically 2–8 weeks; however, cases of infants presenting at birth or after 8 weeks have been described. There are even case reports of hypertrophic pyloric stenosis diagnosed in utero by prenatal ultrasonography. The incidence of the condition is approximately 2–5 cases per 1,000 births per year, and it affects males with a frequency of 4–5 times that of females.

Symptoms and Signs.   The presentation of hypertrophic pyloric stenosis usually consists of one or more of the following:

- Nonbilious vomiting, usually described as "projectile."
- General difficulty feeding, with weight loss and eventual malnourishment.
- Palpable olive-sized mass in the epigastrium or right upper quadrant.
- Visualization of exaggerated gastric peristalsis through the abdominal wall.

Hypertrophic pyloric stenosis diagnosis is not a pediatric emergency, and the diagnosis and documentation of the condition may wait in an overnight situation if necessary.

Hypertrophic pyloric stenosis is an evolving lesion. If initial imaging studies are borderline or negative, but clinical symptoms persist, patients should be reimaged 1–2 weeks later (preferably with ultrasonography).

 ## IMAGING WITH ULTRASONOGRAPHY

Indications.   Ultrasonography is the imaging method of choice, given its degree of accuracy, its ability to directly visualize the anatomy and function of the pylorus, and its lack of ionizing radiation.

Protocol.   Using a linear high-frequency transducer, start with locating the gallbladder in the right upper quadrant, and then turn obliquely sagittal to the body to visualize the pylorus of the stomach in a longitudinal orientation. The pylorus should also then be visualized in the transverse orientation. Once the pyloric sphincter has been visualized, fluid can be given by mouth to assess for pyloric opening, transpyloric flow, and gastric emptying.

Possible Findings (Fig. 40-1)

- Persistent thickening and elongation of the hypertrophied muscle (as opposed to the intermittent thickening in pylorospasm), with "sonolucent donut" on cross-section.
  - Single wall thickness of the pylorus more than 3.5 mm (transverse orientation).

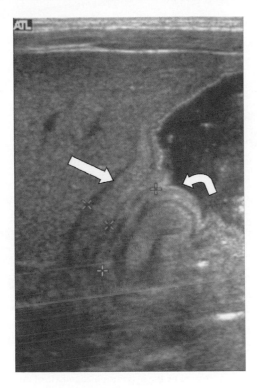

Figure 40-1. Ultrasonography (US) demonstrates elongation of the pyloric canal (>15 mm) and hypertrophy of the muscle (single wall thickness >3 mm). Hypertrophied pylorus muscle (*straight arrow*) appears hypoechoic and the central mucosa appears hyperechoic (*curved arrow*). These findings are compatible with hypertrophic pyloric stenosis.

- Pyloric canal length (longitudinal orientation)
  - Less than 15 mm—normal.
  - 15–17 mm—indeterminate.
  - More than 17 mm—abnormal.
- Hypertrophied pylorus muscle will appear hypoechoic and the central mucosa will appear hyperechoic.
- "Double track sign"—echogenic redundant mucosal lining also hypertrophies and obstructs canal lumen, with numerous sonolucent linear fluid stripes accumulating in the canal.
- Persistent spasm of the pyloric canal, with little fluid passage into the duodenum and decreased gastric emptying.

 IMAGING WITH FLUOROSCOPY

Indications. A barium study is indicated if ultrasonography is not available or if the clinical history is atypical, particularly if bilious vomiting is present suggesting possible malrotation and midgut volvulus.

Technique. Start with an abdominal radiograph to ensure that no pneumoperitoneum is present before beginning the upper gastrointestinal (GI) series. Then give the infant a small amount of barium to drink from a bottle. If the infant is unable or unwilling to drink from a bottle, a nasogastric tube may be inserted and barium injected directly into the stomach. The infant may be placed in the right lateral or right anterior oblique position to facilitate gastric emptying.

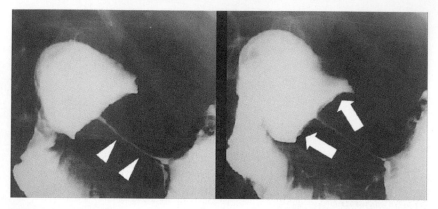

Figure 40-2. Upper gastrointestinal (GI) series demonstrates positive "string sign" with a minimal trickle of barium (*arrowheads*) passing through the pyloric canal. Impression from the on the proximal duodenum (*arrows*) is caused by the hypertrophied muscle of the pylorus. These findings are compatible with hypertrophic pyloric stenosis. Courtesy of Renee Flax-Goldenberg, MD, Johns Hopkins Hospital.

Possible Findings (Fig. 40-2)

■ Gastric hyperperistalsis or "caterpillar stomach," corresponding to the exaggerated peristalsis that may be observed through the abdominal wall on clinical examination.
■ Overdistension of the stomach and delayed gastric emptying.
■ "String sign" with a minimal trickle of barium passing through the pyloric canal.
■ "Beak sign" with a beak-shaped point to the entrance of the pylorus.
■ "Shoulders" impression on the distal antrum, created by the hypertrophied muscle of the pylorus.

 DIFFERENTIAL DIAGNOSIS

■ **Pylorospasm.** This condition typically resolves with time, and one may wait and reimage the infant if necessary to ensure resolution.
■ **Gastroesophageal reflux.** This condition is the etiology of vomiting in two thirds of referrals, and is the presumed diagnosis with a normal ultrasonography given the intermittent nature of vomiting due to gastroesophageal reflux disease (GERD).
■ **Malrotation.** This condition by itself is not an emergency, and may not be discovered until adulthood in an individual with intermittent symptoms. However, malrotation with midgut volvulus is an imaging as well as a surgical emergency, presenting with symptoms of abdominal pain and bilious vomiting, and must be evaluated with an upper GI series.

Further Readings

Cohen HL, Strain JD, Fordham L, et al. Vomiting in infants up to 3 months of age. American College of Radiology appropriateness criteria. *Radiology* 2000;215(suppl):779–786.
Hernanz-Schulman M. Infantile hypertrophic pyloric stenosis. *Radiology* 2003;227: 319–331.
Mandell GA, Wolfson PJ, Adkins ES, et al. Cost-effective imaging approach to the nonbilious vomiting infant. *Pediatrics* 1999;103(6 pt 1):1198–1202.
Swischuk LE. *Imaging of the newborn, infant, and young child.* Philadelphia: Lippincott Williams & Wilkins, 2003.
Tashjian DB, Konefal SH. Hypertrophic pyloric stenosis in utero. *Pediatr Surg Int* 2002;18(5–6):539–540.

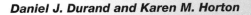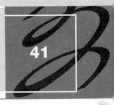

URINARY TRACT INFECTIONS

Daniel J. Durand and Karen M. Horton

41

$\mathcal{U}$rinary tract infections (UTIs) are defined as any microbial colonization of the urine or tissues of the urinary tract. As a result, the term *UTI* encompasses a broad range of pathology ranging from asymptomatic bacteriuria to fulminant pyelonephritis leading to acute renal failure, sepsis, and death. UTIs are a fairly common cause of morbidity, particularly in children and sexually active women. The prompt radiologic detection of uncommon but dangerous complications such as renal abscess allows life-saving interventions such as percutaneous drainage.

 CLINICAL INFORMATION

Etiology. UTI is most commonly caused by bacteria, particularly gram-negative pathogens that normally inhabit the gastrointestinal (GI) tract, such as *Escherichia coli* (*E. coli*) and *Klebsiella* (Table 41-1). Acute pyelonephritis refers to involvement of the renal parenchyma, which can occur due to reflux of infected urine from the bladder, ureteral obstruction or hematogenous seeding during periods of bacteremia (e.g., staphylococcus), or fungemia (e.g., candida). There are many conditions and anatomic defects that put patients at risk for recurrent UTI and pyelonephritis (Table 41-2). Such patients, many of whom are children, are at risk of developing parenchymal scarring, renal failure, and hypertension later in life.

Upper versus Lower. urinary tract infection. The term *lower UTI* is used to describe infection of structures distal to the ureters (bladder, urethra), whereas *upper UTI* refers to infection of the ureters and/or kidneys. The signs and symptoms of UTI often point toward the area and degree of involvement. Isolated bacteriuria is often asymptomatic, while symptoms of external urinary dysuria suggest urethritis. Increased urinary frequency, internal dysuria, suprapubic pain and cloudy urine or hematuria are suggestive of cystitis. Although costovertebral tenderness and flank pain have classically been associated with upper UTI (i.e., pyelonephritis) they are in fact nonspecific findings that commonly accompany lower UTI. When fever, rigors, and other signs of sepsis are also present, all of the symptoms mentioned become much more specific for acute pyelonephritis. Common laboratory findings include pyuria, hematuria, white blood cell (WBC) casts, bacteriuria, leukocytosis, and other signs of acute infection. Elevations in creatinine levels and other signs of renal impairment and hypertension are suggestive of chronic renal pathology (including chronic pyelonephritis), but are unlikely to be caused by acute infection. Children and neonates pose a diagnostic challenge in that they typically present with nonspecific symptoms such as lethargy, irritability, diarrhea, and fever.

Complicated versus Uncomplicated Urinary Tract Infection. "Complicated" cases are those at high risk of failing treatment or developing serious complications, usually due to an underlying condition such as urinary tract obstruction. Generally speaking, an "uncomplicated" UTI is one in a young, healthy, nonpregnant woman and a "complicated" UTI is one occurring in anyone else. It is important to note that most episodes of pyelonephritis represent uncomplicated "upper" UTIs and will respond well to treatment.

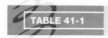

TABLE 41-1   Microbiology of Urinary Tract Infection (UTI) and Pyelonephritis

Pathogen	Comment
Escherichia coli	Responsible for approximately 80% of uncomplicated cases
Staphylococcus saprophyticus	Responsible for 10–15% asymptomatic infections in young women
Klebsiella sp.	Uncomplicated infections
Proteus sp.	Uncomplicated infection, also associated with stone formation and xanthogranulomatous pyelonephritis
Serratia sp.	Often seen in complicated infections
Pseudomonas sp.	Often seen in complicated infections
Staphylococcus aureus	Seen in patients with stones, instrumentation, and bacteremia
Enterobacter	A small percentage of uncomplicated cases
Enteroccocus sp.	Seen in patients with stones, instrumentation, and bacteremia.
Chlamydia trachomatis	Sexually transmitted cause of UTI
Neisseria gonorrhoeae	Sexually transmitted cause of UTI
Ureaplasma urealyticum	Mostly causes cystitis and urethritis
Mycoplasma hominis	Can cause pyelonephritis
Candida sp.	Typically seen in catheterized and diabetic patients
Mycobacterium tuberculosis	Cause of pyelonephritis in immunosuppressed patients (e.g., AIDS)
Pneumocystis carinii	Cause of pyelonephritis in immunosuppressed patients (e.g., AIDS)
Mycobacterium avium-intracellulare	Cause of pyelonephritis in immunosuppressed patients (e.g., AIDS)
Histoplasma sp.	Cause of pyelonephritis in immunosuppressed patients (e.g., AIDS)

AIDS, acquired immunodeficiency syndrome.

Acute versus Chronic Pyelonephritis.   Acute pyelonephritis is typically a clinical diagnosis confirmed by imaging studies, whereas chronic UTI is a radiologic diagnosis based on the demonstration of clubbed calyces associated with focal or diffuse renal scarring. It develops as a result of repeated subacute infection of the renal parenchyma as seen in children with vesicoureteral reflux (VUR). Over the course of multiple infections, the renal parenchyma becomes increasingly scarred, putting the patient at risk for poor renal function and the development of hypertension.

Differential diagnosis includes both upper and lower UTI, urethritis, vaginitis, and nephrolithiasis.

IMAGING OVERVIEW

The primary role of imaging in UTI is to detect correctable complications in order to avoid sepsis and loss of renal function. In addition, radiologic studies can help identify underlying anatomic and functional disorders that may have predisposed the patient to infection, such as VUR in children or benign prostatic hypertrophy in older men. Lastly,

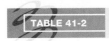

| TABLE 41-2 | Risk Factors for Urinary Tract Infection (UTI) |

General medical issues
Pregnancy
Diabetes
Renal failure
Renal transplant
Immunosuppression
Hospital acquired infection
Multidrug resistant pathogens
Indwelling catheter
Ureteral stent
Nephrostomy tube
Structural abnormalities
  Congenital
    Renal duplication
    Ectopic ureteral insertion
  Renal tract obstruction
    Posterior urethral valves
    Anterior urethral diverticula
    PUJ or VUJ obstruction
    Meatal stenosis
    Renal calculi
    Retrocaval ureter
    Simple and ectopic ureteroceles
  VUR
  Obstruction (acquired)
  Diverticulae
  Fistulae
  Ileal conduits and other urinary diversions
Functional bladder abnormalities
  Neurogenic bladder
  Dysfunctional voiding syndrome
  Prune belly syndrome

PUJ, pelviureteric junction; VUJ, vesicoureteric junction; VUR, vesicoureteral reflux.

acute and follow-up imaging studies are useful to assess the degree of damage and renal scarring.

Although uncomplicated pyelonephritis typically results in findings that are non-specific, some complications (e.g., renal abscess) and some forms of pyelonephritis (e.g., emphysematous pyelonephritis) have a characteristic appearance. For ease of use in reading studies, the following discussion is classified primarily according to imaging modality.

Imaging with Ultrasonography

Indications. Ultrasonography is readily available, inexpensive, and can be especially useful when seeking to minimize radiation exposure to pregnant women and children. Ultrasound is best suited for detecting large fluid collections, as seen in hydronephrosis or renal abscesses, checking for stones, and evaluating the patency of renal vasculature.

Protocol. In assessing for hydronephrosis, be sure the bladder is empty. Try to visualize both the ureteropelvic junction (UPJ) and ureterovesicular junction (UVJ) to look for dilatation and impacted stones.

Possible Findings (Fig. 41-3)

- Acute pyelonephritis. There may be an increase in renal volume with focal or diffuse areas of abnormal echogenicity and loss of corticomedullary differentiation. Although ultrasonography has poor specificity for acute pyelonephritis, this can be improved somewhat with the use of Doppler to demonstrate hypovascularity or absent flow in the involved region.
- Urinary tract obstruction is evidenced by the presence of hydronephrosis and hydroureter. If hydronephrosis is present, try to visualize the proximal ureter, if possible. Also, consider if the hydronephrosis could be chronic—observe if the renal parenchyma is of normal thickness.
- A calculus may be the cause of acute or chronic obstruction and appears as a strongly echogenic focus accompanied by acoustic shadowing. Calculi as small as 3–5 mm may be detected by ultrasonography. Air within the renal collecting system or parenchyma can also appear echogenic but typically demonstrates "dirty" shadowing.
- Abscesses may be seen as abnormal fluid collections within the parenchyma (renal abscesses) or surrounding tissues (perinephric abscess). Renal abscesses are typically well-defined masses with reduced attenuation and a thick, irregular wall. Perinephric extension can occasionally involve the psoas muscle.
- Fungus balls may be visible as nonshadowing echogenic densities which can obstruct the ureter. This is highly suggestive of fungal pyelonephritis.

Imaging with Computed Tomography

Indications. Computed tomography (CT) is not routinely used in the diagnosis of acute pyelonephritis in children due to radiation. In addition, CT has been shown to be less sensitive than functional imaging in diagnosing acute pyelonephritis. However, CT can be a useful adjunct to ultrasonography and dimercaptosuccinic acid (DMSA) scintigraphy in adult patients who require further investigation for a variety of reasons including (1) signs of severe infection or frank sepsis, (2) failed treatment, or (3) findings suggestive of abscess or calculi on ultrasonography.

Protocol. CT urography protocols usually consist of a noncontrast, arterial, and delayed scan with thin slices. The delay time for the arterial phase is 25–30 seconds and with an additional delayed scan at 4 minutes. Other centers wait up to 45–50 seconds for the first phase and perform the delayed scan up to 8 minutes after contrast injection.

Possible Findings (Figs. 41-1–41-3)

- Acute pyelonephritis may exhibit areas of reduced attenuation, which may be uni- or multifocal with areas of poor corticomedullary differentiation. This is best seen on arterial or nephrographic phases.
- Papillary necrosis may be seen as a filling defect in the collecting system on a late contrast-enhanced scan which can also be seen on a radiograph intravenous urography (IVU).
- Renal and perinephric abscesses may also be visible. Renal abscesses are typically well-defined masses with reduced attenuation and a thick, irregular wall. Perinephric extension can occasionally involve the psoas muscle. It is often difficult to distinguish a renal abscess from an infected renal cyst.
- A calculus appears as a hyperdense focus of bone density within the kidney or ureter.
- Hydronephrosis and hydroureter on CT: hydronephrosis appears as dilation of the renal pelvis with clubbing of the calyces in the upper and lower poles. It is often associated with obliteration of renal sinus fat, asymmetric perinephric stranding, and enlargement and hypoattenuation of the entire kidney. Hydroureter appears as a dilated ureter.
- Calcified granulomas, often with cavity formation, are suggestive of renal tuberculosis or infection by other mycobacteria, parasites, or fungi. Such lesions are often seen in acquired immunodeficiency syndrome (AIDS) patients.
- Fungus balls are visible as spherical hyperdense lesions within the collecting system. They are often accompanied by multiple microabscesses of the kidneys.

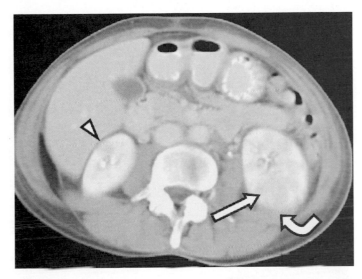

Figure 41-1. Bilateral pyelonephritis on computed tomography (CT). Contrast-enhanced CT demonstrates enlargement of the left kidney, multiple hypodensities (*arrow*), and stranding of perinephric fat (*curved arrow*). These findings are consistent with pyelonephritis. Mild pyelonephritis is also seen in the right kidney (*arrowhead*).

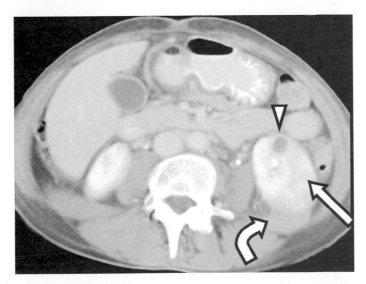

Figure 41-2. This patient developed a left renal abscess (*arrowhead*) as a complication of acute pyelonephritis. Contrast-enhanced computed tomography (CT) scan shows extensive left renal parenchymal hypodensities (*arrow*), and stranding of perinephric fat (*curved arrow*).

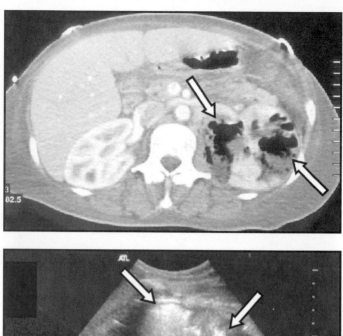

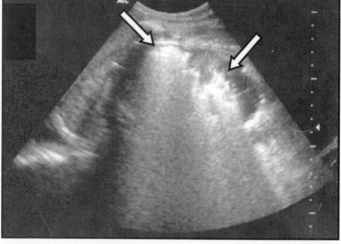

Figure 41-3. Emphysematous pyelonephritis of left kidney. **A:** Contrast-enhanced computed tomography (CT) scan demonstrates gas in the renal parenchyma (*arrows*). **B:** Renal ultrasound (US) in the same patient shows echogenic foci (*arrows*) with dirty shadowing in the renal parenchyma, consistent with gas.

- Xanthogranulomatous pyelonephritis is a rare childhood renal inflammatory disease that results in the destruction of the renal parenchyma and replacement by lipid-laden macrophages. It is associated with calculus formation, obstruction, and infection with *E. coli* and *Proteus* species. CT shows global renal enlargement and multiple, rounded masses of low attenuation representing calyceal dilatation or necrotic tissue (the "bear paw" sign). The walls of these cavities enhance with intravenous (IV) contrast, which is not excreted into the collecting system in the affected kidney.
- Gas bubbles on CT should immediately raise concern for emphysematous pyelonephritis, a life-threatening condition resulting from renal infection by gas-forming microorganisms. The gas bubbles typically overlie the renal fossa or are present within the parenchyma, resulting in an enlarged, mottled kidney. When the gas is limited to the renal

collecting systems it is more likely to represent emphysematous pyelitis, which has a more benign course. Lastly, consider that the gas may have been introduced iatrogenically, by fistula formation or reflux from gas in the bladder.

Functional Imaging with Dimercaptosuccinic Acid Scintigraphy

Indications. In situations where imaging results from ultrasonography and CT are equivocal, functional imaging with DMSA scintigraphy provides the most sensitive method of detecting acute pyelonephritis.

Protocol. ^{99m}Technetium (^{99m}Tc) -DMSA is actively taken up by the renal tubules following IV administration and allows a more quantitative assessment of renal function than that afforded by CT urography. Functional tissue is visible on planar images acquired from the posterior (PA) and PA oblique projections with the patient lying supine.

Possible Findings

■ Focal or diffuse reduction in radiotracer in the affected kidney relative to the healthy kidney may be evidence of either acute pyelonephritis or renal scarring. However, these results can be difficult to interpret if both kidneys are affected or if the patient only has one remaining functional kidney or a congenital duplex kidney. In these cases, other imaging modalities should be performed to confirm the impression.

 STRUCTURAL ABNORMALITIES OF THE URINARY TRACT

Recurrent episodes of acute pyelonephritis or signs of chronic renal scarring should prompt suspicion of an underlying structural or functional abnormality of the urinary tract. A wide variety of such abnormalities are associated with acute UTI and chronic pyelonephritis (Table 41-2). This is especially true of infants and children, who are more likely to have an undiagnosed anatomic abnormality. Ultrasonography is particularly sensitive for these abnormalities and is the test of choice for the primary investigation of UTI in infants and children. In patients with severe infection, ultrasonography can be performed urgently at the bedside, whereas in children with uncomplicated UTI ultrasonography may be performed weeks after treatment as part of follow-up.

VUR occurs in 1–2% of all children and is thought to be due to inadequate length of the intravesicular ureter. In most of these children, VUR will cease spontaneously as the UVJ becomes competent when the intravesicular ureter increases in length with normal growth. The gold standard for detecting VUR is a voiding cystourethrogram (VCUG), although ultrasonography is typically used as a screening tool.

VUR is frequently found in children with UTI, but it is also seen in those with other congenital abnormalities of the renal tract such as dysplastic kidneys and UPV obstruction. Occasionally, cases of VUR can lead to the so-called reflux nephropathy, resulting in ureteral dilation, recurrent episodes of pyelonephritis, and permanent renal damage. Children with VUR who have suffered an episode of pyelonephritis are at increased risk for permanent renal damage, which is best detected with DMSA follow-up imaging 6 months to 2 years after the acute infection.

 TREATMENT AND POSTIMAGING ISSUES

The treatment of UTI and pyelonephritis depends on the severity of the infection. Uncomplicated cases can frequently be managed as outpatients with appropriate antibiotics and follow-up. Patients with "complicated" cases or signs of sepsis or marked debilitation will likely require inpatient treatment with parenteral antibiotics and, in severe cases of obstruction or abscess, percutaneous intervention.

In patients who present with recurrent infections due to the same pathogen within 2 weeks of treatment, a renal ultrasound or CT should be performed to rule out an underlying anatomic abnormality or abscess.

Further Readings

Johansen TE. The role of imaging in urinary tract infections. *World J Urol* 2004;22: 392–398.

Paterson A. Urinary tract infection: an update on imaging strategies. *Eur Radiol* 2004; 14(Suppl 4):L89–100.

Sheth S, Fishman EK. Multi-detector row CT of the kidneys and urinary tract: techniques and applications in the diagnosis of benign diseases. *Radiographics* 2004;24:e20.

Stamm WE, Schaeffer AJ. The state of the art in the management of urinary tract infections. *Am J Med* 2002;113(Suppl A1):1S–84S.

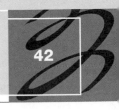

BLADDER AND URETERAL INJURY
Visveshwar Baskaran

42

ladder injuries are, in most cases, associated with motor vehicle accidents or with pelvic fracture. Ureteral injuries are rare and more often iatrogenic than due to penetrating trauma or crush injuries. Ureteral laceration or avulsion occurs more commonly in children.

CLINICAL INFORMATION

Mechanisms.   **Bladder injuries** overwhelmingly involve a distended bladder. A distended bladder is no longer protected by its usual low-lying position in the pelvis, so compression of the bladder can occur against the spine. Severity of bladder injury ranges from contusion to frank rupture. Rupture can be intraperitoneal, usually involving the fundus or posterior bladder wall, or extraperitoneal, usually involving the anterior or lateral wall, near the bladder neck. Penetrating injuries to the bladder usually result in intraperitoneal rupture, whereas ruptures associated with pelvic fractures are commonly extraperitoneal.

Ureteral injuries are most commonly iatrogenic, often complications related to gynecologic surgery, urologic procedures, or vascular surgery. Most noniatrogenic cases are the result of penetrating trauma, generally involve the upper one third of the ureter, and are almost always associated with injuries to adjacent organs. Ureteral contusion may result from projectiles producing a "blast effect" in the region of the ureter. Ureteral laceration or avulsion usually occurs in the setting of a deceleration or crush injury (i.e., automobile tire), often resulting in disruption of the ureter at the ureteropelvic junction (UPJ). Combination injuries involving the upper and lower genitourinary tract are very rare, and when present, nearly universally associated with fatality.

Complications.   Complications of bladder injury include urine peritonitis, in the case of intraperitoneal rupture, and tissue necrosis, and abscess or phlegmon formation in the case of extraperitoneal rupture. Ureteral injury can be complicated by urinoma, abscess, fistula, ureteral stricture, or hydronephrosis.

Symptoms and Signs.   Symptoms and signs are variable. The degree of hematuria does not appear to correlate with the severity or nature of the bladder injury but is seen in almost all cases. Blood at the urethral meatus is suggestive of a urethral injury.

- **Ureteral Injuries.** Hematuria may not be present if complete transection has occurred. Bilateral ureteral damage can cause anuria. Symptoms and signs are nonspecific and include those of infection, peritonitis, or urinary obstruction. If the condition remains undiagnosed, urine may be seen at the entrance or exit wounds after 7–10 days.
- **Intraperitoneal Rupture.** Patients describe urgency to void but an inability to do so. Hypotension and tachycardia may be present, with signs of toxicity and generalized peritonitis appearing after 24–72 hours.
- **Extraperitoneal Rupture.** The patient can void, with great discomfort, small amounts of sanguineous urine. Blood or urine may cause a suprapubic or pelvic mass. Urine can dissect up as far as the kidneys or into the thighs or buttocks.

IMAGING WITH RADIOGRAPHS

Indications.   Routinely performed as initial evaluation of abdominal trauma.

Protocol.   Supine anteroposterior (AP) film of the abdomen.

Possible Findings

- Pelvic ring disruption, often identified as diastasis of the symphysis pubis or frank fractures of the pubic rami. Up to 15% of patients with pelvic fractures have bladder trauma, whereas 70% of those with bladder rupture have a pelvic fracture.
- Diffusely increased radiodensity within the pelvis, caused by a hematoma.
- Adynamic ileus, which may be associated with an intraperitoneal bladder rupture.
- Displacement of the obturator fat line due to pelvic hematoma.

IMAGING WITH CONVENTIONAL RETROGRADE CYSTOGRAPHY

Indications.   Conventional retrograde cystography is equivalent to computed tomographic (CT) cystography and may be performed if urethral trauma is absent and if CT scanning of the abdomen is deemed unnecessary. Conventional retrograde cystography can be positive when intravenous pyelography (IVP) is negative, especially with small, flaplike bladder tears. The study is contraindicated if the IVP demonstrates extravasation.

Protocol.   Before placement of a Foley catheter in the male urethra, the urethra must be demonstrated to be intact by retrograde urethrography. If IVP or CT is to be done, these studies should be performed first because any extravasated contrast on the retrograde cystogram could obscure the kidneys and ureters. Diluted (30%) water-soluble contrast is infused by gravity into the bladder using a Foley catheter, preferably under fluoroscopy. Infusion is stopped immediately when extravasation is identified. A minimum of 300 mL of contrast must be used to ensure adequate distension of the bladder. Five views of the bladder should be obtained on 14- × 17-inch film: AP, lateral, both obliques, and postvoid view. The postvoid film is essential; it is the only film to show extravasation in approximately 10% of cases.

Possible Findings

- **Bladder contusion and interstitial injury.** The contrast-filled bladder usually appears normal in bladder contusion. CT may be more sensitive. In interstitial injury, a bladder wall defect is present without evidence of contrast extravasation.
- **Intraperitoneal bladder rupture** (Fig. 42-1). Contrast outlines the paracolic gutters and bowel loops and fills the pelvic peritoneal recesses. Extravasated contrast appears above a line joining the acetabular roofs.
- **Extraperitoneal bladder rupture** (Fig. 42-2). Extravasated contrast-laden urine appears as streaks in the perivesical space. Contrast may also spread into soft tissue planes around the pelvis but does not surround bowel loops and appears below a line joining the acetabular roofs.
- **Perivesical hematoma.** A "teardrop" bladder may be seen as a result of hematoma compressing the bladder walls.

IMAGING WITH EXCRETORY UROGRAPHY (INTRAVENOUS PYELOGRAPHY)

Indications.   IVP will almost always demonstrate ureteral injury and may obviate further evaluation of the bladder as well. However, a negative IVP does not rule out bladder rupture, because only a small percentage of bladder ruptures are demonstrated on IVP. In these cases, conventional retrograde cystography or CT cystography is indicated. If findings are equivocal for ureteral injury, retrograde ureterography may be performed.

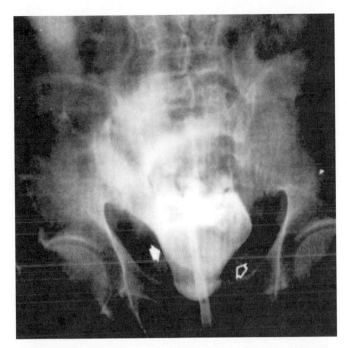

Figure 42-1. Anteroposterior (AP) film from a conventional retrograde cystogram shows an intraperitoneal bladder rupture with contrast material outlining several small bowel loops. There is also mass effect on the bladder from pelvic hematomas (*arrows*). (Lang EK. Chapter 111: trauma of the urinary tract. In: Taveras JM, Ferrucci JT, eds. *Radiology: diagnosis/imaging/intervention*, Vol. 4. Philadelphia: JB Lippincott Co, 1991:18. Figure 25.)

Protocol.   A contrast dose of 1–1.5 mL/lb to compensate for the aggressive fluid hydration such patients often receive. Delayed films can be useful in identifying slow or intermittent intraperitoneal extravasation.

Possible Findings

■ **Ureteral injury.** Contrast extravasation, usually into a urinoma, is seen in ureteral laceration or avulsion. The distal ureter may not be visualized. Contrast may flow superiorly and surround the kidney, which in some cases may mimic a renal laceration. Even minimal hydronephrosis should increase suspicion of trauma to the ipsilateral ureter.

■ Other findings are the same as for retrograde cystography.

IMAGING WITH COMPUTED TOMOGRAPHY

Indications.   CT is routinely performed as part of an evaluation for abdominal and pelvic trauma. When ureteral injury is suspected, excretory phase contrast-enhanced CT allows for rapid assessment of ureteral integrity. Retrograde ureterography may be performed in equivocal cases. Recent studies demonstrate that with adequate retrograde bladder distension with dilute contrast, conventional cystography and CT cystography are equivalent. CT cystography can easily be performed during routine CT evaluation of the trauma patient and has the advantage of not requiring patients with fractures and other

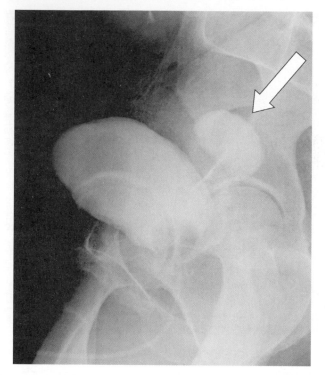

Figure 42-2. Oblique film from a conventional retrograde cystogram demonstrates a collection of contrast (*arrow*) posterior to the bladder compatible with extraperitoneal bladder rupture.

potentially unstable injuries to be moved during the study. A disadvantage, however, is the additional radiation exposure required.

Protocol.   IV contrast is extremely useful for the evaluation of ureteral and bladder trauma and is required to rule out concurrent solid organ injury. Excretory phase CT is obtained if needed by scanning 3–5 minutes after contrast injection. For bladder trauma, CT cystography is performed after retrograde bladder distension using Foley catheter with at least 300 mL of dilute water-soluble contrast (50 mL of contrast/500 mL of saline). Postdrainage scans may also be acquired.

Possible Findings

- **Ureteral injury.** Contrast extravasation, often into a urinoma, is seen along the expected course of the ureter in the setting of a ureteral laceration or avulsion. Contrast extravasation typically occurs in the inferior medial perinephric space.
- **Bladder contusion and interstitial injury.** An intramural hyperdensity (hemorrhage) or contrast collection may be present without evidence of extravasation.
- **Intraperitoneal bladder rupture.** Contrast collects in peritoneal spaces such as Morrison's pouch and the paracolic gutters, between mesenteric folds, and in pelvic recesses. It is important to inspect the rectum, small bowel, and pelvic vasculature for additional injuries.
- **Extraperitoneal bladder rupture** (Fig. 42-3). Contrast leaks into the perivesical space. The perirectal and presacral spaces can also be affected in more complex ruptures.
- **Perivesical hematoma.** An "hourglass" appearance of the bladder may be seen.

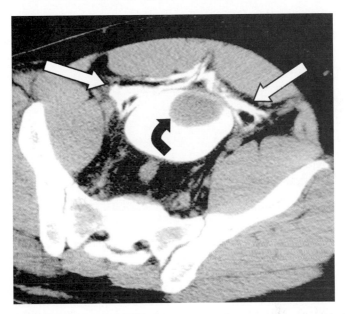

Figure 42-3. Extraperitoneal bladder rupture on retrograde computed tomographic (CT) cystogram. There is contrast extravasation into the perivesicular space (*straight arrows*). Blood clot seen within the bladder (*curved arrow*).

Further Readings

Dunnick NR, Sandler CM, Newhouse JH, et al. *Textbook of uroradiology*, 3rd ed. Philadelphia: Lippincott Williams & Wilkins, 2003:451–483.

Jeffrey RB. Multidetector CT in blunt thoracoabdominal trauma. In: Fishman EK, Jeffrey RB, eds. *Multidetector CT: principles, techniques, and clinical applications.* Philadelphia: Lippincott Williams & Wilkins, 2004:533–547.

Mirvis SE. Injuries to the urinary system and retroperitoneum. In: Mirvis SE, Shanmuganathan K, eds. *Imaging in trauma and critical care*, 2nd ed. Philadelphia: WB Saunders, 2003:483–517.

Morey AF, Iverson AJ, Swan A, et al. Bladder rupture after blunt trauma: guidelines for diagnostic imaging. *J Trauma* 2001;51:683–686.

Rosenstein D, McAninch JW. Urologic emergencies. *Med Clin N Am* 2004;88:495–518.

Schneider RE. Genitourinary system. In: Marx JA, Hockberger RS, Walls RM, eds. *Rosen's emergency medicine: concepts and clinical practice*, 5th ed. St. Louis: Mosby, 2002:437–456.

Vaccaro JP, Brody JM. CT cystography in the evaluation of major bladder trauma. *Radiographics* 2000;20:1373–1381.

Zagoria RJ. *Genitourinary radiology: the requisites*, 2nd ed. Philadelphia: Mosby, 2004: 201–255.

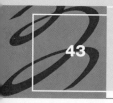

ECTOPIC PREGNANCY
Claire S. Cooney and Loralie D. Ma

CLINICAL INFORMATION

Etiology and Epidemiology. Ectopic pregnancy is the implantation of a fertilized ovum outside of the endometrial cavity. The incidence of ectopic pregnancy plateaued in the early 1990s at approximately 19 per 1,000 pregnancies, by the most recent estimates from the Centers for Disease Control and Prevention. The death rate from ectopic pregnancy has declined by approximately 90% since 1979 likely due to earlier detection. The cause of ectopic implantation of the zygote is hypothesized to be delayed transit of the zygote secondary to abnormal fallopian tubes, which may have abnormal angulation or adhesions from inflammation or previous surgery. Risk factors include previous pelvic surgery, history of pelvic inflammatory disease, previous ectopic pregnancy, diethylstilbestrol (DES) exposure, prior tubal ligation, ovulation induction, *in vitro* fertilization, and intrauterine device. In most ectopic pregnancies, rupture occurs at or before the eighth week of gestation. Rupture in cornual (interstitial) pregnancies and abdominal pregnancies can occur later (8–10 weeks), often with life-threatening hemorrhage.

Location

■ **Tubal:** 95% of ectopic pregnancies (ampullary + isthmic = 92%)
  • Ampullary portion—closest to the ovary.
  • Isthmic portion—middle portion of the fallopian tube.
  • Cornual or interstitial portion—at or near the junction of the fallopian tube with the uterus (3%).

■ **Other:** 5% of ectopic pregnancies
  • Abdominal.
  • Ovarian.
  • Interligamentary.
  • Cervical.

Symptoms and Signs. The classic presentation, seen in less than 50% of patients, consists of (1) abnormal vaginal bleeding (75%), (2) pelvic pain, and (3) palpable adnexal mass in the setting of a positive ß-human chorionic gonadotropin (ß-hCG). Other clinical signs include secondary amenorrhea, a positive ß-hCG that does not rise greater than 66% in 48 hours (with intrauterine pregnancy [IUP], levels roughly double every 48 hours), and falling hematocrit or shock.

IMAGING WITH ULTRASONOGRAPHY

Indications. Initial evaluation for suspected ectopic pregnancy (vaginal bleeding with or without pelvic pain) in a patient with a positive ß-hCG.

Protocol. Transabdominal scan with full bladder, then endovaginal examination after bladder is emptied. A Foley catheter may be placed to facilitate adequate bladder filling.

Possible Findings. The main question to be answered is whether an IUP is present. Some normal sonographic "milestones" are given in Table 43-1. The following is a list of

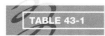

	Sonographic Milestones Expected in Normal Pregnancy (Endovaginal Examination)	
Finding	**May be seen**	**Must be seen**
Intrauterine gestation sac	Quantitative serum ß-hCG ≥800 IU	Quantitative serum ß-hCG ≥1,800 IU
Yolk sac	Gestational sac ≥4 mm	Gestational sac ≥10 mm
Fetal pole	Gestational sac ≥8 mm	Gestational sac ≥18 mm
Heartbeat	Crown-rump length >2 mm	Crown-rump length ≥5 mm

ß-hCG, ß-human chorionic gonadotropin.

the possible sonographic appearances and the meaning of each, given a positive ß-hCG (unless otherwise indicated, all mean sac diameters in the subsequent text refer to the endovaginal examination):

- **Normal pelvic ultrasonography (US) with no IUP or adnexal masses.** Differential diagnosis includes ectopic pregnancy, early IUP, or complete spontaneous abortion (if vaginal bleeding is present). A negative US result does not rule out ectopic pregnancy. Follow-up with serial ß-hCG and possibly follow-up US should be suggested. ß-hCG doubles every 2–3 days in early pregnancy (first 60 days) with a normal gestation, and rises less for ectopic pregnancy, and decreases following spontaneous abortion. If the quantitative serum ß-hCG is equal to or greater than 1,800 IU (Second International Standard), a gestational sac should normally be seen within the uterus (Table 43-1). Endovaginal visualization of the fetus is possible as early as 4.5 weeks after last menstrual period (LMP).
- **Decidual reaction.** Refers to the endometrial thickening that normally occurs in pregnancy. Unless an IUP is identified, the differential diagnosis of this finding is the same as that for a normal pelvic US, as discussed in the preceding text. Decidual reaction with anechoic fluid in the center from bleeding may mimic a gestational sac ("pseudogestational sac"). In approximately 85% of normal pregnancies, the three layers of the decidual reaction can be seen forming the "double decidual ring" appearance. Again, this does not influence the differential diagnosis unless an IUP is identified.
- **Saclike structure within uterus without an IUP.** The differential diagnosis is early IUP, ectopic pregnancy, or incomplete abortion. The latter two diagnoses are favored if the sac is distorted. A fetal pole should be visualized by transabdominal US when the sac size is 25 mm or by endovaginal US when the sac size is 18 mm. Watch out for the pseudogestational sac.
- **IUP.** Is confirmed if a yolk sac, fetal pole, or fetal heart motion is identified within a gestational sac. An IUP effectively rules out ectopic pregnancy, although it is possible for ectopic and IUP to coexist (incidence 1:7,000).
- **Cul-de-sac fluid.** Moderate cul-de-sac fluid, especially if the fluid is complex, raises the suspicion of a ruptured ectopic pregnancy, even if no mass is seen. In such cases, it is useful to check for ascites and determine the extent of intraperitoneal fluid. A small amount of cul-de-sac fluid is not unusual in normal patients.
- **Adnexal mass.** Given a positive ß-hCG, is highly suspicious for ectopic pregnancy. Even higher suspicion and specificity should be expressed if the adnexal mass is associated with pelvic fluid, an anechoic center, apparent gestational sac, or fetal heart motion (Fig. 43-1). Fetal heart motion within an adnexal mass is the only sign with 100% specificity, but it is not commonly seen in an ectopic pregnancy.
- **Eccentrically placed gestational sac near cornu.** If a gestational sac is near the junction of the uterus and fallopian tube and is incompletely surrounded by the myometrial muscle layer, interstitial ectopic pregnancy must be considered. This entity is important to recognize because it often presents later (up to 17 weeks gestational age) with life-threatening hemorrhage due to its relationship to the uterine blood supply.

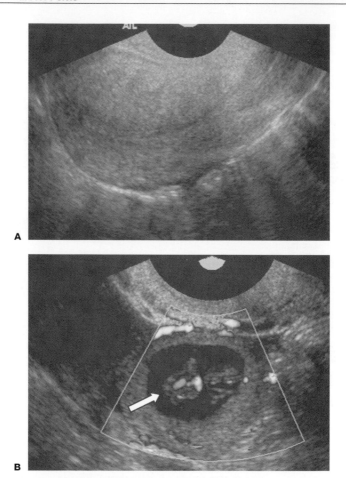

A

B

Figure 43-1. **A:** Endovaginal ultrasonography (US) demonstrates absence of an intrauterine pregnancy. **B:** Power Doppler endovaginal examination of right adnexa shows a vascular cystic lesion with a fetal pole (*arrow*), compatible with ectopic pregnancy, corresponding to location of pain.

- **Complete extrauterine fetus and placenta** indicate an abdominal ectopic pregnancy. In these rare cases, the uterus is externally compressed by the gestation and the uterine wall cannot be seen to separate the gestation from the bladder or abdominal wall.
- **Doppler US findings.** Increased blood flow around an adnexal or pelvic mass is highly suggestive of ectopic pregnancy.

DIFFERENTIAL DIAGNOSIS

- **Spontaneous abortion:** especially if there has been heavy bleeding and cramping, and the pelvic US is essentially normal with no IUP, adnexal mass, or significant free fluid. The patient is usually followed up with serial quantitative ß-hCG, which should decrease, and possibly a followup US.
- **Incomplete abortion/abortion in progress:** an intrauterine gestation that appears abnormally low within the uterus, especially if the cervical canal is open, or if the IUP contents

appear abnormal. Usually this is followed clinically with serial quantitative ß-hCG and follow-up US.

- **Embryonic or fetal death in utero:** An IUP without fetal heart motion. There may be obvious breakdown of fetal tissue. Treatment is with dilatation and curettage (D&C). In the past, this condition was poorly termed a *missed abortion*. Fetal demise is indicated by the following: crown-rump length (CRL) greater than 5 mm and no cardiac activity; mean sac diameter equal to or greater than 10 mm and no yolk sac; mean sac diameter equal to or greater than 18 mm and no embryo; or absent yolk sac in the presence of embryo. Additionally, if the heart rate is less than or equal to 85 bpm at 5–8 weeks, a spontaneous abortion is likely.
- **Anembryonic gestation or blighted ovum:** Gestational sac without development of a fetal pole. Usual treatment is with D&C.
- **Fluid within small bowel loops:** Watch for peristalsis!
- **Eccentrically placed IUP in a retroflexed or fibroid uterus.**
- Many other entities, such as hemorrhagic corpus luteum, ruptured or torsed ovarian cyst, endometrioma, or hydrosalpinx, can have similar presentations and sonographic findings as ectopic pregnancy, but all of these are *not* associated with a positive ß-hCG.

 PITFALLS

Although heterotopic pregnancies (concomitant IUP and ectopic) are rare, occurring in 1 in 7,000 pregnancies, the incidence is increasing due to assisted reproductive techniques.

An early IUP can present with a corpus luteum (which may look like an ectopic) and no intrauterine findings. Correlate with serial ß-hCG levels and possibly follow-up US. If a diagnosis of ectopic pregnancy is made, the patient will be treated with methotrexate and will lose the pregnancy.

Up to 56% of ectopic pregnancies treated with methotrexate may present for follow-up US with enlarging ectopic gestational masses. In asymptomatic women with declining ß-hCG levels, these findings are believed to represent hematomas rather than persistent trophoblastic tissue.

 ISSUES AFTER IMAGING

Medical Treatment.   Methotrexate has become the treatment of choice for early, uncomplicated ectopic pregnancies. The success rate in appropriately selected women ranges from 86–94%. Women with the most success from medical therapy are asymptomatic with ß-hCG levels less than 5,000 IU, ectopic size less than 3–4 cm, and no fetal cardiac activity. Contraindications to medical therapy include ß-hCG level greater than 15,000 IU, fetal cardiac activity, and ruptured ectopic. However, one recent study has shown medical therapy success in cases with fetal heartbeat.

Surgical Treatment.   Laparoscopic salpingostomy is the surgical treatment of choice if the patient is not a candidate for medical therapy. Salpingectomy should be performed if there is uncontrolled bleeding, recurrent ectopic in the same fallopian tube, severely damaged tube, or tubal pregnancy larger than 5 cm.

Further Readings

Campbell J. *Clinical sonography: a practical guide*, 2nd ed. Boston: Little Brown and company, 1991:69–87.

Lipscomb GH, Stovall TG, Ling FW. Nonsurgical treatment of ectopic pregnancy. *N Engl J Med* 2000;343:1325–1329.

Middleton W, Kurtz A, Hertzberg B. *The requisites: ultrasound*, 2nd ed. Missouri: Mosby, 2004:357–371.

Yao M, Tulandi T. Current status of surgical and non-surgical treatment of ectopic pregnancy. *Fertil Steril* 1997;67:421.

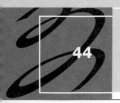

OVARIAN TORSION
Claire S. Cooney

Ovarian torsion is the twisting of the ovary on its ligamentous attachments causing vascular compromise. It is an uncommon event, but accounts for 3% of all gynecologic operative emergencies and can have significant adverse sequelae. Symptoms can be vague, and therefore imaging is crucial for prompt diagnosis and treatment to avoid irreparable damage to the ovary.

 CLINICAL INFORMATION

Etiology. Twisting of the ovarian pedicle leads to compromise of lymphatic and venous drainage, causing the ovary to become enlarged and edematous. Next, ovarian ischemia can occur due to compromise of arterial flow, resulting in infarction, necrosis, and hemorrhage. Risk factors include an ovarian mass, pregnancy, and ovarian hyperstimulation syndrome.

Symptoms and Signs. The classic clinical scenario is a woman of childbearing age who presents with acute onset of lower abdominal pain associated with nausea and vomiting. The clinical presentation can include one or more of the following:

- Unilateral pelvic or lower abdominal pain (right more common than left), possibly intermittent, and usually acute in onset (in contrast to slowly developing migratory pain of appendicitis).
- Nausea and vomiting can occur during episodes of pain.
- Peritoneal signs.
- Ascites—hemorrhagic, inflammatory, or transudative.
- Fever—rare and may be due to ovarian necrosis.

Clinical workup must include a careful pelvic examination before imaging, as the presence of an adnexal mass dramatically increases possibility of torsion. ß- human chorionic gonadotropin (ß-hCG) is required for premenopausal patients.

Differential Diagnosis. If the ß-hCG is positive, ectopic pregnancy must be considered. If it is negative, appendicitis, pelvic inflammatory disease, tubo-ovarian abscess, endometriosis, degenerating fibroid, hemorrhagic cyst, gastroenteritis, intussusception, diverticulitis, and menstrual cramping are in the differential diagnosis.

 IMAGING WITH ULTRASONOGRAPHY

Indications. Ultrasonography is the examination of choice for the diagnosis of ovarian torsion because it can accurately and rapidly differentiate ovarian torsion from other pelvic disorders that have the same nonspecific clinical presentation.

Protocol. Transabdominal scan with full bladder, then endovaginal examination with color Doppler after bladder is emptied. A Foley catheter may be placed to facilitate adequate bladder filling. Both adnexa should be examined.

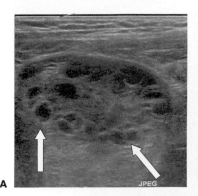
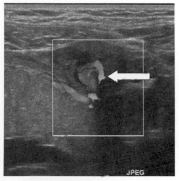

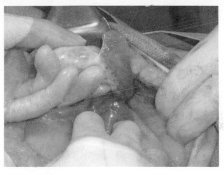

Figure 44-1. **A:** Transabdominal ultrasonography (US) demonstrates enlarged left ovary that was tender during the examination. Multiple peripheral follicles (*arrows*) were seen in the ovary, suggesting edema. **B:** Doppler US demonstrates "twisted pedicle sign" (*arrow*) consistent with torsion. **C:** Diagnosis was confirmed during laparotomy.

Possible Findings (Fig. 44-1)

- Enlarged hypoechoic ovary due to congestion, edema, and interstitial hemorrhage. If the ovary is normal in size (2 × 3 × 4 cm) and echogenicity, torsion is very unlikely.
- Mass in ovaries or adnexa, often greater than 4 cm.
- Prominent peripheral follicles due to ovarian parenchymal edema.
- Diminished or absent venous and arterial flow on color Doppler.
- "Twisted pedicle" sign on color Doppler, showing distended twisting vessels leading to the ovary.
- Abnormal location of the ovary.
- Hyperechoic areas in ovary due to hemorrhage.
- Free fluid in the pelvic cul-de-sac.
- Normal or hyperemic ovary in intermittent torsion.

 IMAGING WITH COMPUTED TOMOGRAPHY

Indications. Computed tomography (CT) should not be used as the primary imaging modality in evaluation for ovarian torsion. However, it is commonly used for evaluation of acute abdominal pain and therefore may suggest presence of ovarian torsion.

Protocol. Intravenous (IV) and oral contrast are typically used as part of a standard abdominal CT protocol and are useful in the evaluation for other pathology.

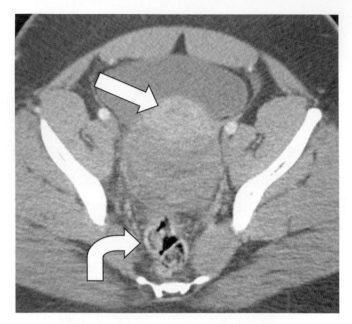

Figure 44-2. Contrast-enhanced computed tomography (CT) scan demonstrates a hypodense mass between the uterus (*straightarrow*) and the rectum (*curved arrow*). This is a common location and appearance of torsed ovary. Courtesy of Kenneth Wang, MD, Johns Hopkins Hospital.

Possible Findings (Fig. 44-2)

- Mass in the ovary or adnexa.
- Enlarged (>2 ×3 × 4 cm), hypodense ovary due to edema.
- Engorged blood vessels.
- Stranding surrounding the ovary.
- Absence of enhancement of the affected ovary due to vascular compromise.
- Abnormal location of the ovary.
- Ascites.
- Hematoma (attenuation dependent on age).

 IMAGING WITH MAGNETIC RESONANCE

Indications.   Magnetic resonance imaging (MRI) should not be used for evaluation of suspected ovarian torsion. However, MRI plays an important role in evaluation of ovarian masses and may suggest presence of ovarian torsion.

Protocol.   Typical pelvic MRI protocols include axial T1-weighted; axial, coronal, and sagittal T2-weighted sequences. Fat suppressed T1- and T2-weighted sequences can help differentiate blood products from fat in dermoids. Pre- and postgadolinium axial T1-weighted imaging can help detect malignancy or inflammatory disease.

Possible Findings

- Mass in the ovary or adnexa.
- Enlarged ovary (>2 ×3 × 4 cm).
- Edema adjacent to the ovary (high T2 and low T1 signal).

- Thick, straight vessels draping around the affected ovary.
- Absence of enhancement of the affected ovary.
- Abnormal location of the ovary.
- Ascites.
- Hemorrhage (signal characteristics depend on age).

 ## PITFALLS

Ovarian blood flow on color Doppler ultrasound is not a reliable marker for definitive diagnosis of torsion. Diminished or absent flow on Doppler ultrasound increases the likelihood of torsion. The presence of arterial flow does not exclude torsion.

With intermittent torsion, the ovaries may appear normal on ultrasonography, CT, or MRI. Additionally, color Doppler may show a hyperemic ovary compared to the contralateral side.

 ## ISSUES AFTER IMAGING

Ovarian torsion is a surgical emergency. If the torsed ovary is not necrotic, surgical detorsion and oophoropexy should be performed.

Further Readings

Cohen HL, Sivit CJ. *Fetal and pediatric ultrasound*. McGraw-Hill, 2001:516–519.

Dolgin SE. Acute ovarian torsion in children. *Am J Surg* 2002;183–195.

Kimura I, Togashi K, Kawakami S, et al. Ovarian torsion: CT and MR imaging appearances. *Radiology* 1994;190:337–341.

Semelka RC. *Abdominal—pelvic MRI*. New York: Wiley-Liss, 2002.

Sivit CJ. Imaging children with acute right lower quadrant abdominal pain. *Pediatr Clin North Am* 1997;44:586.

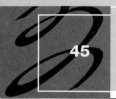

PELVIC FRACTURES
Visveshwar Baskaran

45

$\mathcal{T}$raumatic injuries of the pelvis encompass a heterogeneous group of lesions, which vary widely in mechanism. Rapid recognition of bony and soft tissue abnormalities, determination of pelvic stability, and classification of injury pattern is essential in guiding appropriate therapeutic intervention.

 CLINICAL INFORMATION

Mechanisms. Pelvic fractures resulting from high-energy trauma such as motor vehicle accidents are increasingly common and can result in disruption of the pelvic ring at multiple sites. Earlier classification systems attempted to separate stable injuries from unstable injuries. Recently, classification systems based on mechanism have been advocated, dividing fractures into those due to anteroposterior (AP) compression, lateral compression, or vertical shear (Fig. 45-1). Acetabular fractures often occur with traumatic posterior hip dislocations (i.e., knee striking dashboard) or lateral compression injury, and are divided into elementary or associated fracture types (Fig. 45-2). Isolated pelvic fractures may occur from sports injuries (avulsion or direct pelvic impact). Avulsion fractures result from intense sudden pulling of a tendon on its apophyseal insertion site, such as the anterior superior iliac spine (sartorius), anterior inferior iliac spine (rectus femoris), ischial tuberosity (hamstring muscles), and pubis (adductors). Insufficiency fractures occur in elderly osteoporotic patients, most commonly affecting the pubis and sacral ala.

Symptoms and Signs. In the setting of acute massive blunt trauma, pelvic ring disruptions should be suspected if the following are present:

- Physical examination findings such as lacerations, contusions, evidence of crush injury, or pelvic ring instability on palpation.
- Hemodynamic instability from pelvic hemorrhage.
- Blood at urethral meatus—genitourinary injury often associated with anterior pelvic fracture.
- Pelvic pain.
- Gait abnormality.
- Neurologic deficits from injury to lumbosacral plexus, most commonly L5 and S1.

Differential Diagnosis. The major differential diagnosis is soft tissue trauma and hemorrhage without fracture. All of the secondary signs listed in the preceding text may be present even when a fracture is not present.

 IMAGING WITH RADIOGRAPHS

Indications. Excellent initial examination before proceeding to computed tomography (CT); identifies nearly all *clinically important* fractures and dislocations; can be performed while patient is being stabilized.

Protocol. AP pelvis. Inlet and outlet views (allows identification of subtle pubic or sacral neural foraminal fractures). Coned oblique views of ilium or obturator ring (if suspected

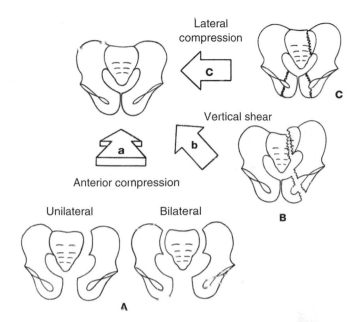

Figure 45-1. Mechanisms of pelvic fracture. *Arrows a,b,* and *c* denote external forces and diagrams *A, B,* and *C* denote resultant fractures. (Reprinted with permission from Rogers LF, Hendrix RW. Chapter 121: fractures of the pelvis. In: Taveras JM, Ferrucci JT, eds. *Radiology: diagnosis/imaging/intervention,* Vol. 5. Philadelphia: JB Lippincott Co, 1991:2. Figure 1.)

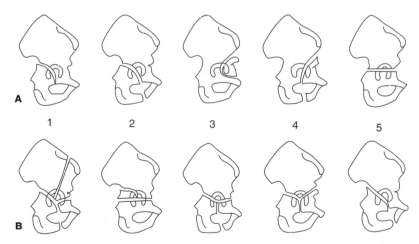

Figure 45-2. Classification of acetabular fractures. Top row **(A)** depicts elementary fractures: 1 = posterior wall fracture, 2 = posterior column fracture, 3 = anterior wall fracture, 4 = anterior column fracture, 5 = transverse fracture. Bottom row **(B)** depicts associated fractures: 1 = two-column fracture, 2 = transverse-posterior wall fracture, 3 = T-type fracture, 4 = anterior wall posterior hemitransverse fracture, 5 = posterior column posterior wall fracture. (Reprinted with permission from Neumann NH, Verdon JP, Moushine E, et al. Traumatic injuries: imaging of pelvic fractures. *Emerg Radiol* 2002;12:1324, Springer-Verlag. Figure 23.)

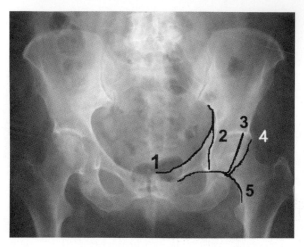

Figure 45-3. Pelvic Line: (1) Iliopectenial, (2) Ilioischeal, (3) Anterior acetabular rim, (4) Posterior acetabular rim, (5) Shenton's arcuate line.

fracture not seen on previous views). Coned AP, lateral, caudad, and cephalad angled views of sacrum (if sacral fracture suspected but not seen on previous views). Coned AP and Judet (right and left posterior oblique) views of acetabulum (if acetabular fracture suspected).

Possible Findings

■ Cortical discontinuity and loss of normal lines and contours (Fig. 45-3).
  • Iliopectineal line—from sciatic notch to pubic symphysis along superior pubic ramus.
  • Ilioischial line—from sciatic notch to medial margin of ischium.
  • Obturator ring.
  • Pelvic "teardrop" at medial margin of acetabulum.
■ Thickening of obturator muscle due to hematoma.
■ Soft tissue density in pelvis (fluid or blood) displacing bowel loops superiorly.
■ Pelvic ring disruption (multiple fractures common in ring structures such as the pelvis).
■ Diastasis of the symphysis pubis (normal <5 mm).
■ Diastasis of sacroiliac joints (normal 2–4 mm).
■ Loss of symmetric sacral arcuate lines due to fracture of bony neural foramina.
■ Acetabular fracture (Fig. 45-4).
  • Elementary. Anterior column, posterior column, anterior wall, posterior wall, and transverse.
  • Associated. Two-column, transverse-posterior wall, T-type, anterior column posterior hemitransverse, posterior column posterior wall.
  • Most common. Posterior wall, transverse with posterior wall, and two-column fractures.

IMAGING WITH COMPUTED TOMOGRAPHY

Indications. CT can identify fractures that are not seen on plain radiographs or can further define the extent of fractures diagnosed on radiograph.

Other Specific Situations

■ Inadequate history or physical examination.
■ Suspicion of sacral fracture or sacroiliac joint diastasis.

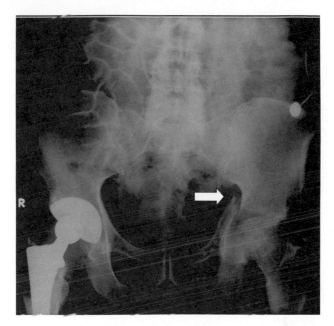

Figure 45-4. Anteroposterior (AP) radiograph of the pelvis demonstrates anterior column acetabular fracture (arrow).

- Suspicion of unstable pelvic fracture.
- Hip dislocations.
- Acetabular fractures.
- Single pelvic ring fracture.

Protocol. Noncontrast axial CT of the pelvis with coronal and sagittal reconstructions should be performed. Three-dimensional (3D) volume rendering techniques can be helpful for surgical planning. Noncontrast CT is sufficient for detection of pelvic fractures; however, if vascular injury is suspected, pelvic CT arteriography may be performed at the same time. Oral or rectal (water soluble) contrast may be used if gastrointestinal tract injury is suspected.

Possible Findings

- Cortical discontinuity or irregularity in pelvic ring.
- Diastasis of symphysis pubis or sacroiliac joints.
- Paired fractures of pelvic ring.
- Acetabular fracture—elementary and associated fracture patterns as noted in the preceding text.
- Hematoma associated with fractures.
- Perforation of bowel or urinary tract with extraluminal contrast or air.
- Other soft tissue injury or solid organ laceration.

 OTHER IMAGING TESTS

- **Arteriography indications.** (1) Hemodynamic instability despite external pelvic fixation or fluid resuscitation, (2) other bleeding sources (intra-abdominal, intrathoracic, and intracranial) excluded, or (3) treatment by embolization desired. Most commonly, the hemorrhage is from the superior gluteal, iliolumbar, pudendal, or obturator arteries.

■ **Retrograde urethrography indications.** (1) Severe anterior pelvic trauma; (2) blood at urethral meatus or at vaginal introitus in women; or (3) before Foley catheterization (see Chap. 42, "Bladder and Ureteral Injury" and Chap. 60, "Retrograde Urethrogram").

■ **Conventional retrograde or CT cystography indications.** Suspicion of bladder injury. Small bladder tears are best seen on early filling views and slow bladder leaks are best seen on delayed views (see Chap. 42, "Bladder and Ureteral Injury" and Chap. 61, "Voiding Cystourethrogram (VCUG)").

■ **Excretory urography (intravenous pyelogram [IVP]) indications.** Suspicion of bladder, ureteral, or renal trauma not already diagnosed. The IVP should follow retrograde urethrography or cystography (see Chap. 42, "Bladder and Ureteral Injury").

Further Readings

Buckwalter KA, Farber JM. Application of multidetector CT in skeletal trauma. *Semin Musculoskelet Radiol* 2004;8:147–156.

Cwinn AA. Pelvis. In: Marx JA, Hockberger RS, Walls RM, eds. *Rosen's emergency medicine: concepts and clinical practice*, 5th ed. St. Louis: Mosby, 2002:626–642.

Hak DJ. The role of pelvic angiography in evaluation and management of pelvic trauma. *Orthop Clin N Am* 2004;35:439–443.

Jeffrey RB. Multidetector CT in blunt thoracoabdominal trauma. In: Fishman EK, Jeffrey RB, eds. *Multidetector CT: principles, techniques, and clinical applications.* Philadelphia: Lippincott Williams & Wilkins, 2004:533–547.

Mirvis SE. Injuries to the urinary system and retroperitoneum. In: Mirvis SE, Shanmuganathan K, eds. *Imaging in trauma and critical care*, 2nd ed. Philadelphia: WB Saunders, 2003:483–517.

Mirza A, Ellis R. Initial management of pelvic and femoral fractures in the multiply injured patient. *Crit Care Clin* 2004;20:159–170.

Schaefer-Prokop C, vonSmekal U, van der Molen AJ. Musculoskeletal system. In: Prokop M, Galanski M, eds. *Spiral and multislice computed tomography of the body.* Stuttgart: Thieme Medical Publishers, 2003:962–967.

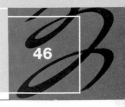

TESTICULAR TORSION

46

Karen M. Horton and George P. Kuo

$\mathcal{T}$esticular torsion is a surgical emergency. Infarction can occur as soon as 4 hours after the onset of symptoms; however, if the degree of torsion is low, the testes can stay viable for as long as 24 hours. In general, surgical intervention within 6 hours of the onset of symptoms is preferred.

CLINICAL INFORMATION

Etiology and Epidemiology. The normal testis (Fig. 46-1) is surrounded by the tunica vaginalis which is anchored posteriorly to the epididymis and scrotal wall. The testicular artery, the major blood supply to the testicle, runs in the spermatic cord. However, in some males, the tunica vaginalis surrounds the entire testis and inserts high on the spermatic cord. This anomaly is called a *bell clapper deformity* (Fig. 46-2) and predisposes to rotation of the testis within the tunica vaginalis, thereby twisting the spermatic cord and compromising blood flow to the testicle. Although testicular torsion can occur at any age, most cases occur in males around puberty (age 12–18). There is a second peak in early childhood.

Clinical History. Acute onset of severe unilateral scrotal pain, often accompanied by nausea and vomiting. The pain can be referred to the lower abdomen or thigh. The vast majority of cases of testicular torsion occur spontaneously. History of possible precipitating events such as strenuous exercise or trauma is elicited in <5% of cases. There is sometimes a history of similar episodes in the past that are presumably related to previous torsion and spontaneous resolution.

Laboratory Studies. Urinalysis almost always negative. There is usually no leucocytosis early on. Possible low-grade fever.

Physical Examination. Early on, the testis is firm and often located high within the scrotal sac. The epididymis is usually not located in its usual posterior position, unless the testicle has torsed 360 or 720 degrees. Later, the hemiscrotum swells and becomes erythematous. If not diagnosed and surgically corrected, torsion leads to ischemic necrosis and atrophy of the testicle. The unaffected testis may be positioned transversely within the scrotum, indicating a bell clapper deformity.

    Differential diagnosis of acute scrotal pain includes testicular torsion, torsion of the testes appendage (müllerian duct remnant), epididymitis, orchitis, and less commonly incarcerated inguinal hernia, vasculitis, and tumor. Testicular torsion and torsion of the appendage testes account for more than 90% of cases of acute onset of scrotal pain in the appropriate age group. Epididymitis and orchitis are the most common causes of painful scrotal swelling in an adult and are typically gradual in onset and accompanied by fever, urethral discharge, urinary tract symptoms, and a positive urinalysis. They typically result from an ascending infection of the urinary tract, sexually transmitted disease in younger men, and prostatitis in older men.

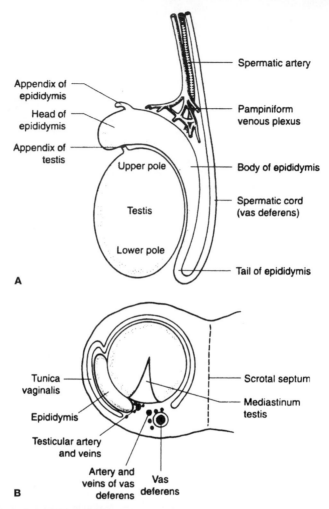

Figure 46-1. Anatomy of the testis and scrotum. Anatomy is shown in **(A)** longitudinal section and **(B)** transverse section. (Reprinted with permission from Ryan SP, McNicholas MMJ. *Anatomy for diagnostic imaging*. Philadelphia: WB Saunders, 1994:223, Fig. 6.16.)

 IMAGING WITH COLOR DOPPLER ULTRASOUND

Indications.   Ultrasonography is a fast, accurate, noninvasive imaging modality which allows direct visualization of the testicle and its blood flow. Sensitivity is 80–90% and specificity is 90–100%.

Protocol.   High-frequency linear transducer (7.5 or 10 MHz). Support the scrotum with your hand or a towel. Image the testicle in both the longitudinal and transverse planes. Try to obtain a coronal view of both testicles simultaneously, with and without color Doppler, in order to compare echotexture and blood flow.

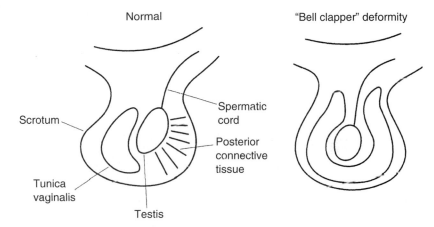

Figure 46-2. "Bell clapper" deformity. Normally, the testis is tethered posteriorly by connective tissue. In the "bell clapper" deformity, the tunica vaginalis surrounds the testis, allowing the testis and spermatic cord to swing freely. (Reprinted with permission from Datz H *Handbook of nuclear medicine*, 2nd ed. St. Louis: Mosby-Year Book, 1993:179, Fig. 6-2.)

Possible Findings

- Enlarged hypoechoic heterogeneous testis and epididymis (Fig. 46-3). A normal testis measures approximately 3 × 5 cm and is homogeneously echogenic; the normal epididymis is located posteriorly and is a relatively echopenic tubular structure.
- Decreased or absent color Doppler signal in comparison to the normal contralateral testis (Fig. 46-4). Check both arterial and venous flow, as venous flow may be compromised first.
- Rim of hypervascularity around the torsed testis due to preserved flow to the scrotal wall through pudendal artery branches.
- Enlarged spermatic cord.
- Scrotal skin thickening.
- Infarcted testicle will appear small and echogenic without detectable flow.
- Hydrocele.

Imaging Tips for Ultrasonography

- Optimize the machine settings by examining the normal testicle first.
- Make sure the Doppler gain and velocity scale is set exactly the same when comparing the testicles.
- The asymptomatic contralateral testicle is not always normal because the bell clapper deformity is bilateral. Occasionally, the patient will have evidence of old torsion or infarction on the contralateral side.
- Ultrasonographic findings of an enlarged hypoechoic testis with decreased blood flow may be indistinguishable from a hypoechoic tumor involving the entire testicle. The clinical presentation and physical examination are helpful in distinguishing torsion from tumor.
- *Missed* torsion refers to a situation where symptoms have been present for more than 24 hours and the testicle is irreversibly damaged. The opportunity to save the testis has been "missed."
- A testicle needs to twist 540 degrees to compromise both arterial and venous flow acutely. A twist <540 degrees will primarily compress veins. This has been referred to as a *partial torsion*. However, a partial torsion will become complete when distended veins compress arterial flow.

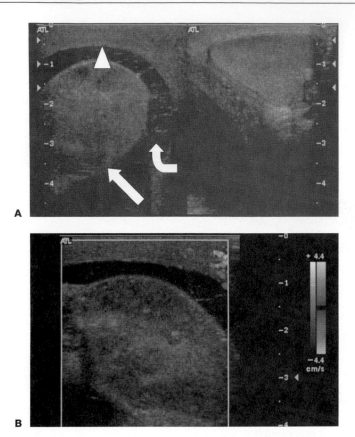

A

B

Figure 46-3. A: Ultrasonography (US) demonstrates enlarged heterogeneous right testicle (*arrow*), complex hydrocele (*curved arrow*), and right scrotal skin thickening (*arrowheads*) suggestive of torsion. However, similar appearance may be seen in infection or tumor. **B:** Absence of vascular flow on color Doppler is highly suggestive of testicular torsion. Testicular infarction due to orchitis can occasionally have the same appearance. Courtesy of Katarzyna Macura MD, Johns Hopkins Hospital.

- In acute epididymitis, the epididymis appears enlarged and more echopenic with increased vascularity. In chronic epididymitis, the epididymis will be small and echogenic, and may contain calcifications.
- Orchitis is an infection of all or part of the testicle and results in an enlarged and less echogenic testicle with increased vascularity.
- Fractured testis following trauma have irregular borders with echopenic regions throughout. Echogenic blood (hematocele) will also be present.

 IMAGING WITH NUCLEAR MEDICINE

Indications. Accurate and relatively fast imaging method used to detect decreased blood flow to a torsed testis. Sensitivity is 96% and specificity is 98%.

Protocol. Adult dose is 20–30 mCi ^{99m}Technetium (^{99m}Tc) pertechnetate given intravenously. Place a lead shield below the scrotum to decrease background activity from the

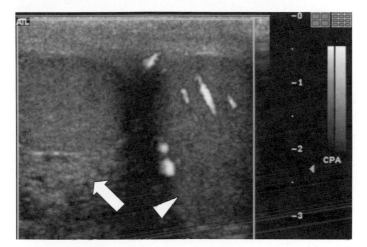

Figure 46-4. There is reduced perfusion of the right testicle (*arrow*) in comparison to the other side (*arrowhead*) on power Doppler ultrasound (US) cleavage view. This is compatible with torsion. Normal echogenicity of the torsed testicle increases likelihood of viability. Courtesy of Katarzyna Macura MD, Johns Hopkins Hospital.

thighs. Tape the penis cephalad to the lower abdominal wall so that its vascularity will not be superimposed on the scrotum. Center γ-camera on scrotum. Following injection, take immediate dynamic anterior scrotal images every 2 seconds for 1 minute to assess perfusion. Take static anterior scrotal images every 5 minutes for approximately 20 minutes to assess the blood pool and soft tissue uptake.

Possible Findings

- **Perfusion phase:** decreased tracer activity on the affected side compared with the normal testicle (perfusion can be normal early on).
- **Soft tissue phase:** central decreased tracer activity surrounded by rim of increased activity due to preserved flow to the scrotal wall through internal pudendal artery branches.
- Nubbin sign: linear increased activity with abrupt cut-off extending medially from iliac vessels; this represents increased blood flow in spermatic cord above the torsion.

Imaging Tips for Nuclear Medicine

- False positives can occur if a hydrocele or scrotal hernia is present and overlying the testicle.
- Normal or increased testicular perfusion does not rule out the possibility of incomplete torsion or torsion with spontaneous resolution.
- Certain stages of testicular abscess or tumor can have similar findings of decreased central tracer activity with a rim of increased activity.
- Orchitis will appear as diffusely increased radiotracer activity throughout the testicle.
- Epididymitis appears as focally increased activity in the region of the epididymis (often appears comma-shaped).

 ISSUES AFTER IMAGING

Prompt surgical management is indicated to reduce the torsion. Bilateral orchiopexy is performed to prevent future torsion of either testicle. Viability of a torsed testicle is more than 80% if surgical intervention takes place within 4–6 hours of the onset of symptoms.

If the testicle is nonviable at the time of surgery, an orchiectomy of the infarcted testicle is performed followed by orchiopexy of the healthy contralateral testicle.

Further Readings

Datz FL. *Handbook of nuclear medicine*, 2nd ed. St. Louis: Mosby-Year Book, 1993: 176–185.

Mettler FA, Guiberteau MJ. *Essentials of nuclear medicine imaging*, 4th ed. Philadelphia: WB Saunders, 1998.

Middleton WD, Kurtz AB, Hertzberg BS. *Ultrasound: the requisites*, 2nd ed. St. Louis: Mosby, 2004:167–173.

Prater JM, Overdorf BS. Testicular torsion: a surgical emergency. *Am Fam Physician* 1991;44:834–840.

Sanders RC. Possible testicular mass: pain in the testicle. In: Sanders RC, ed. *Clinical sonography: a practical guide*. Philadelphia: Lippincott Williams & Wilkins, 1998:365–372.

Sidhu PS. Clinical and imaging features of testicular torsion: role of ultrasound. *Clin Radiol* 1999;6:343–352.

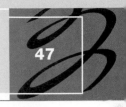

TUBO-OVARIAN ABSCESS

Aimee Lynn Maceda and Satomi Kawamoto

47

*T*ubo-ovarian abscess (TOA) is a serious complication of pelvic inflammatory disease (PID). Rupture of a TOA may cause generalized peritonitis and/or septic shock and is an indication for immediate surgical intervention.

CLINICAL INFORMATION

Mechanism.   PID occurs due to ascending infection from the cervix extending through the endometrial cavity into fallopian tubes and adnexa. The initial infection is usually caused by *Chlamydia trachomatis* or *Neisseria gonorrhoeae*, with subsequent colonization by anaerobes, gram-negative bacteria, and streptococci. Predisposing factors include history of sexually transmitted disease or PID, multiple sexual partners, and presence of intrauterine device (IUD). TOA can be unilateral or bilateral, independent of IUD use.

Signs and Symptoms.   Presentation of TOA is nonspecific and similar to PID, including abdominal or pelvic pain (>90%), fever and leukocytosis (60–80%), vaginal discharge, vaginal bleeding, nausea, cervical motion tenderness, and palpable pelvic mass. Some patients with TOA may be asymptomatic or have mild symptoms. Absence of fever or leukocytosis does not exclude the diagnosis of TOA. Seventy percent of women with PID are younger than 25 years. A white blood cell (WBC) and β-human chorionic gonadotropin (hCG) should be obtained in all patients suspected of having TOA.

Differential Diagnosis.   Differential diagnosis includes hydro- or pyosalpinx, ectopic pregnancy, endometriosis, ovarian neoplasm/cyst, ovarian torsion, appendicitis, and diverticulitis.

IMAGING WITH ULTRASONOGRAPHY

Indication.   Diagnosis of PID should be made on the basis of symptoms, clinical examination, and laboratory tests, not imaging. Imaging is indicated in patients with suspected PID who have a palpable mass, are severely ill and need inpatient therapy, are failing to respond to antibiotic therapy, or whose discomfort prevents an adequate pelvic examination. The primary goal of imaging is to differentiate between TOA and uncomplicated PID, which requires establishing the presence or absence of an inflammatory adnexal mass. Ultrasonography is the imaging test of choice for evaluation of TOA with up to 93% sensitivity and up to 98% specificity.

Protocol.   Transabdominal and endovaginal ultrasonography should be performed. Endovaginal examination has a greater sensitivity and specificity than transabdominal examination alone and must be performed unless the patient's symptoms are unbearable.

Possible Findings in PID without TOA

- Are nonspecific.
- Uterus is slightly enlarged with a prominent endometrial echo. Fluid or purulent material in the uterus may be seen (endometritis).

255

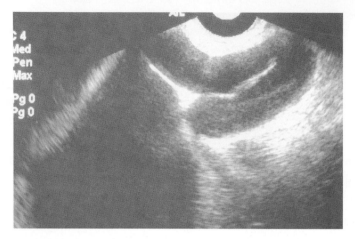

Figure 47-1. Fallopian tube is thickened on endovaginal pelvic ultrasound (US), consistent with salpingitis. Courtesy of Joel Fradin, MD, Johns Hopkins Bayview Hospital.

■ Fallopian tube wall thickening (≥5 mm) and/or hyperemia on color Doppler suggest presence of salpingitis (Fig. 47-1).
■ Fallopian tube dilatation commonly occurs in chronic PID (Fig. 47-2). The dilated tube may contain clear anechoic fluid (hydrosalpinx) or echogenic debris due to pus (pyosalpinx). If the dilated tube is viewed in cross-section, thickened endosalpingeal folds may resemble the "cogwheel sign", seen in up to 86% of patients with acute disease (Fig. 47-3).
■ Fluid in the pelvic cul-de-sac. Complex pelvic fluid with internal echoes, septations, and fluid–fluid levels signify fluid that may be due to infection or hemorrhage.
■ Pelvic pain associated with endovaginal probe motion which may be severe.
■ Ovaries may be enlarged with numerous small cysts (referred to as *polycystic ovary appearance*).

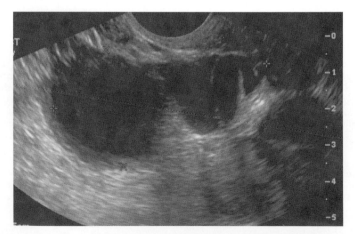

Figure 47-2. Endovaginal pelvic ultrasonography (US) demonstrates dilated tortuous tubular structure consistent with hydrosalpinx. There are minimal internal echoes consistent with minimal debris. Courtesy of Daniel Mollura, MD, Johns Hopkins Hospital.

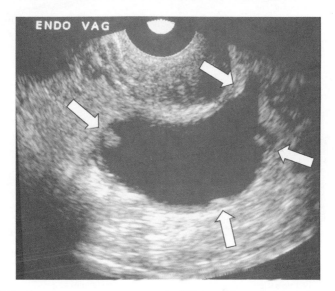

Figure 47-3. Endovaginal pelvic ultrasonography (US) demonstrates dilated tubular structure with "cogwheels" (*arrows*) consistent with hydrosalpinx. Courtesy of Joel Fradin, MD, Johns Hopkins Bayview Hospital.

Possible Findings in Pelvic Inflammatory Disease with Tubo-Ovarian Abscess

- Ultrasonography identifies a mass in greater than 90% of clinically diagnosed TOAs and approaches 100% sensitivity in surgically confirmed TOAs.
- Complex adnexal mass, which can be either unilocular or multilocular. These are typically hypoechoic with acoustic enhancement, irregular borders and thick, ill-defined walls (Fig. 47-4). The sonographic appearance is highly variable—the mass may be predominately cystic or solid. Delineation between the ovary and fallopian tube may become impossible.
- Anechoic and hypoechoic collections usually represent pus.
- Cellular debris with fluid–fluid level, septations, or even gas (dirty shadowing).

 IMAGING WITH COMPUTED TOMOGRAPHY

Indications. CT is not typically used to diagnose TOA and PID. However, CT is commonly performed for evaluation of acute abdominal pain and may suggest presence of TOA or hydrosalpinx. Also, CT can be used for patients in whom ultrasonography fails to provide adequate information, especially to look for other abscess in the abdomen.

Protocol. Intravenous (IV) and oral contrast are used when evaluating possible abdominal or pelvic pathology.

Possible Findings in PID without TOA

- Are nonspecific.
- Cystic tubular adnexal lesions due to hydrosalpinx or pyosalpinx.
- Pelvic inflammatory changes including stranding, haziness/obscuration of pelvic fascial planes, abnormally enhancing and polycystic appearing ovaries, fluid in the endometrial canal, or enlarged, abnormally enhancing cervix.

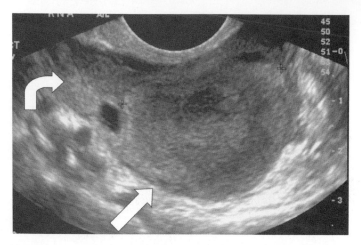

Figure 47-4. Endovaginal pelvic ultrasonography (US) demonstrates a heterogeneous mass (*straight arrow*) with enhanced through transmission, in patient with clinical symptoms of pelvic inflammatory disease (PID), compatible with tubo-ovarian abscess (TOA). The ovary (*curved arrow*) is displaced by the mass. Courtesy of Janet Sailor, MD, Johns Hopkins Hospital.

- Fluid (usually complex) in the pelvic cul-de-sac.
- Adjacent bowel loops may be dilated and fluid filled due to adynamic ileus resulting from inflammation.
- Inflammatory stranding along the right paracolic gutter and inferior right lobe of the liver due to spread of bacteria superiorly from the pelvis, that is, Fitz-Hugh-Curtis syndrome.

Possible Findings in Pelvic Inflammatory Disease with Tubo-Ovarian Abscess

- Tubular or spherical soft tissue mass with central areas of lower attenuation and a thick irregular wall.
- Obliteration of fat planes between the mass and other pelvic structures (involvement of ureter, rectosigmoid colon, urinary bladder, or small bowel). Ipsilateral ureterectasis seen in 56%.
- Abscesses-fluid collections with enhancing peripheral rim, which may contain internal septations, fluid-debris levels, and sometimes gas.

 IMAGING WITH MAGNETIC RESONANCE

Indications.   Magnetic resonance imaging (MRI) can be used as a secondary to help to differentiate TOA and hydrosalpinx from other cystic pelvic masses.

Protocol.   Typical pelvic MRI protocols include axial T1-weighted sequence and axial and coronal T2-weighted sequences. Fat suppressed T1- and T2-weighted sequences can help to differentiate blood products from fat in dermoids. Pre- and postgadolinium axial T1-weighted sequences can help to detect malignancy or inflammatory disease.

Possible Findings in PID without TOA

- Are nonspecific.
- Cystic tubular adnexal lesions due to hydrosalpinx (thin walls) or pyosalpinx (thickened walls) (Fig. 47-5).

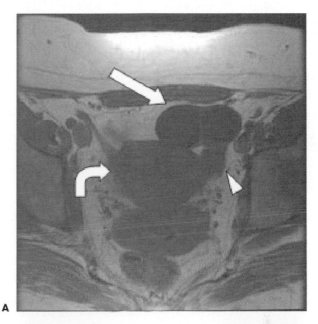

A

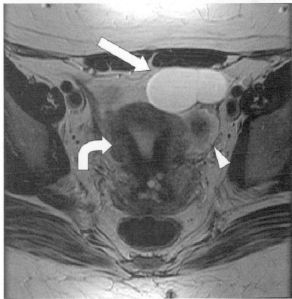

B

Figure 47-5. **A:** T1-weighted and **(B)** T2-weighted axial magnetic resonance imaging (MRI) of the pelvis demonstrate T1 dark and T2 bright tubular structure (*straight arrow*) compatible with hydrosapinx. Uterus (*curved arrow*) and left ovary (*arrowhead*) are seen adjacent to the dilated fallopian tube. Courtesy of David Grand, MD, Johns Hopkins Hospital.

- Pelvic inflammatory changes including soft tissue edema (low T1, high T2 signal), abnormally enhancing and polycystic appearing ovaries, fluid in the endometrial canal, or enlarged, abnormally enhancing cervix.
- Pelvic fluid (usually complex).

Possible Findings in Pelvic Inflammatory Disease with Tubo-Ovarian Abscess

- Ill-defined adnexal mass with thick, irregular walls containing fluid (occasionally internal septa or gas).
- Fluid collections with enhancing peripheral rim, which may contain internal septations and fluid-debris levels.

 ## ISSUES AFTER IMAGING

If clinically stable, patients can be treated with broad-spectrum antibiotics that include anaerobic coverage. Medical therapy is successful in up to 75% of cases. Surgery should be performed if medical therapy fails or if there is evidence of rupture (i.e., peritonitis or sepsis). Ultrasonographic-guided drainage may also play a role in selected cases.

Further Readings

Horrow Mindy. Ultrasound of pelvic inflammatory disease. *Ultrasound Q* 2004;20: 171–179.

Lambert MJ. Tubo-ovarian abscess. *Emergency Med Clin Am* 2004;22:683–696.

Livengood CH. Tuboovarian abscess. In: UpToDate. www.uptodate.com. Version 13.2, 2006.

Mudgil, Shikha. Pelvic Inflammatory Disease/Tubo-ovarian Abscess. EMedicine. www.emedicine.com 2007.

Sam JW, Jacobs JE, Birnbaum BA. Spectrum of CT findings in acute pyovenic pelvic inflammatory disease. *Radiographics* 2002;22:1324–1327.

Timor-Tritsch IE, Lerner JP, Monteagudo A, et al. Transvaginal sonographic markers of tubal inflammatory disease. *Ultrasound of obstetrics and gynecology* 1998;12:56–66.

Tukeva TA, Aronen HJ, Karjalainen PT, et al. MR imaging in pelvic inflammatory disease: comparison with laparoscopy and US. *Radiology* 1999;210(1):209–216.

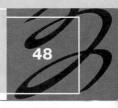

RETAINED PRODUCTS OF CONCEPTION

Laura Amodei

48

etained products of conception (RPOC) can be a troublesome complication of spontaneous or induced abortion and childbirth. The retained tissue can cause persistent bleeding, pain, and endometritis. However, overdiagnosis should be avoided because the standard treatment is curettage, which itself is associated with potential complications, including cervical laceration, uterine perforation, and uterine synechiae—in up to 7% of cases. There are also potential complications from the required anesthesia.

CLINICAL INFORMATION

Clinial History and Presentation. RPOC can occur after spontaneous or induced abortion, transvaginal delivery, or cesarean section, and can be discovered as late as several months after delivery. Common presenting complaints include persistent postpartum vaginal bleeding, pelvic pain, and fever. These symptoms are nonspecific and can also be seen after a normal delivery. Patients may have anemia due to persistent bleeding or leukocytosis in the setting of superimposed infection. Physical examination is not reliable for detection of RPOC.

IMAGING WITH ULTRASONOGRAPHY

Indication.   Ultrasonography is the modality of choice for evaluation of RPOC.

Technique.   In the patient who is immediately postpartum, transabdominal imaging may be adequate, although endovaginal imaging can generally be tolerated and should be performed. In the patient who is postabortion or who is in the later postpartum period, endovaginal ultrasonography adds to the sensitivity of transabdominal imaging and should always be performed. A few studies have suggested that hysterosonography may help distinguish between blood clots and RPOC but this is not yet standard of care.

Possible Findings (Fig. 48-1).

- Gestational sac definitively establishes the diagnosis of RPOC.
- Endometrial mass, defined as a focal heterogeneous or echogenic area within the endometrium.
- Blood flow within the endometrium on Doppler imaging is highly suggestive of RPOC. However, RPOC can be present without Doppler flow (possibly because of minimal or slow flow, technical limitations, or sonographer inexperience) and can lead to a false-negative examination. Also immediately after delivery, "normal" blood flow in involuting vessels at the placental implantation site can appear to be endometrial and can lead to a false-positive examination.
- Endometrial thickening greater than 10 mm.
- Complex endometrial fluid.

A negative pelvic ultrasonographic examination essentially excludes RPOC in the postpartum or postabortion period (negative predictive value up to 100%). However, depending on the criteria used, positive predictive value is surprisingly low, especially in

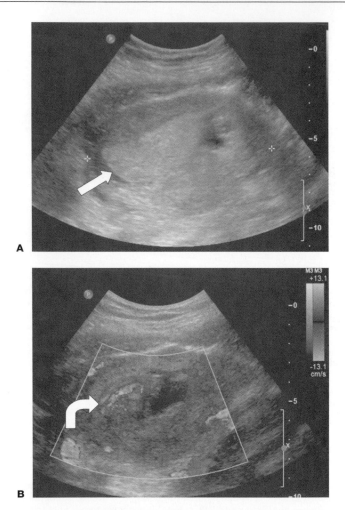

Figure 48-1. A: Transverse ultrasonographic (US) view demonstrates an endometrial mass (*arrow*) in a patient following elective abortion. **B:** Color Doppler shows increased flow in the mass (*curved arrow*) consistent with retained products of conception. Courtesy of Katarzyna Macura, MD, Johns Hopkins Hospital.

the postabortion patient with published estimates of false-positive rates for sonographic diagnosis of RPOC in the range of 15–50%. False-positive examinations may be due to normal postabortion or postpartum findings such as endometrial thickening, complex endometrial fluid, and endometrial "masses" representing blood clots, hyperechoic foci due to air, and even Doppler flow from involuting vessels at the placental implantation site. False positives will decrease as the time since abortion or delivery increases. For example, in the first postpartum week, an endometrial "mass" can be seen in up to half the number of patients and the endometrium may measure greater than 10 mm, even without RPOC. Over time, endometrial thickening resolves and the endometrium appears as a thin white line by 8 weeks postpartum. Thickened, irregular, or heterogeneous endometrium is commonly seen in the first week after dilatation and curettage (D&C), but the presence of these findings after several weeks should raise suspicion of RPOC. The most specific findings for

RPOC are presence of a gestational sac, endometrial mass, and possibly blood flow within the endometrium. An endometrial mass with significant blood flow is definitely concerning for RPOC.

IMAGING WITH MAGNETIC RESONANCE

Magnetic resonance imaging (MRI) is not routinely performed for evaluation of RPOC. Possible findings include variably enhancing soft tissue masses, but this appearance is nonspecific and differential considerations include arteriovenous malformation, multiple endometrial polyps, and trophoblastic disease. MRI may also be helpful in identifying other postpartum causes of a patient's symptoms, such as ovarian vein thrombosis, when conventional studies have been inconclusive or nondiagnostic.

ISSUES AFTER IMAGING

All unstable patients and most symptomatic patients with RPOC will be managed surgically with dilatation and evacuation/curettage. However, particularly in the postabortion period, even when RPOC are present, stable patients may be managed expectantly or medically.

Further Readings

Brown DL. Pelvic ultrasound in the postabortion and postpartum patient. *Ultrasound Q* 2005;21(1):27–37.

DiSalvo DN. Sonographic imaging of maternal complications of pregnancy. *J Ultrasound Med* 2003;22:69–89.

Durfee SM, Frates MC, Luong A, et al. The sonographic and color Doppler features of retained products of conception. *J Ultrasound Med* 2005;24(9):1181–1186. quiz 1188–1189.

Edwards A, Ellwood DA. Ultrasonographic evaluation of the postpartum uterus. *Ultrasound Obstet Gynecol* 2000;16:640–643.

Leyendecker JR, Gorengaut V, Brown JJ. MR Imaging of maternal diseases of the abdomen and pelvis during pregnancy and the immediate postpartum period. *Radiographics* 2004;24:1301–1316.

Mulic-Lutvica A, Bekuretsion M, Bakos O, et al. Ultrasonic evaluation of the uterus and uterine cavity after normal, vaginal delivery. *Ultrasound Obstet Gynecol* 2001;18(5): 491–498.

Noonan JB, Coakley FV, Qayyum A, et al. MR imaging of retained products of conception. *Am J Roentgenol* 2003;181(2):435–439.

Sadan O, Golan A, Girtler O, et al. Role of sonography in the diagnosis of retained products of conception. *J Ultrasound Med* 2004;23(3):371–374.

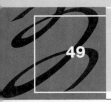

DEEP VENOUS THROMBOSIS
49
Christopher L. Smith

$\mathcal{D}$eep venous thrombosis (DVT) is defined as a localized area of thrombus within the deep venous system of the lower or upper extremities. The most severe and life-threatening complication of DVT is pulmonary embolism (PE). Ninety percent of pulmonary emboli originate in the deep venous system of the lower extremities and pelvis. Accurate diagnosis and treatment of DVT are necessary to prevent the high morbidity and mortality associated with PE.

 ## CLINICAL INFORMATION

Etiology

Risk factors for the development of DVT include history of previous thromboembolic disease, prolonged immobility, obesity, and recent surgery involving the lower extremities and pelvis. Additional risk factors include varicose veins, fracture, trauma, malignancy, autoimmune disorders (e.g., systemic lupus erythematosus [SLE]), heart failure, diabetes mellitus, polycythemia vera, hypercoagulable disorders (e.g., antiphospholipid antibody syndrome), pregnancy, oral contraceptives, estrogen replacement, and smoking. These risk factors are all related to the three pathogenic factors for thromboembolism described by Virchow's triad: venous endothelial damage, hypercoagulability of blood, and decreased blood flow or stasis.

The most common locations for development of DVT include the dorsal veins of the calf, iliofemoral veins, internal iliac veins, and occasionally in the ovarian veins (gonadal veins). DVT has been found to occur more commonly in the left leg than in the right, which is possibly due to the left common iliac vein being slightly compressed by the right common iliac artery as they cross just distal to the bifurcation. Before 1970, DVT of the upper extremity was much rarer (<2). However, the incidence of upper extremity DVT has been increasing since that time because of the increased use of long-term indwelling venous catheters and dialysis shunts.

Symptoms and Signs.   The clinical appearance of DVT is neither sensitive nor specific. It is estimated that 50% of DVT are clinically silent. When present, clinical findings include leg swelling (especially if asymmetric or unilateral), warmth, erythema, pain, tenderness, a positive Homans' sign, fever, and leukocytosis.

Differential Diagnosis.   Entities that can mimic the clinical appearance of DVT include cellulitis, Baker's cyst (especially if acutely dissecting), superficial thrombophlebitis, arterial insufficiency, "compartment syndromes," and myositis.

 ## IMAGING WITH ULTRASONOGRAPHY

Indications.   When available, ultrasonography is the initial study of choice for the detection of DVT in the thigh and popliteal veins. This modality is also useful for evaluation of thrombus within the upper extremities. It is a noninvasive test with no radiation exposure and has been found to be accurate with a high sensitivity (97%) and specificity (95%) for thrombus above the knee. It is less sensitive for the small veins in the calf for which treatment with anticoagulation is controversial and is usually not performed.

Protocol. Lower extremity—a high frequency linear array transducer should be used (5 MHz). The patient is positioned supine with the leg slightly externally rotated and the knee slightly flexed. The femoral vein is located in the groin (medial to the femoral artery) and is then followed down the thigh to the popliteal vein, with the examination including the common femoral vein, superficial femoral vein, popliteal vein, profunda femoral vein, and greater saphenous vein. Additionally, both external iliac veins are imaged (even if the study is a unilateral lower extremity evaluation). If thrombosis is detected in the femoral veins, the common iliac veins and inferior vena cava (IVC) should be imaged in order to determine the extent of thrombus. The veins are examined in both longitudinal and transverse planes with graded compression and Doppler images. Furthermore, a spectral waveform is also obtained, typically in conjunction with augmentation. This is performed by manually squeezing the patient's calf while imaging with the pulsed Doppler cursor in the vein. Augmentation should not be performed if thrombus is visualized, as this maneuver can cause a thrombus to embolize.

A similar technique is used when evaluating the upper extremity veins for DVT. The venous structures typically evaluated include the internal jugular, brachiocephalic (to the extent that it can be visualized), subclavian, axillary, brachial, cephalic, and basilic veins.

Possible Findings (Fig. 49-1)

- Intraluminal thrombus. The thrombus may be occlusive (complete absence of flow) or nonocclusive (partial or mural thrombus).
- Lack of compressibility. A normal vein is highly compliant and will collapse with direct external compression by the ultrasound transducer. If a thrombus is present, the vein will not compress completely.
- Absence of flow. Decreased or absent signal within the vein using color Doppler and measured with the pulsed Doppler cursor. Attention should be paid to the color scale used, as a scale that is too high may not show signal when in fact there is no thrombus present, merely slow flow.
- Absence of augmentation. This maneuver transiently increases flow within the vein and should result in a concordant "spike" in the Doppler spectral waveform. Absence of this finding suggests thrombosis.
- Absence of phasicity. The iliac veins normally demonstrate a triphasic waveform. Lack of this phasicity (a monophasic waveform) can indicate a more central thrombus in the IVC.
- Chronic thrombus often has a heterogeneous/echogenic echotexture. Chronic thrombus may be partially occlusive and may be accompanied by collateral vessels and intimal thickening. However, it is typically difficult to determine the age of a thrombus. Without these signs of chronicity, any sonographic evidence of thrombosis is presumed to be acute in the presence of acute symptoms.

Imaging Tips for Ultrasonography

- Do not confuse the greater saphenous vein, part of the superficial venous system, with the deep femoral veins. However, depending on the extent of thrombus within the vein and the proximity to the junction with the deep venous system, some clinicians will either opt to follow this thrombus with repeated imaging or treat depending on the severity.
- Do not rely solely on clot visualization. Some clots may be echopenic. Therefore the importance of including Doppler images and spectral waveform in the examination.
- The superficial femoral vein is part of the deep venous system. Recently some experts have advised to change the name of the vein to "femoral vein" in order to avoid confusion.
- Increased pulsatility of the spectral waveform suggests heart failure, usually right sided.

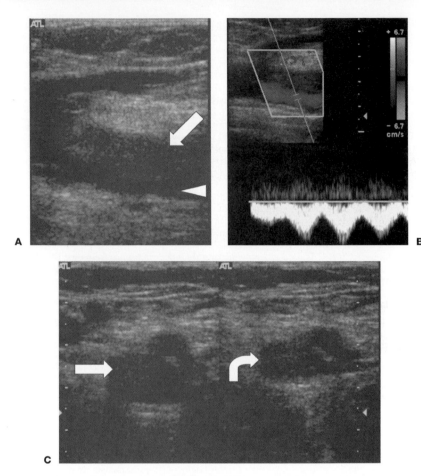

Figure 49-1. Partial deep venous thrombosis (DVT) on ultrasonography (US). **A:** Longitudinal US view demonstrates echogenic material in the lumen of common femoral vein (*straight arrow*), consistent with partial thrombosis. The patent portion on the lumen is hypoechoic (*arrowhead*). **B:** Doppler US confirms partial patency of the lumen. **C:** Transverse US images demonstrate echogenic material in the lumen of the common femoral vein (*straight arrow*), consistent with thrombus. The vessel does not fully compress during pressure with transducer (*curved arrow*), confirming presence of DVT.

 IMAGING WITH COMPUTED TOMOGRAPHY

Indications.   Computed tomographic venography (CTV) has recently been studied as an alternative to ultrasonography for the diagnosis of DVT. In the lower extremities, CTV is usually performed as an adjunct examination following a computed tomography (CT) pulmonary angiogram, but should not be performed in women of childbearing age due to high gonadal radiation dose. However, recent studies have shown that CTV is not as sensitive as ultrasonography for lower extremity DVT. For the upper extremities, CTV can be a useful alternative for evaluation of the central brachiocephalic veins that are usually difficult to evaluate with ultrasonography. CTV is also useful for evaluation of the

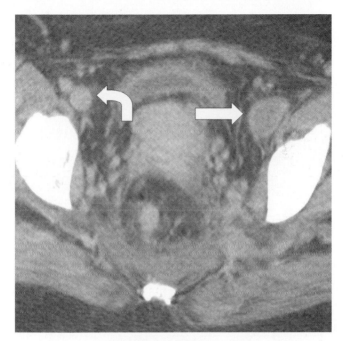

Figure 49-2. Deep venous thrombosis (DVT) on computed tomography (CT). Three-minute delayed phase of contrast-enhanced CT demonstrates enlargement and absence of luminal enhancement of left external iliac vein (*arrow*) consistent with thrombosis. Compare to the left external iliac vein (*curved arrow*). There is minimal enhancement of the thrombosed vessel wall, which is supplied by vasa vasorum.

central venous system, including the superior vena cava (SVC) and IVC, especially if SVC syndrome is suspected. Additionally, CTV is usually more useful than ultrasonography in cases of suspected ovarian/gonadal vein thrombotic disease. If there is concern about an extrinsic mass compressing the venous system leading to secondary thrombosis, CT with CTV would be indicated.

Protocol. Two to 3 minutes after administration of intravenous contrast CT scan of the anatomic area of interest is performed. When performing CTV following CT pulmonary angiography, suggest scanning from iliac crests to the popliteal fossa.

Possible Findings (Fig. 49-2)

- Intraluminal filling defect (should be seen on numerous contiguous slices).
- Abrupt cutoff of an opacified vein.
- Indirect signs. Nonvisualization of an anatomic vein, collateral veins present, inadequate filling of the common femoral, external iliac, and common iliac veins. Extrinsic mass causing compression.

 IMAGING WITH MAGNETIC RESONANCE IMAGING

Indications. Similar to CTV. Magnetic resonance (MR) venography can be performed as an alternative to CTV when there is a contraindication to administering iodinated contrast (e.g., renal failure or transplant) or where radiation dose is to be limited (e.g., pregnancy). Findings are similar to CTV.

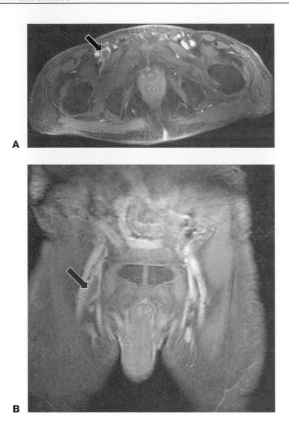

Figure 49-3. Deep venous thrombosis (DVT) on magnetic resonance imaging (MRI). **A:** Axial and **(B)** coronal T1-weighted fat saturation gadolinium enhanced images demonstrate a filling defect (*arrows*) with enlargement of the right common femoral vein.

Protocol.   One-and-a-half to 2 minutes after administration of intravenous gadolinium contrast, perform a 3D T1-weighted acquisition. To optimize venous filling/visualization, inflate blood pressure cuff around the proximal portion of the extremity.

Possible Findings.   Findings are similar to CT (Fig. 49-3). Magnetic resonance imaging (MRI) can also depict soft tissue and muscle edema secondary to impaired venous drainage.

 ISSUES AFTER IMAGING

Once a patient is diagnosed with a DVT, the current clinical standard of care is to treat the patient with anticoagulation for at least 3 months to decrease the risk of PE and further propagation of the clot. This treatment does not directly cause the clot that is present to resolve. Direct catheter-based intravenous thrombolysis with thrombolytic agents (such as urokinase and tissue plasminogen activator [TPA]) can also be performed. The current belief is that catheter-directed thrombolysis is able to preserve deep venous valves, thereby reducing the rate of future varicose veins. Studies are currently under way to determine the efficacy and risks of this treatment option and to fully define the clinical indications of this therapy. If anticoagulation is contraindicated, an IVC filter can be placed. Anticoagulation to treat venous thrombosis below the knee is controversial.

Further Readings

Baarslag HJ, van Beek EJ, Koopman MM, et al. Prospective study of color duplex ultrasonography compared with contrast venography in patients suspected of having deep venous thrombosis of the upper extremities. *Ann Intern Med* 2002;136(12):1–30.

Katz DS, Loud PA, Hurewitz AN, et al. CT venography in suspected pulmonary thromboembolism. *Semin Ultrasound CT MR* 2004;25(1):67–80.

Koopman MMW, van Beek EJR, ten Cate JW. Diagnosis of deep venous thrombosis. *Prog Cardiovasc Dis* 1994;37:1–12.

Kristo DA, Perry ME, Kollef MH. Comparison of venography, duplex imaging, and bilateral impedance plethysmography for diagnosis of lower extremity deep venous thrombosis. *South Med J* 1994;87:55–60.

Matzdorff AC, Green D. Deep venous thrombosis and pulmonary embolism: prevention, diagnosis, and treatment. *Geriatrics* 1992;47:48–63.

Peterson DA, Kazerozni EA, Wakefield TW, et al. Computed tomographic venography is specific but not sensitive for diagnosis of acute lower-extremity deep venous thrombosis in patients with suspected pulmonary embolus. *J Vasc Surg* 2001;34(5):798–804.

Putman CE, Ravin CE, eds. *Textbook of diagnostic imaging*, 2nd ed. Philadelphia: WB Saunders, 1994:546–562.

Sanders RC. Pain and swelling in the limbs: rule out limb or mass, Baker's cyst; possible aneurysm. In: Sanders RC, ed. *Clinical sonography: a practical guide*, 2nd ed. Boston: Little Brown and Company, 1991:395–401.

Taffoni MJ, Ravenel JG, Ackerman SJ. Prospective comparison of indirect CT venography versus venous sonography in ICU patients. *Am J Roentgenol* 2005;185(2):457–462.

Washington L, Goodman LR, Gonyo MB. CT for thromboembolic disease. *Radiol Clin North Am* 2002;40(4):751–771.

Weinmann EE, Salzman EW. Deep-vein thrombosis. *N Engl J Med* 1994;331:1630–1641.

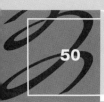

OSTEOMYELITIS
50 *Rick W. Obray, Cathleen F. Magill, and Oleg M. Teytelboym*

Osteomyelitis is most commonly caused by bacterial organisms with *Staphylococcus aureus* accounting for approximately 85% of infections. The infection can occur due to hematogenous seeding, contiguous spread from a soft tissue infection or septic arthritis, or direct contamination from surgery or trauma. Three stages of osteomyelitis are identified: acute, subacute, and chronic. The hallmark of subacute osteomyelitis is the development of Brodie's abscess, a central area of suppuration and necrosis that is walled off by granulation tissue that forms a fibrous capsule. Chronic osteomyelitis develops in patients with acute osteomyelitis that has not been adequately treated. Osteomyelitis has a bimodal distribution, occurring most frequently in children and in adults older than 50 years. Risk factors in the latter group include compromised immunity and typical causes of bacteremia including injection drug use, central lines, dialysis, indwelling urethral catheters, and subacute bacterial endocarditis. In children, the femur, tibia, and humerus are the bones most commonly affected. Vertebral, sacroiliac, and sternoclavicular bones are the most commonly involved in adults.

 CLINICAL INFORMATION

Signs and Symptoms. Presentation of osteomyelitis depends on the clinical stage of disease and can be quite variable. With acute osteomyelitis, patients typically experience fever, local bone pain, redness, tenderness, warmth and swelling, with gradual onset over several days to a week. These symptoms are less likely to occur with osteomyelitis of the hip, pelvis, and vertebrae. In contrast, patients with subacute osteomyelitis experience less severe pain, swelling, and constitutional symptoms, with a far more insidious onset. Leukocytosis and elevated erythrocyte sedimentation rate (ESR) and C-reactive protein (CRP) levels are commonly present in acute osteomyelitis, but not in chronic osteomyelitis.

Differential Diagnosis. Fracture, cellulitis, septic arthritis, crystal-induced arthropathies, tumor (Ewing's sarcoma, osteosarcoma, metastatic lesion), amyloid, Legg-Calve-Perthes (hip), transient osteoporosis of the hip, avascular necrosis, eosinophilic granuloma, osteoid osteoma, and myositis ossificans.

 IMAGING WITH RADIOGRAPHS

Indications. All evaluations of suspected osteomyelitis should begin with radiographs. However, because the bony abnormalities of acute osteomyelitis take 10–14 days to manifest themselves, negative radiographs do not exclude the diagnosis, requiring further evaluation with advance imaging modalities.

Protocol. At least two views of the area of interest should be obtained. Coned views should be obtained when possible. Comparative views of the contralateral extremity are often helpful in discerning early, subtle findings.

Possible Findings

Acute Infection, Less Than 2 Weeks
- Soft tissue swelling with contiguous spread of infection.

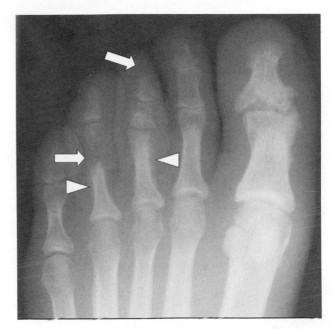

Figure 50-1. Subacute osteomyelitis on radiographs. There are multiple bony erosions (*arrows*), periosteal reaction (*arrows*), and soft tissue swelling. Courtesy of William Scott Jr, MD, Johns Hopkins Hospital.

- Swelling is absent early on with hematogenous spread, and becomes detectible 3–10 days after infection.
- Osteopenia is not recognizable until the bone mineral content decreases by 35–50%, which usually takes 10–14 days to develop after the onset of bone infection.

Subacute Infection, 2–6 Weeks (Fig. 50-1)
- Lytic lesion with or without sclerosis.
- Periosteal reaction.
- Brodie's abscess that is commonly seen in children and has been classified into four types by Gledhill et al. Type 1 is characterized by the presence of a metaphyseal lucency only. In type 2, there is associated cortical destruction. Types 3 and 4 progress to involve the diaphysis, with the presence of cortical hyperostosis in type 3 and an "onion skin" subperiosteal reaction in type 4.

Chronic Infection, Greater Than 6 Weeks (Fig. 50-2)
- Extensive sclerosis.
- Periosteal or endosteal reaction.
- Sequestrum, which represents a fragment of necrotic bone embedded in the inflammatory process and isolated from its vascular supply.
- Involucrum, which represents formation of periosteal new bone around necrotic bone. The involucrum may contain cloacae, which are fistulous tracts to the adjacent subcutaneous tissue.

Vertebral Osteomyelitis
- Loss of disk height.
- Vertebral end plate erosions and osteopenia.

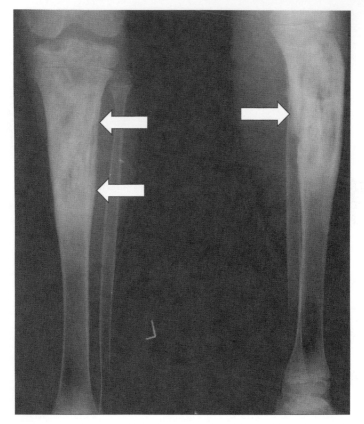

Figure 50-2. Chronic osteomyelitis on radiographs. Frontal and lateral views of the tibia demonstrate sclerosis involving the proximal epiphysis, metaphysis, and diaphysis, with periosteal reaction (*arrows*). Courtesy of William Scott Jr, MD, Johns Hopkins Hospital.

- Vertebral body collapse in advanced disease.
- Can be difficult to differentiate from degenerative changes.

 IMAGING WITH MAGNETIC RESONANCE

Indications. Magnetic resonance imaging (MRI) is the modality of choice for definitive evaluation of osteomyelitis with 82–100% sensitivity and 75–96% specificity. MRI permits early detection, and can accurately evaluate the extent of disease. Radiographs are important for correlation with MRI findings and should always be performed before MRI.

Protocol. MRI should include T1, short T1 inversion recovery (STIR) or T2-weighted sequences, and possibly fat-suppressed T1-weighted sequence after gadolinium. Nonfat suppressed T1-weighted sequence is crucial for evaluation of bone marrow replacement.

Possible Findings (Fig. 50-3)

- Low T1 bone marrow signal (lower than muscle) implies bone marrow replacement and is required for definitive diagnosis of osteomyelitis on MRI.

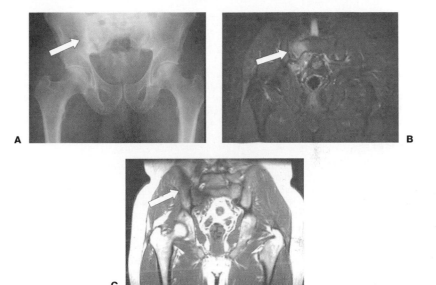

Figure 50-3. Sacroiliitis with osteomyelitis on radiograph and MRI. **A:** Anteroposterior (AP) view of the pelvis shows sclerosis surrounding right sacroiliac joint (*arrow*) consistent with sacroiliitis and osteomyelitis. **B:** Coronal T2-weighted image demonstrates edema surrounding right sacroiliac joint (*arrow*). **C:** Coronal T1-weighted image shows dark T1 signal (*arrow*) corresponding to area of edema, definitively confirming presence of superimposed osteomyelitis. Courtesy of Kevin Chang, MD, Johns Hopkins Hospital.

- High T2 bone marrow signal implies presence of edema, which may be due to infection, trauma, infarction, or postoperative changes (present for several months after surgery). Edema from adjacent soft tissues, ligaments, or tendons can sometimes diffuse into the bone resulting in increased T2 signal in marrow. Without low T1 signal, bone marrow edema is nonspecific.
- Bone marrow enhancement is present in osteomyelitis, but it is nonspecific because anything that is bright on T2 will enhance because gadolinium essentially reflects distribution of water.
- Intraosseous abscess can be differentiated from bone marrow edema by presence of enhancement only in the periphery of the abscess.
- Sequestrum is dead bone and will be low signal on T1 and T2 sequences.
- Cortical destruction is best visible on T1 sequences.
- Sinus tract is bright on T2, isointense on T1, and enhances after administration of gadolinium.

Pitfalls

- Low T1 marrow signal may not be present during the earliest phase of infection, necessitating a broad differential if high T2 marrow signal is present. Follow-up may be necessary to establish the diagnosis.
- Neuroarthropathy in diabetic foot may be difficult to differentiate from osteomyelitis because low T1 marrow signal may be present in both. Both disorders may also coexist.
  - Enhancement is present in osteomyelitis, but not in neuroarthropathy.
  - Osteomyelitis typically occurs secondary to ulcers at the pressure points (distal metatarsals and calcaneus). Neuroarthropathy is primary centered at the joints (ankle).
  - Osteomyelitis may cause cortical destruction. Neuroarthropathy causes bone fragmentation and malalignment.

IMAGING WITH NUCLEAR MEDICINE

Bone Scan

Indications. Bone scan provides an alternative to MRI for early detection of osteomyelitis and can be performed when MRI contraindications are present (pacemaker, claustrophobia, etc.). Disadvantages include limited spatial resolution, impairing the ability to delineate complex anatomy, and the potential for ineffective delivery of isotopes to the extremities of patients with peripheral vascular disease.

Protocol

1. Three-phase bone scan is performed after injection of 15–25 mCi of ^{99m}Technetium (^{99m}Tc)-methylene diphosphonate (MDP).
2. Flow phase is obtained immediately after injecting the radiotracer with dynamic images. Imaging of the contralateral side is recommended for comparison.
3. Blood pool phase is acquired 10–20 minutes after injection.
4. Bone phase is acquired 4 hours after injection. Single photon emission computed tomography (SPECT) and particularly SPECT/CT computed tomography (CT) are superior to planar images.
5. Delayed images at 24 hours are recommended for patients with peripheral vascular disease, in whom there may be delayed transit of the radiotracer to the extremities.

Possible Findings

■ Increased uptake on all three phases (flow, blood pool, and bone phases) is required for diagnosis of osteomyelitis. The diagnosis can be made within 24–72 hours of infection onset.

Pitfalls

■ Low sensitivity in distal extremities due to poor spatial resolution.
■ Low specificity because trauma, neuroarthropathy, and reflux sympathetic dystrophy also demonstrate increased uptake on all three phases of bone scan.
■ Bone phase uptake can persist for up to 3 years after surgery or fracture.

Gallium Scan

Gallium scanning is performed when osteomyelitis is still highly suspected despite a negative bone scan, or one with nonspecific findings. This test has improved specificity (67%) over the three-phase bone scan alone, with imaging typically performed 48 hours after injection. False positives can occur secondary to tumor uptake, fractures, and marked excretion through the gastrointestinal tract. Sensitivity, however, is poor at 25–80%. In contrast to the bone scan, gallium is not dependent on vascular flow, making it more useful in patients with peripheral vascular disease.

White Blood Cell Scan

Indications. White blood cell (WBC) scan allows specific visualization of infection. WBC scan is not helpful in spine or pelvis due to physiologic bone marrow uptake.

Protocol. For *in vitro* labeling of WBCs with ^{111}Indium (^{111}In) or ^{99m}Tc-hexamethylpropyleneamine oxime (HMPAO), 50 mL of the patient's blood is required. The labeling takes approximately 2 hours. The imaging is performed 24 hours after reinjection of the labeled WBCs. SPECT and particularly SPECT/CT are superior to planar images.

Possible Findings

■ Focally increased uptake is consistent with infection.

Pitfalls

■ Inability to differentiate soft tissues from bone due to poor spatial resolution limiting. This is particularly problematic in the distal extremities.

■ False positives due to physiologic bone marrow uptake in distal extremities of patients with diabetes. This problem can be solved by correlation with ^{99m}Tc sulfur colloid bone marrow scan.

 IMAGING WITH COMPUTED TOMOGRAPHY

CT is not a part of routine osteomyelitis workup because of poor specificity. Because CT imaging provides excellent spatial and contrast resolution of bones and soft tissues, it is superior to MRI in detecting cortical bone destruction, periosteal reaction, gas in the bone, involucra, sequestra, and foreign bodies that may be serving as a nidus of infection. CT may be used for guiding percutaneous aspirations and biopsies needed for diagnosis.

 ISSUES AFTER IMAGING

Osteomyelitis is treated with at least a 4- to 6-week course of parenteral antibiotic therapy. Infected hardware must be removed. In selected cases, implantation of antibiotic-impregnated beads can be performed. Amputation may be necessary with osteomyelitis of the feet in patients with diabetes and severe peripheral vascular disease.

Further Readings

Abernathy L, Carty H. Modern approach to the diagnosis of osteomyelitis in children. *Br J Hosp Med* 1997;58:464.

Blickman JG, van Die CE, de Rooy JWJ. Current imaging concepts in pediatric osteomyelitis. *Eur Radiol* 2004;14:L55–L64.

Buhne KH, Bohndorf K. Imaging of postraumatic osteomyelitis. *Semin Musculoskelet Radiol* 2004;8(3):199–204.

Kaplan PA, Helms CA, Dussalt R, Anderson MW, Major NM. *Muskuloskeletal MRI.* WB Saunders, 2001.

Karwowska A, Davies H, Jadavji T. Epidemiology and outcome of osteomyelitis in the era of sequential intravenous-oral therapy. *Pediatr Infect Dis* 1998;17:1021.

Restrepo CS, Gimenez CR, McCarthy K. Imaging of osteomyelitis and musculoskeletal soft tissue infections: current concepts. *Rheum Dis Clin North Am* 2003;29:89–109.

Schauwecker Dwarnings. The scintigraphic diagnosis of osteomyelitis. *Am J Roentgenol* 1992;158:9–18.

Stoller DW, Tirman PFJ, Bredella MA. *Diagnostic imaging orthopedics,* 1st ed. Salt Lake City: Amirsys Inc., 2004:38–41.

Tehranzadeh J, Wong E, Wang F, et al. Imaging of osteomyelitis in the mature skeleton. *Radiol Clin North Am* 2001;39:223–250.

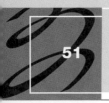

PERIPHERAL VASCULAR INJURY
Christopher L. Smith

51

eripheral vascular injury occurs in 25–35% of patients with penetrating trauma. Arterial injury carries major morbidity and complications and further diagnostic imaging is indicated when a projectile's path is suspected to be near a major vessel.

 CLINICAL INFORMATION

Etiology.   Peripheral vascular injury is most commonly the result of penetrating trauma, but it may also occur with blunt trauma, especially if there is an associated fracture or joint dislocation. For example, in 50% of cases of posterior knee dislocation, there is a popliteal artery injury making further diagnostic evaluation mandatory in this setting. Catheter angiography can also be a cause of arterial injury.

Arterial injury can lead to arterial thrombosis or can result in an expanding hematoma, which can compress adjacent blood vessels and cause peripheral ischemia. Sequelae of arterial injury include formation of a pseudoaneurysm or development of an arteriovenous fistula. Pseudoaneurysms can continue to expand and rupture at any time. With active hemorrhage peripheral arterial injury can even lead to exsanguination and death.

Symptoms and Signs

- **Signs of hemorrhage.** Pulsatile external bleeding, an expanding or pulsating hematoma, unexplained hypotension with Hct less than 30% or rapid Hct drop (15% drop within 2 hours).
- **Signs of ischemia.** Severe pain, loss of peripheral pulses, progressive swelling of an extremity, coolness or pallor of an extremity, cyanosis, poor capillary refill.
- **Altered flow.** Bruit, palpable thrill (with arteriovenous fistula), ipsilateral dilated veins (with arteriovenous fistula).
- **Associated deficits.** Loss of peripheral neurologic function, fracture, joint dislocation (especially the knee).

Physical Examination.   It is vital to palpate the appropriate peripheral pulses, both proximal and distal: carotid in the neck; axillary, brachial, radial for the upper extremity; and femoral, popliteal, posterior tibial, and dorsalis pedis for the lower extremity. Auscultation should be performed to assess for murmurs and bruits. A standard clinical Doppler is often useful for examining the distal pulses and especially when peripheral pulses are nonpalpable.

If physical signs are present, then the rate of positive findings with further diagnostic imaging increases dramatically. For example, arteriography demonstrates arterial injury in 90% of cases with absent distal pulses and in 50% of those with diminished peripheral pulses.

 IMAGING WITH COMPUTED TOMOGRAPHIC ANGIOGRAPHY

Indications.   The use of computed tomographic angiography (CTA) for the evaluation of lower extremity vascular pathology has been well described in the literature. This modality is useful in the evaluation of both peripheral vascular disease and traumatic arterial injuries of the lower and upper extremities. Recently many have suggested that CTA is preferable to conventional arteriography for the initial evaluation of traumatic arterial injuries because it is noninvasive, rapid to perform, nearly universally available, and provides information about surrounding structures/injuries.

Protocol. Best performed using multidetector computed tomography (CT) (at least 16 rows). The examination is typically performed with the smallest slice thickness available to improve the resolution and to allow for multiplanar and 3D reconstructions. Studies are performed with nonionic intravenous contrast usually injected at rate of 3 mL/second. Scan delay to data acquisition is approximately 25 seconds with scans obtained in a proximal to distal orientation. Scans of the upper extremities are performed with the patient's arms stretched over the chest, by the side, or extended over the head. Lower extremity scans can be performed with the patient in the normal supine position. If possible, symmetry should be maintained because comparison is often useful. Once the data sets are generated, they are sent to a freestanding workstation where maximum intensity projection (MIP), multiplanar reconstruction (MPR) and 3D maps are evaluated.

Possible Findings (Fig. 51-1)

- **Arterial occlusion.** Nonvisualization of the artery especially when compared to adjacent arteries in the same and contralateral extremity. It is important to compare nearby arteries in the same extremity to ensure that the nonvisualization is not a result of a poor contrast bolus. Occasionally, a low-density intraluminal-filling defect that represents a thrombus can be seen.
- **Arterial dissection.** Often an intimal flap will be seen. The false lumen may or may not fill with contrast depending on the presence of thrombosis and the chronicity of the injury. A sharply tapering, often angulated artery, which then becomes occluded, can also be a sign of a dissection.
- **Arterial injury.** Direct arterial injury can result in active contrast extravasation from the vessel into an adjacent hematoma. Direct arterial injury can also result in a pseudoaneurysm, which is demonstrated by a small focal outpouching, usually surrounded by hematoma, adjacent to the vascular lumen, which fills with contrast. As arteries are a

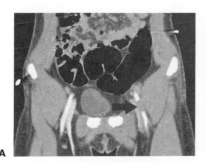
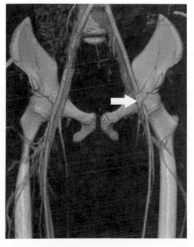

Figure 51-1. A: Coronal oblique reconstruction and **(B)** Three-dimensional (3D) volume rendered reconstructed images demonstrate absence of flow in a segment of left common femoral artery (*arrow*). This patient fell on a bicycle handlebar, causing a dissection of the vessel.

high-pressure system, there is usually a large hematoma associated with arterial injury. Arterial narrowing secondary to spasm can also be a secondary sign of an arterial injury.

■ **Arteriovenous malformations and fistulas.** early filling with contrast of a dilated adjacent vein can be seen with arteriovenous malformations or fistulas. Confirmation can be obtained with comparison to the contralateral side, which will demonstrate an unopacified venous system. The level of the fistula can be surmised based on the opacified/unopacified junction within the vein.

IMAGING WITH ULTRASONOGRAPHY

Indications.   If the mechanism of injury is suspected to be related to a recent catheterization, ultrasonography of the affected vessel can be performed as the initial study of choice, especially because ultrasonography can be performed in a portable manner. However, if major blunt or penetrating trauma has occurred, CTA or digital subtraction angiography (DSA) should usually be considered first.

Protocol.   The clinically suspected injured vessel is directly evaluated using both gray-scale and Doppler imaging. Cine clips and spectral waveforms are useful and almost always obtained. If possible, a high frequency linear array transducer (5 MHz) should be used.

Possible Findings (Figs. 51-2 and 51-3)

■ **Arterial occlusion.** Absence of power or color Doppler flow within a vessel is the sine qua non of arterial occlusion. If no Doppler flow is visualized within the vessel, scan parameters should be optimized in order to detect slow flow within the vessel before concluding that the vessel is occluded. The flow proximal to the occlusion can be to and fro in appearance with cyclic reversal of flow on color Doppler imaging.

■ **Arterial dissection.** An intimal flap can be seen on gray scale imaging. The false lumen may or may not demonstrate flow on Doppler imaging depending on the presence of thrombosis and the chronicity of the injury. Additionally, the flow of the false and true lumens will often have different velocities and the flow in the false lumen can occasionally be reversed when compared to the true lumen.

■ **Arterial injury.** Direct arterial injury can result in direct visualization of Doppler flow through the vessel wall and extending beyond the vessel into an adjacent complex fluid collection representing the hematoma. Often the region of the defect can be seen or surmised based on the Doppler images. Direct arterial injury can also result in a

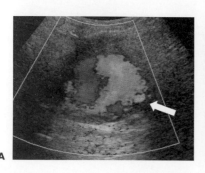

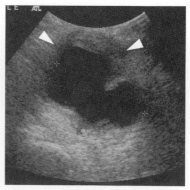

A

B

Figure 51-2. A: Pseudoaneurysm on Doppler ultrasound shows a classic "yin-yang" pattern of flow (*arrow*). **B:** Gray scale ultrasonographic image demonstrates hypoechoic hematoma around the pseudoaneurysm (*arrowheads*).

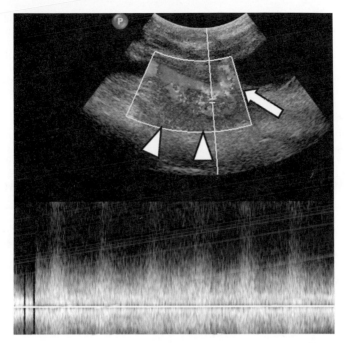

Figure 51-3. Arteriovenous fistula with Doppler ultrasound demonstrates extensive aliasing (*arrowheads*) in the region of superficial femoral vein and artery. Mixed arterial and venous waveform is noted in this area, confirming presence of arteriovenous fistula. Pseudoaneurysm is also present (*arrow*).

pseudoaneurysm which is demonstrated by a swirling appearance of the color Doppler flow in a focal outpouching adjacent to the vessel. This appearance can be referred to as a *Yin-Yang* flow pattern. With a pseudoaneurysm, it is important to define the neck as this has treatment ramifications.

■ **Arteriovenous malformations and fistulas.** Arterialization of the venous flow (pulsatile waveform within a vein) on Doppler imaging suggests an arteriovenous fistula. Additionally the feeding artery will usually have a low-resistance flow pattern with high systolic and diastolic flow and decreased S/D ratio. Additionally, the loss of the normal triphasic arterial flow can also be seen. Comparison with adjacent arteries is important for confirmation.

IMAGING WITH MAGNETIC RESONANCE ARTERIOGRAPHY

Indications. Similar to CTA; however, not usually performed in the setting of acute trauma. Magnetic resonance imaging (MRI) could be performed as an alternative to CTA when there is a contraindication to administering iodinated contrast (e.g., renal failure or transplant) or where radiation dose is to be limited (e.g., pregnancy). Findings are similar to CTA.

Protocol. Magnetic resonance arteriography (MRA) of the extremities is tailored to the specific extremity being imaged; therefore, one should confirm the protocol before proceeding. However, most facilities when imaging the lower extremities use a multistation approach (usually a total of three stations) in which both lower extremities with a defined field of view are imaged in a stepwise manner usually proximal to distal. Precontrast images are acquired to be used as a mask (3D time of flight [TOF] spoiled gradient recalled echo [SPGR]). This is then followed by administration of a Gadolinium-based contrast agent (usually 20–40 mL depending on the size of the patient) at 2 mL/second. Then postcontrast images are acquired in a multistation approach using the same sequence as the mask images (3D TOF SPGR). The multistation approach allows one to maximize the signal to noise ratio and is also used to improve the resolution and avoid off-field effects. A 3D acquisition improves the temporal acquisition times.

Possible Findings

Similar to CTA, with the additional advantage of possible evaluation of flow characteristics using phase-contrast imaging.

IMAGING WITH DIGITAL SUBTRACTION ANGIOGRAPHY

Indications.   DSA has long been seen as the reference standard for evaluation of suspected peripheral vascular injury. If the mechanism of injury was a posterior knee dislocation, the current standard of care is still to perform direct catheter angiography. Arteriography is more invasive than CTA or MRA and exposes the patient to radiation risk. However, if the CTA or MRA are equivocal or if an emergent therapeutic intervention (such as embolization) is being considered, DSA should be performed. Arteriography is usually performed following an abnormal finding on CTA or secondary to an associated physical examination finding. In cases of absent pulses, arteriography or immediate operative intervention should be performed.

Protocol.   See Chapter 53, "Arteriography Primer".

Possible Findings

Similar to CTA, with the additional advantage of dynamic imaging and higher resolution. Dynamic imaging allows for evaluation of flow characteristics, such as flow dynamics between the artery and vein and the rate of active extravasation.

Further Readings

Abrams HL. *Abrams angiography: vascular and interventional radiology*, 3rd ed. Boston: Little Brown and company, 1983.

Busquets AR, Acosta JA, Colon E, et al. Helical computed tomographic angiography for the diagnosis of traumatic arterial injuries of the extremities. *J Trauma* 2004;56(3):625–628.

Fishman EK, Neyman EG, Smith CL, et al. *Evaluation of utility of upper extremity cta using 16 and 64 multi-detector ct with 3d volume rendering*. Poster Presentation RSNA 12/2004.

Johnstrude IS, Jackson DC, Dunnick NR. *A practical approach to angiography*, 2nd ed. Boston: Little Brown and company, 1987:165–166.

Kadir S. *Diagnostic angiography*. Philadelphia: WB Saunders, 1986.

Kim D, Orron DE. *Peripheral vascular imaging and intervention*. St Louis: Mosby-Year Book, 1992:155–164.

Portugaller HR, Schoellnast H, Hausegger KA, et al. Mulitslice spiral CT angiography in peripheral arterial occlusive disease: a valuable tool in detecting significant arterial lumen narrowing? *Eur Radiol* 2004;14(9):1681–1687.

Reimer P, Landwehr P. Non-invasive vascular imaging of peripheral vessels. *Eur Radiol* 1998;8(6):858–872.

Soto JA, Munera F, Morales C, et al. Related articles, focal arterial injuries of the proximal extremities: helical CT arteriography as the initial method of diagnosis. *Radiology* 2001;218(1):188–194.

Weissleder R, Rieumont MJ, Wittenberg J. *Primer of diagnostic imaging*. St Louis: Mosby, 1997:646–649.

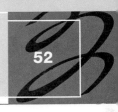

SEPTIC ARTHRITIS
Rick W. Obray and Cathleen F. Magill

52

CLINICAL INFORMATION

Etiology and Epidemiology. Septic arthritis occurs in all age-groups. In pediatric patients, the hip, knee, and ankle are the most commonly affected joints. In adults, the knee is by far the most commonly affected joint, followed by the hip and shoulder. Patients with a history of intravenous drug abuse (IVDA) often present with involvement of the sternoclavicular and sacroiliac joints, as well as the spine.

Septic arthritis most commonly results from hematogenous seeding of the highly vascular synovial membrane in the context of bacteremia. Much less common etiologies include penetrating trauma, nonpenetrating trauma to a joint, and introduction of bacteria during joint procedure.

Neisseria gonorrhoeae is the most common cause of septic arthritis in the United States, with the highest prevalence among young sexually active adults and homosexual men. Of all nongonococcal cases, *Staphylococcus* is the most frequent etiologic agent, and is particularly represented in patients with a history of diabetes or rheumatoid arthritis. Other common bacterial agents include *Streptococcus species*, *Pseudomonas aeruginosa*, and *Escherichia coli*. Although *Hemophilus influenzae* formerly accounted for a large share of cases in children younger than 2 years, the advent of the *Hemophilus influenzae* type b (Hib) vaccine has reduced the number of cases to near extinction.

Easy hematogenous ingress of bacteria is facilitated by the absence of a limiting basement membrane under the highly vascular synovium. Once inside this space, egress is difficult, and rapid destruction of the joint space occurs. Risk factors for septic arthritis include unprotected sexual intercourse, diabetes, cancer, chronic liver disease, chronic alcoholism, corticosteroid therapy, IVDA, sickle cell disease, previous joint damage, and hypogammaglobulinemia.

Symptoms and Signs. Most patients present with the acute onset of a warm, erythematous, edematous, painful joint with associated fever and malaise. In 80–90% of patients, septic arthritis is monarticular. When it is polyarticular, usually only two to three joints are involved.

The diagnosis of septic arthritis is usually made clinically. Leukocytosis is often present in children, but not as commonly in adults. Erythrocyte sedimentation rate (ESR) and C-reactive protein (CRP) levels are also frequently elevated. The primary tool for analysis of septic arthritis is the joint aspirate (Gram stain, cell count, and culture). Most clinicians perform aspiration of the knee joint at the bedside. Aspiration of the hip and shoulder often requires fluoroscopic guidance by a radiologist.

Differential Diagnosis. The differential diagnosis should be tailored based on each patient's risk factors and comorbidities. A general differential includes all of the inflammatory arthritides—rheumatoid arthritis, gout, calcium pyrophosphate dihydrate deposition (CPPD) syndrome, Reiter's syndrome, arthritis associated with inflammatory bowel disease and psoriatic arthritis. However, in contrast with septic arthritis, these arthritides tend to be polyarticular. Synovial osteochondromatosis and pigmented villonodular synovitis are also in the differential diagnosis. The differential diagnosis in children should be expanded to include trauma (epiphyseal fracture, child abuse), Legg-Calve-Perthes disease, leukemia, slipped capital femoral epiphysis, and transient synovitis.

IMAGING WITH RADIOGRAPHS

Indications.   It is reasonable to initiate any evaluation of an acute articular process with radiographs. In children, they are especially important for ruling out trauma.

Protocol.   Obtain standard orthogonal views of the affected joint. In the absence of trauma, evaluation of the hip in children should include anteroposterior (AP) views of the pelvis with both hips in the neutral and frog-leg lateral positions.

Possible Findings (Figs. 52-1 and 52-2)

■ Radiographs are often normal in the first few days of infection.
■ The most important finding is the presence of a joint effusion, with associated displacement of the para-articular fat pads, swelling of the capsule and surrounding soft tissue, and joint space widening and obliteration of soft tissue planes because of edema.
■ Late findings often indicate irreversible damage and include osteomyelitis, periosteal elevation, joint space narrowing/osteoarthritis due to cartilage destruction, and bony erosion of the articular surfaces.
■ Radiographs are generally good at revealing effusions of the elbow, knee, and ankle, but are less useful in examining most other joints for effusions.

 IMAGING WITH ULTRASONOGRAPHY

Indications.   Ultrasonography is a sensitive test for identifying joint effusions as small as 1–2 mL and can help guide joint aspiration and drainage procedures. It has the added benefits of being noninvasive, safe, inexpensive, and relatively easy to use. Ultrasonography is especially useful for detection of an effusion in a child's hip.

Possible Findings (Fig. 52-1)

■ If an effusion is present in the hip, fluid will be visualized anterior and lateral to the femoral head and neck.
■ Any fluid detected in the joint should be aspirated with sonographic guidance.

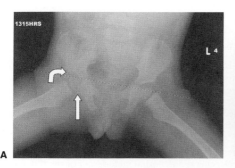 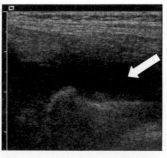

Figure 52-1. **A:** Anteroposterior (AP) view of the pelvis shows lateral displacement of the right femoral head straight (*straight arrow*), raising suspicion of joint effusion. There is subtle erosion of the right acetabulum (*curved arrow*). **B:** Right hip ultrasonography (US) demonstrates large effusion (*arrow*), raising suspicion of septic arthritis. The diagnosis was confirmed with US-guided hip aspiration. Courtesy of Renee Flax–Goldenberg, MD, Johns Hopkins Hospital.

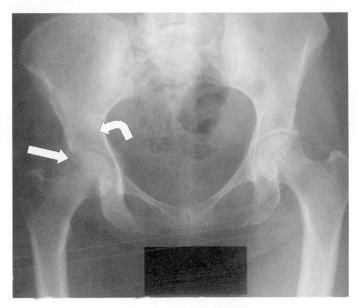

Figure 52-2. Anteroposterior (AP) view of the pelvis shows osteopenia in the right femoral head (*straight arrow*) and right acetabulum (*curved arrow*). This is compatible with septic arthritis because the process involves both sides of the joint. Joint aspiration and culture showed tuberculosis as the underlying organism. Courtesy of William Scott Jr, MD, Johns Hopkins Hospital.

 IMAGING WITH MAGNETIC RESONANCE

Indication. Magnetic resonance imaging (MRI) is not typically needed to diagnose septic arthritis. However, it can be very useful in the diagnosis of ambiguous cases, and to determine the extent of bone and soft tissue infections. MRI usually detects abnormalities with 24 hours of the onset of the infection.

Protocol. The protocol usually depends on the joint of interest. However, it typically includes T1, T2, short T1 inversion recovery (STIR), and postcontrast T1-weighted imaging in multiple planes.

Possible Findings (Fig. 52-3)

■ Synovial enhancement, perisynovial edema, and joint effusion are the most reliable findings for diagnosis of septic joint.
■ Low T1 marrow signal (lower then skeletal muscle) is suggestive of osteomyelitis.

Pitfalls

■ Joint effusion is absent in 30% of patients with septic arthritis.
■ Noninfectious inflammatory arthritis can have similar MRI appearance as septic arthritis.
■ Reactive marrow changes are commonly present in septic arthritis and can include high T2 signal and enhancement due to marrow edema. Low T1 signal (lower then muscle) is required for definitive diagnosis of osteomyelitis.

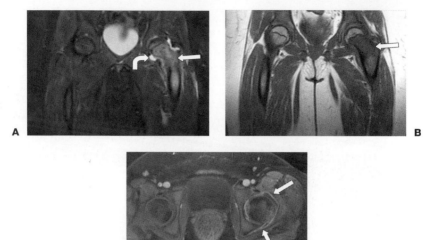

Figure 52-3. Septic arthritis on magnetic resonance imaging (MRI). **A:** Coronal T2-weighted image demonstrates left hip joint effusion (*curved arrow*) and edema of left proximal femur (*straight arrow*). **B:** Coronal T1-weighted image shows dark T1 signal in the left proximal femur (*arrow*) corresponding to area of edema, definitively confirming presence of superimposed osteomyelitis. **C:** Axial fat suppressed postcontrast T1-weighted image shows enhancement of left femoral head and adjacent soft tissues (*arrows*), confirming presence of inflammation. Courtesy of David Grand, MD, Johns Hopkins Hospital.

Further Readings

Jaramillo D, Treves ST, Kasser JR, et al. Osteomyelitis and septic arthritis in children: appropriate use of imaging to guide treatment. *Am J Roentgenol* 1995;165(2):399–403.

Karchevsky M, Schweitzer ME, Morrison WB, et al. MRI findings of septic arthritis and associated osteomyelitis in adults. *Am J Roentgenol* 2004;182:119–122.

Learch TJ, Farooki S. Magnetic resonance imaging of septic arthritis. *J Clin Imaging* 2000;24:236–242.

Shirtliff ME, Mader JT. Acute septic arthritis. *Clin Microbiol Rev* 2002;15(4):527–544.

Wysoki M, Shah R. Osteomyelitis and septic arthritis in children: guidelines for the use of imaging. *AJR Am J Roentgenology* 1995;166(2):399–403.

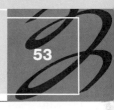

ARTERIOGRAPHY PRIMER
Kevin A. Smith

53

INDICATIONS FOR EMERGENT ARTERIOGRAPHY

- Aortic dissection.
- Gastrointestinal bleeding.
- Ischemic bowel.
- Ischemic extremity.
- Penetrating neck trauma.
- Peripheral vascular injury with decreased pulses, distal ischemia, bruit, or expanding hematoma.
- Renal artery injury.
- Subarachnoid hemorrhage to evaluate for cerebral aneurysm.
- Thoracic and abdominal aorta injury.

Note. Because of the increased speed and availability of computed tomographic (CT) scanners, many of these conditions are initially evaluated with CT/computed tomographic angiography (CTA). In many cases, CT scanning can obviate the need for more invasive arteriography or be used to guide subsequent intervention.

PREPROCEDURE CONSULT INFORMATION

- Medical history.
- Allergies.
- Current medications (e.g., Coumadin, heparin, aspirin, sedatives).
- Laboratory values: creatinine, hematocrit, platelets, prothrombin time (PT), partial thromboplastin time (PTT).
- Pulses: femoral, posterior tibial, and dorsalis pedis bilaterally. If absent, check upper extremities. If necessary, document with portable Doppler.
- Informed consent.
- Intravenous (IV) access.

PATIENT MANAGEMENT DURING PROCEDURE

- Monitors: blood pressure, continuous electrocardiogram (ECG), oxygen saturation.
- Oxygen through nasal cannula for oxygen saturation below 95%.
- Premedication:
  - Fentanyl 25–50 μg IV (adult dose) for analgesia
    - Reversed with naloxone 0.1–0.2 mg increments IV.
  - Midazolam 0.5–1 mg IV (adult dose) for sedation
    - Reversed with flumazenil 0.2 mg IV, maximum 1 mg
- After assessing hemodynamic and respiratory status, sedation can be continued throughout the procedure as needed in aliquots of 0.5–1 mg midazolam IV and 25–50 μg fentanyl IV.

FEMORAL ARTERY PUNCTURE

Preparation.   Make sure distal pulses (posterior tibial and dorsalis pedis) have been documented. Prep both groins. The artery is first localized by palpation for point of maximum impulse. Staying below the inguinal ligament ensures the puncture will be extraperitoneal. The inguinal crease can be an unreliable landmark, particularly in obese patients. In these patients, a fluoroscopic image of the hip can be used to establish landmarks for needle placement. Optimal artery entry site is at level of mid-femoral head. Skin entry should be at inferior margin of the femoral head to allow 45-degree needle entry into artery. A blunt metal instrument can be used to mark the anticipated site of skin entry. Anesthetize the skin and superficial soft tissues with 1–2% lidocaine. Use a number 11 scalpel to make a 5-mm a dermatotomy (skin nick).

Puncture.   Using the nondominant hand, palpate the arterial pulse with middle finger above and index finger below the skin puncture site. The point of maximal arterial pulsation should be between these two fingers. Insert the needle into the dermatotomy with bevel up and the hub at a 45-degree angle from the skin surface.

Single Wall Puncture Technique.   Advance an 18-gauge needle slowly until there is pulsatile blood return. Stabilize the needle with the nondominant hand and carefully advance the guidewire (e.g., 0.035-in. Bentson or 3 J long taper), making sure that it advances easily into the vessel with no resistance. Using fluoroscopy, confirm wire placement and advance the wire into the lower abdominal aorta.

Double Wall Puncture Technique.   Advance the needle slowly, looking for blood return in the well or feeling for arterial pulsations at the end of the needle; when either is detected, advance the needle with a quick, firm thrust to penetrate both walls of the vessel (usually contacting the underlying femoral head). Remove the stylet. Decrease the angle of the needle from the skin surface and slowly pull the needle back. When there is pulsatile blood return, carefully advance the guidewire (such as 0.035-in. Bentson or 3 J long taper), making sure that it advances easily into the vessel with no resistance. Using fluoroscopy, confirm wire placement and advance the wire into the lower abdominal aorta.

Sheath Catheter.   Withdraw the needle over the guidewire. As the needle is withdrawn by the dominant hand, use the thumb and index finger of the nondominant hand to hold the wire firmly in place, and use the remaining fingers of that hand to apply pressure over the projected arterial entry site of the wire (not necessarily the skin entry site). Holding pressure at this point is important in preventing soft tissue hematoma (because the needle has made a hole slightly larger than the wire). Wipe the wire with wet gauze, and advance a vascular sheath into the artery over the wire, working close to the skin entry site. Once the sheath is in place, catheters can be advanced and exchanged through the sheath. Always advance straight or angled catheters with guidewire and direct fluoroscopic visualization. Type of catheter and technique will vary depending on indication for procedure.

Imaging Protocols (Table 53-1).

HEMOSTASIS

After removing the catheter, apply 15 minutes of moderate compression with the fingers just above the puncture site while palpating the pulse. Pulsations should not be obliterated. Gently reduce pressure over 5 minutes for a total compression time of 20 minutes. If bleeding recurs, repeat the compression. A variety of closure devices are available to reduce or eliminate postprocedure arterial compression time.

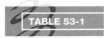

| TABLE 53-1 | Imaging Protocols |

Study (catheter position)	Total volume and rate	Image acquisition	Useful projections
Abdominal aortogram (above celiac axis)	50 mL @ 25/s	3/s × 2 s 1/s × 2× Two delays	Lateral view to demonstrate mesenteric vessel origins
Thoracic aortogram (ascending aorta)	70 mL @ 35/s	3/s × 3 s 1/s × 2 s	AP and steep (70 degrees) RPO to open arch
Bilateral lower extremity runoff (distal aorta)	60–80 mL @ 6–8/s	0 for 4 s 1/s × 3 s, pelvis 1/s × 2 s, thigh 1/s × 4 s, knee 4 delays, calf	Common iliac bifurcation — ipsilateral posterior oblique 45 degrees (side of interest down) Common femoral bifurcation — contralateral posterior oblique 45 degrees (side of interest up)
Unilateral renal arteriogram (proximal renal artery)	12 mL @ 6–8/s	3/s × 2 s 1/s × 2 s Two delays	Left renal artery origin — 15 degrees RPO Right renal artery origin –15 degrees LPO
SMA (selective)	50–60 mL @ 6–8/s	1/s × 9 s Six delays	Lateral best to rule out proximal lesions AP view better for distal branches

AP, anteroposterior; RPO, right posterior oblique; LPO, left posterior oblique; SMA, superior mesenteric artery.

POSTPROCEDURE MANAGEMENT

- Check pulses in groin and both feet, puncture site for hematoma, and vital signs.
- Flat bed rest (head may be slightly elevated) with leg straight for 4–6 hours, 2 hours of a closure device is used.
- PO or IV fluids, depending on clinical status.
- Resume preprocedure diet and medications.

Further Readings

Baum S, Pentecost MJ. *Abrams' angiography: interventional radiology*, 2nd ed. Philadelphia: Lippincott Williams & Wilkins, 2005.

Dahnert W. *Radiology review manual*, 6th ed. Philadelphia: Lippincott Williams & Wilkins, 2007.

Ferrucci JT, Taveras JM, eds. *Radiology*. Philadelphia, PA: Lippincott Williams & Wilkins, 2002 (CD-ROM version).

Kandarpa K, Aruny JE. *Handbook of interventional radiologic procedures*, 3rd ed. Philadelphia: Lippincott Williams & Wilkins, 2002.

Kaufman JA, Lee MJ. *Vascular and interventional radiology: the requisites*. Philadelphia: Mosby, 2004.

Weissleder R, Wittenberb J, Harisinghani MG. *Primer of diagnostic imaging*, 3rd ed. Philadelphia: Mosby, 2003.

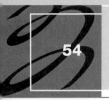

 MATERIALS

- Spinal needle, 20- or 22-gauge, 3.5-in. length (approximately).
- Lidocaine 1%.
- Syringes, 10 and 20 mL, with short extension tubing.
- Saline, sterile nonbacteriostatic.
- Nonionic contrast, 20 mL (approximately), Omnipaque 300 or 360 or equivalent.

Indications. Suspected septic arthritis (for aspiration), trauma, loosening or infection of hip joint prosthesis, hip dysplasias, and some synovial disorders. Steroid injection for pain management.

Consent. Risk of procedure is mainly due to possible allergy to contrast or local anesthetic. Bleeding or introducing infection is a remote possibility.

Scout Films. Anteroposterior (AP) and lateral views of hip.

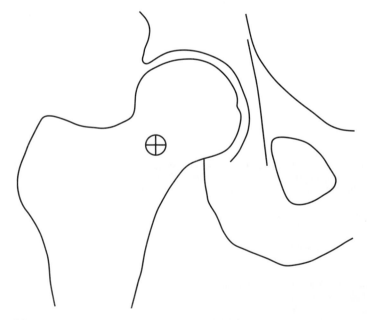

Figure 54-1. Landmarks for needle placement in hip arthrography.

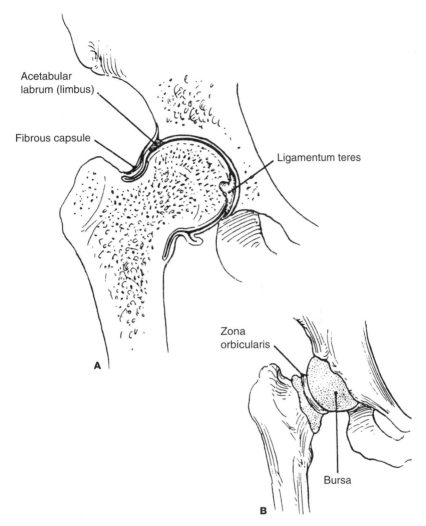

Figure 54-2. Anatomy of hip joint capsule. **A:** Coronal section and **(B)** distended synovial bursa. (Arndt RD, Horns JW, Gold RH. *Clinical arthrography*, 2nd ed. Baltimore: Williams & Wilkins, 1985:130, Fig. 3-1.)

Patient Position.   Supine with affected hip in neutral rotation. Tape toes together (feet pointing up) to keep femoral vessels medial to procedure. If a pendulous abdomen overlies the hip, tape the abdomen out of the way.

Landmarks.   Palpate femoral pulse. Begin at skin 1 cm lateral to femoral artery and 2 cm inferior to inguinal crease. Aiming for the center of the femoral neck, mark exact skin position with a radiopaque marker using fluoroscopy (Fig. 54-1).

Preparation.   Make a skin indentation or indelible mark at desired puncture site. Prepare and drape the area using sterile technique. Administer local anesthetic.

Insert Needle.   Using fluoroscopic guidance, advance needle perpendicular to table with stylet in place until it strikes the femoral neck. Attempt to aspirate joint fluid. Optional: If none returns, attempt to inject saline (~10 mL). The needle is in the joint capsule if fluid can be aspirated or the saline can be injected easily. If evaluating for infection, save all aspirated material for bacteriologic analysis.

Test Injection.   To confirm intra-articular position, do a "test" injection (ideally <1 mL) of contrast under fluoroscopic observation. Contrast should be observed flowing freely away from the needle tip but remain confined to the joint. If the needle tip is extra-articular, contrast will pool around the tip. A few drops of contrast in the joint space will not affect subsequent bacteriologic analysis.

Inject Contrast.   After confirming intra-articular position and if arthrography is desired, inject contrast to fill the joint space (Fig. 54-2). This requires an average of 15–20 mL.

Radiographs.   Remove needle and exercise hip (actively or passively) for a few moments to distribute the contrast. Overhead films are taken: AP hip in neutral, internal, and external rotation; lateral view.

Joint Prosthesis.   Aim for the medial edge of the metallic neck of the prosthesis. The skin location is more superior than for a normal hip. The puncture could also be performed directly over the prosthetic neck, but fluoroscopic guidance would be obscured. The needle is advanced until it strikes the metal of the prosthesis. The capacity of the prosthetic hip joint can vary from 5 mL to more than 30 mL.

Steroid Injection.   If procedure is performed for pain management, inject steroid mixture (e.g., triamcinolone 40 mg and 5 mL bupivacaine 0.5%) after confirming intra-articular position with test injection of contrast.

Further Readings

Arndt RD, Horns JW, Gold RH. *Clinical arthrography*, 2nd ed. Baltimore: Williams and Wilkins, 1985.

Berg TD, El-Khoury GY. Needle procedures in the peripheral musculoskeletal system. In: *Essentials of musculoskeletal imaging*. Churchill Livingstone, New York, 2003: 690–697.

Freiberger RH, Kaye JJ, Spiller J. *Arthrography*. New York: Appleton-Century-Crofts, 1979.

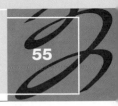

MATERIALS

- Spinal needle, 20- or 22-gauge, 3.5-in. length (approximately)
- Lidocaine 1%.
- Syringes, 10 and 20 mL, with short extension tubing.
- Saline, sterile nonbacteriostatic.
- Nonionic contrast, 20 mL (approximately), Omnipaque 300 or 360 or equivalent.

Indications. Suspected rotator cuff tear, adhesive capsulitis, loose bodies. Injection of magnetic resonance (MR) contrast for MR arthrography.

Consent. Risk of procedure is mainly due to possible allergy to contrast or local anesthetic. Bleeding and introducing infection are remote possibilities.

Scout Films. Anteroposterior (AP) films of shoulder in internal and external rotation; axillary view.

Patient Position. Patient lies supine with injured shoulder toward operator, arm supinated and palm up (externally rotated). Slight elevation of the shoulder with a pillow may help to rotate the glenoid labrum out of needle's path to joint space.

Landmarks. Begin at skin 1 cm inferior and 1 cm lateral to coracoid process. Aiming for the center of the joint, mark exact skin position with a radiopaque marker using fluoroscopy (Fig. 55-1). Under fluoroscopy, the glenoid should be facing slightly anteriorly and not seen in tangent; otherwise, the glenoid labrum will be in the way.

Preparation. Make a skin indentation or indelible mark at desired puncture site. Prepare and drape the area using sterile technique. Administer local anesthetic.

Insert Needle. Using fluoroscopic guidance, direct needle into joint space with needle absolutely perpendicular to table. Advance needle until resistance is encountered (presumably against glenoid) and pull back 1–2 mm. Optional: Gently attempt to inject saline. The needle is in the joint capsule when the saline can be injected easily, and especially if some fluid can be aspirated.

Test Injection. Do a "test" injection (ideally <1 mL) of contrast under fluoroscopic observation. Contrast should be observed flowing freely away from the needle tip and beginning to outline the joint; if the needle tip is extra-articular, contrast will pool around the tip. (A little extra-articular contrast does not affect the study.) There should be very little resistance to injection, if any.

Inject Contrast. After intra-articular position is confirmed, inject contrast to fill the joint space until patient begins to feel discomfort from distension of the joint capsule. This requires an average of 12 mL. Under fluoroscopic observation, contrast usually moves into

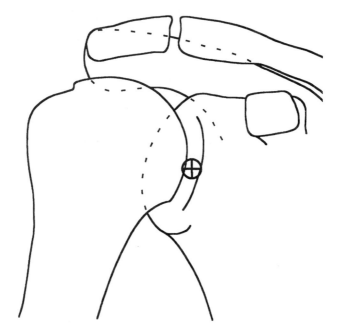

Figure 55-1. Landmarks for needle placement in shoulder arthrography.

the axillary recess first (Fig. 55-2), then medially into the subscapular recess and laterally across the humeral neck with outlining of the articular surfaces; visualization of the latter further confirms correct intra-articular position of the needle.

Films. Remove needle and exercise shoulder (actively or passively) for a few moments to distribute the contrast. Overhead films are taken: AP shoulder in neutral, internal, and external rotation; axillary view; tangential view of the glenoid fossa (optional).

Normal Contrast Distribution. The glenohumeral joint normally communicates with the subscapularis bursa (located inferior to the coracoid process) and with the synovial sheath of the long head of the biceps (Fig. 55-2). The subacromial bursa, located just inferior to the acromion, does not normally communicate with the glenohumeral joint.

Rotator Cuff Injury. The joint space and articular surfaces should normally appear as a thin line of contrast paralleling the cortex of the humeral head and ending at the medial border of the greater tuberosity. Any contrast superior or lateral to this line is abnormal and usually the result of a rotator cuff injury.

 MAGNETIC RESONANCE ARTHROGRAPHY

If procedure is being performed for MR arthrography, a 1:200 dilution of gadolinium contrast is injected into the joint. This solution can be made by instilling 0.1 mL of gadolinium contrast from a tuberculin syringe into a 20-mL syringe filled with sterile saline. Alternatively, the gadolinium contrast can be diluted in iodinated contrast so that filling of the joint can be monitored fluoroscopically.

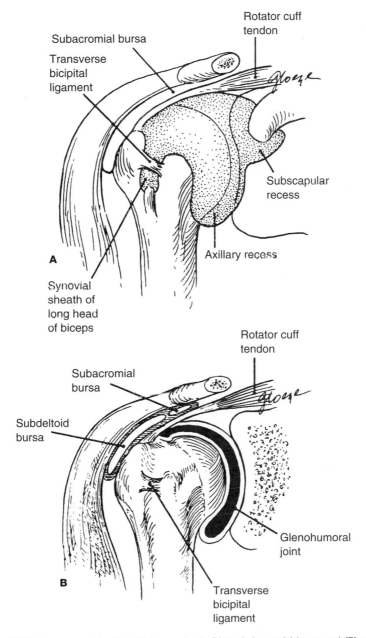

Figure 55-2. Anatomy of shoulder joint capsule. **A:** Distended synovial bursa and **(B)** coronal section. (Arndt RD, Horns JW, Gold RH. Clinical arthrography, 2nd ed. Baltimore: Williams & Wilkins, 1985;82, Fig. 2-1.)

Further Readings
Arndt RD, Horns JW, Gold RH. *Clinical arthrography*, 2nd ed. Baltimore: Williams and Wilkins, 1985.
Elentuck D, Palmer WE. Direct magnetic resonance arthrography. *Eur Radiol* 2004;14: 1956–1967.
Freiberger RH, Kaye JJ, Spiller J. *Arthrography*. New York: Appleton-Century-Crofts, 1979.

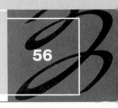

BARIUM STUDIES – UPPER GASTROINTESTINAL TRACT

Double-Contrast Upper Gastrointestinal Tract Series (Table 56.1)

Indications. Possible indications include (1) dyspepsia, (2) weight loss, (3) upper abdominal mass, (4) gastrointestinal (GI) hemorrhage, and (5) partial upper GI obstruction.

Contraindications. Complete large bowel obstruction.

Patient Prep. NPO for 6 hours.

Premedication. Some radiologists use glucagon 0.1–0.3 mg IV, given slowly over 30 seconds, p.r.n to slow gastric emptying.

Caution. Use water-soluble iodinated contrast if perforation is suspected. Use nonionic water-soluble contrast if aspiration is also likely. Nonionic contrast agents are less likely than Gastrografin to cause chemical pneumonitis if aspirated.

Single-Contrast Upper Gastrointestinal Tract Series (Table 56.2)

Indications. Indications for this study are essentially the same as for the double-contrast study. Advantage: requires less patient mobility. Disadvantage: purely mucosal lesions are not well visualized.

Contraindications. Complete large bowel obstruction.

Patient Prep. NPO for 6 hours.

Premedication. See double-contrast study.

Caution. Use water-soluble iodinated contrast if perforation is suspected. Use nonionic water-soluble contrast if aspiration is also likely. Nonionic contrast agents are less likely than Gastrografin to cause chemical pneumonitis if aspirated.

Pediatric Upper Gastrointestine Series (Table 56.3)

Indications. In the pediatric population, the common indications include major causes of persistent vomiting: (1) gastroesophageal (GE) reflux, (2) pyloric obstruction, (3) GI malrotation.

Patient Prep. NPO for 4 hours if less than or equal to 2 years old; NPO for 6 hours if older than 2 years.

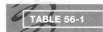

TABLE 56-1	Double-Contrast Upper Gastrointestinal (GI) Protocol[a]

Start		
Standing		*Give:* gas pills, water; fluoro for position; drink 2–3 gulps *thick* barium (hold cup in L hand near L shoulder)
Spot filming — thick barium		
Stand	LPO	– **2/1 air esophagram** (include gastroesophageal junction [GEJ]), two exposures
Coat		– Finish at least 3/4 of barium, face table, bring table down with patient prone, then position L lateral, then supine.
Supine	AP	– **1/1 body** stomach (in air)
	LPO	– **1/1 antrum** stomach (in air); try air bulb[b]
	RPO	– **1/1 Schatzki view** and **body** stomach (include lesser curve)
R lateral		– **1/1 anterior wall** and **GEJ** (in air) and duodenal **bulb**
Prone	PA	– **1/1 body** and **antrum** stomach (over bolster)
	RAO	– **2/1 antrum, bulb** and **C-sweep** (with compression)
[L lateral][b]		
Spot filming — thin barium		
Prone	RAO	Fluoro: observe single big swallow of *thin* barium from thoracic inlet to GEJ; observe stripping wave
		2/1 drinking esophagram [over bolster] (include GEJ), two exposures
Supine	AP	Check for GE reflux, document level if present
[Supine LPO][b]		
Stand	LPO	**1/1 fundus** stomach[b]
		4/1 bulb, antrum (with compression), two exposures
	AP	**4/1 proximal** and **distal stomach** (with compression), one to two exposures
Finish up		
		Overheads: routine

[a]Spot film (9" × 9") formats:

 1/1   2/1   4/1

[b]**2/1** Opportunities to image the duodenal bulb in air ("air bulb"); make two exposures (include antrum and bulb, then bulb and C-sweep). (Trick: Try turning patient prone LAO to drain excess barium from the duodenal bulb and to fill it with air; then turn patient back to supine LPO for spot film.)

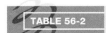

TABLE 56-2	Single-Contrast Upper GI Protocol[a]

Spot filming

Prone	RAO	– **2/1 drinking esophagram** (include GE junction)
		– **1/1** or **2/1** gastric **antrum;** duodenal **bulb** and **C-sweep** ± compression paddle
Supine	RPO	– **1/1 Schatzki view** and **GE junction**
		– [**4/1**] [duodenal **bulb** in profile]
Supine	AP	– **1/1 stomach**
		– Check for GE reflux
Semierect		– **4/1 stomach** quadrants with compression
		– [**1/1**] [gastric **fundus** and **GE junction** in air]
Supine	I PO	– **1/1** or **2/1** duodenal **bulb** and gastric **antrum** in air (attempt)

[a]Spot film (9" × 9") formats:

```
 ___        ___        ___
|   |      | | |      |_|_|
|___|      |_|_|      |_|_|

 1/1        2/1        4/I
```

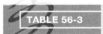

TABLE 56-3	Pediatric Upper GI Protocol[a]

Start

Be especially attentive to **collimate** as much as possible. A rough outline is given in the subsequent text; pediatric studies are usually highly tailored for the clinical question.

Position	Film	View/Maneuver
L lateral and supine AP	2/1	Drinking esophagram Allow stomach to empty; try not to overfill stomach to avoid obscuring ligament of Treitz later in examination
R lateral or supine RAO	4/1	Duodenal bulb Follow contrast (starting from stomach on lateral view, show contrast moving slightly superiorly to duodenal bulb, then inferiorly in second portion duodenum)
Supine AP	1/1	Stomach, C-loop, and ligament of Treitz (show contrast crossing to left of midline) Fill stomach fully, look for GE reflux (child should not be crying) Consider water siphon test if study is to rule out GE reflux

Finish up

Overhead: consider one AP abdominal film afterwards for an overall picture of the upper GI tract, including the proximal small bowel.

[a]Spot film (9" × 9") formats:

```
 ___        ___        ___
|   |      | | |      |_|_|
|___|      |_|_|      |_|_|

 1/1        2/1        4/1
```

Caution. Use water-soluble iodinated contrast if perforation is suspected. Use nonionic water-soluble contrast if aspiration is also likely. Nonionic contrast agents are less likely than Gastrografin to cause chemical pneumonitis if aspirated. Nonionic contrast agents also cause less shift of body fluids into the bowel lumen and should be used in all infants (especially neonates and preoperative patients) requiring water-soluble contrast.

"WHIPPLE" STUDY (Figs. 56-1 and 56-2 for relevant anatomy.)

- Goal of study is to rule out (r/o) obstruction or extravasation at the various surgical anastomoses.
- T-tube cholangiogram to evaluate choledochojejunostomy; try to demonstrate pancreaticoduodenostomy (use gravity).
- Limited Gastrografin upper gastrointestinal (UGI) for gastrojejunostomy.

BARIUM STUDIES – LOWER GASTROINTESTINAL TRACT

Double-Contrast Barium Enema (Table 56.4)

Indications. Possible indications include (1) change in bowel habit, (2) lower abdominal pain, (3) abdominal mass, (4) occult blood in stools, and (5) colon obstruction.

Contraindications. Contraindications include (1) toxic megacolon, (2) pseudomembranous colitis, and (3) recent rectal biopsy (within 3–7 days) through rigid sigmoidoscope. Biopsies performed with flexible endoscopy are not a contraindication.

Patient Prep. Modify for inpatients. Use caution if patient is diabetic. Alternative for outpatients: Fleet Prep Kit no.1 from drugstore, follow instructions for "12-hour prep."

1. Light lunch.
2. Two glasses water or juice in afternoon.
3. One bottle magnesium citrate before supper (10 oz).

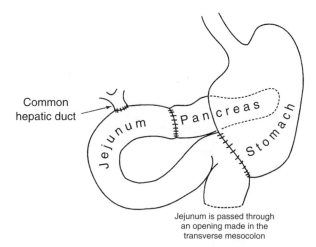

Common hepatic duct

Jejunum is passed through an opening made in the transverse mesocolon

Figure 56-1. Standard pancreaticoduodenectomy (Whipple procedure). (Drawn from Cameron JL. Current status of the Whipple operation for periampullary carcinoma. *Surg Rounds* 1988 (September):77–87, Fig.1).

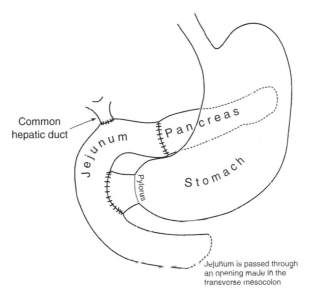

Figure 56-2. Pylorus-preserving pancreaticoduodenectomy. (Drawn from Cameron JL. Current status of the Whipple operation for periampullary carcinoma. *Surg Rounds* 1988 (September):77–87, Fig. 2).

4. Clear liquid supper.
5. Two glasses water or juice after supper.
6. Two Dulcolax tablets before bed (swallow whole).
7. NPO after midnight except medications.
8. One glass water or juice in the morning.
9. One Dulcolax suppository or water enema in the morning.

Premedication. Some radiologists use glucagon 1 mg IV, given slowly over 30 seconds, p.r.n colon spasm from diverticulitis or other cause.

Caution. Use water-soluble contrast if perforation is suspected. If an obstruction or tight stricture is found, advance only a *small* amount of barium past the narrowing to define its upper margin. Advancing more barium risks causing an impaction.

Single-Contrast Barium Enema Series (Table 56.5)

Indications. Indications for this study are essentially the same as for the double-contrast study. Advantage: requires much less patient mobility. Disadvantage: purely mucosal lesions are not well visualized.

Contraindications. See double-contrast study.

Patient Prep. See double-contrast study.

Premedication. See double-contrast study.

Caution. Use water-soluble contrast if perforation is suspected. If an obstruction or tight stricture is found, advance only a *small* amount of barium past the narrowing to define its upper margin. Advancing more barium risks causing an impaction.

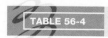 **TABLE 56-4** Double-Contrast Barium Enema Protocol[a]

Start		
L lateral		– Use thick barium
		– Do rectal examination (helpful to have patient bring knees toward chest)
		– Insert tube
		– Inflate balloon, but not if rectal disease is suspected; tape in place if necessary
Coat		– Prone [Trendelenburg] [LAO]: run barium gently to splenic flexure, clamp enema tube
		– [Reverse Trendelenburg]: lower barium bag and drain barium from rectosigmoid colon
		– Prone flat: pump air gently, get barium to cross spine (watch for air leaking back back into the barium bag!!)
		– R lateral: pump air, get barium to hepatic flexure
		– Supine: check coating (but keep patient prone and try to drain barium again if too much is in R colon)
Spot filming		
Supine	LPO	– **1/1 sigmoid** colon ("unwind" the sigmoid with spot films before cecum fills!) (sometimes try LAO to unwind)
	RAO	– **1/1 sigmoid** colon (go to overheads if contrast begins refluxing into cecum or if patient likely to "lose" enema, then do the remaining spot films)
Standing		– Run barium to cecum [drain L colon again]
	RPO	– **1/1 splenic flexure**
	AP	– **1/1 transverse colon**
	LPO	– **1/1 hepatic flexure**
		– [**1/1 cecum**]
Supine	AP	– **1/1 cecum** (if filled, try Trendelenburg or RPO)
L lateral		– Drain rectum again [pump more air]
		– **1/1 rectum**
Prone	PA	– **1/1 rectum**
Finish up		
		Overhead films, then postvoid film

[a]Spot film (9" × 9") formats:

1/1 2/1 4/1

 COLOSTOMY ENEMA

Indications.   Essentially the same as for the double-contrast study.

Contraindications.   Same as double-contrast study.

TABLE 56-5		Single-Contrast Barium Enema Protocol[a]

Start		
L lateral		– Use thin barium
		– Do rectal examination (helpful to have patient bring knees toward chest)
		– Insert tube
		– Inflate balloon, but *not* if rectal disease is suspected; tape in place if necessary
		Run barium slowly, observing the leading edge
		Stop barium flow during each spot film
Spot filming		
L lateral		– **1/1 rectum**
Supine	LPO	– **1/1 sigmoid** colon (try L lateral or even slight *LAO* to "unwind" the sigmoid on the spot films)
	RPO	– **1/1 sigmoid** colon
		– **1/1 splenic floxure**
	AP	= **I/1 transverse colon**
	LPO	– **1/1 hepatic flexure**
"Supine"		– **2/1 cecum** and **terminal ileum** with and without compression (two exposures)
Finish up		
		Fluoro colon while compressing with paddle; spot film with compression any suspicious areas
		Overheads (with tube, then postvoid)

[a]Spot film (9" × 9") formats:

    1/1   2/1   4/1

Patient Prep. Clean skin around ostomy site, put a spare ostomy bag over site, cut hole in bag. Examine ostomy with little finger; if possible—define direction. Insert lubricated cone enema tip, have patient hold in place.

Caution. Single-contrast examination with thin barium. Include a lateral view of ostomy.

Hypaque Enema Recipe. Hypaque sodium powder: 1 can (250 g) in 1,300 mL water.

BARIUM STUDIES – MISCELLANEOUS

Small Bowel Series (Table 56.6)

Indications. Possible indications include (1) assess the severity of small bowel obstruction, (2) diagnose/assess severity of inflammatory bowel disease, (3) detect small bowel masses.

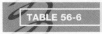

TABLE 56-6	Small Bowel Series[a]

Start
1. Drink two cups thin barium (one cup if after Upper GI), drink at once; R lateral position to help gastric emptying [optional KUB centered high after first cup].
2. 20 min KUB.
3. Follow-up films p.r.n., spot film 1/1 with compression paddle any abnormal small bowel loops (average transit time to terminal ileum 45–90 min).

Spot filming

Terminal ileum — 2/1 distended with contrast and with compression paddle (patient LPO)

Barium filled loops — 1/1 in all four quadrants

Hints

To separate pelvic small bowel loops, try turning patient prone with pelvis on top of bolster or inflated compression paddle and taking spot films or angled overhead film. If still having trouble separating loops, try turning patient while fluoroscoping in realtime.

[a]Spot film (9" × 9") formats:

    1/1   2/1   4/1

Contraindications.   Complete large bowel obstruction.

Patient Prep.   NPO for 6 hours except for medications.

Enteroclysis

Indications.   Same as for small bowel series. Enteroclysis is significantly better for detection of small bowel masses.

Contraindications.   Complete large bowel obstruction.

Patient Prep.   NPO for 6 hours except for medications.

Caution.   Methylcellulose is an emetic when it comes into contact with the stomach.

Cantor Tube Placement
1. Obtain informed consent (mention risk of bowel rupture, mucosal damage). (Give metoclopromide [Reglan] 10 mg PO p.r.n to promote peristalsis.)
2. Wet a stiff teflon-coated wire and mark distance equal to the length of the tube. Test the tube's balloon, if any.
3. Ask patient if one side of nose is more patent than the other. Swab nasal passage with plenty of lidocaine gel and have patient sniff. Use cotton-tipped applicator dipped in small cup filled with the gel. Spray throat with lidocaine spray.
4. Warm tube with water to soften. Lubricate tube with lidocaine gel. Position patient upright (preferably) or semi-upright. Advance tube into nasopharynx. Have patient start sucking on lemon swabs and advance tube into stomach. Fluoro to check position.

5. Position patient semi-upright left posterior oblique (LPO) and advance tube along greater curvature of stomach (this guides tube tip to pylorus).
6. Insert wire into tube and advance tip to within 4 inches of end of tube to maintain tube position along greater curvature. Slide tube over wire into duodenum (patient supine or right posterior oblique [RPO]), keeping wire stationary, then advance to ligament of Treitz (patient LPO). Torque tube as necessary. Wire must remain in stomach and inside tube. Sucking on lemon swabs may help tube advancement by promoting peristalsis.
7. Air may be injected into stomach to define anatomy. Use manual collimation to limit exposure. Limit fluoro time to 15 minutes. If tube tip is left near pylorus, it may go in on its own.

Enteroclysis Protocol
1. Inflate catheter balloon (≥20 mL) to prevent reflux of methylcellulose back into stomach (an emetic).
2. Barium: 200–250 mL @ 50–100 mL/minute, or enough to see barium column cross the left sacroiliac joint. Fluoro the leading edge.
3. Methylcellulose: 10–12 syringes (50 mL each) @ 50–100 mL/minute. Spot film 1/1 distended loops.
4. Overheads: anteroposterior (AP) (and both obliques).
5. Include a lateral view of any ostomy present.

T-Tube Cholangiogram Series (Table 56.7)
Indications. Look for obstruction or extravasation.

Swallowing Study Screening Series (Table 56.8)
Indications. Possible indications include (1) dysphagia, (2) aspiration, (3) suspected esophageal perforation.

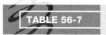

TABLE 56-7	T-tube Cholangiogram

Start
1. Scout film RUQ.
2. Connect three-way stopcock between T-tube and drainage bag; connect sideport to 50 mL syringe filled with water-soluble contrast (such as Renografin).
3. Remove air from T-tube, if possible.

Position	Film	View/Maneuver
Trendelenburg [LPO]	1/1	Inject contrast gently, fill intrahepatic ducts by gravity. (Can even try turning patient prone if not immediately post-op).
Reverse Trendelenburg	1/1	Fill distal CBD, demonstrate passage of contrast into duodenum.
Supine, RPO, LPO	1/1	spot films of CBD

Finish Up
Turn off stopcock — obtain 10 min delayed KUB to demonstrate drainage of contrast into duodenum.

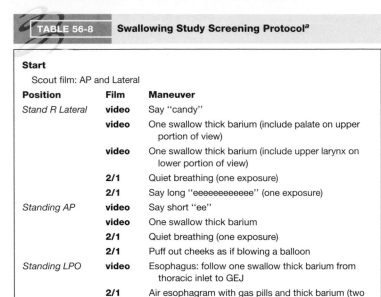

TABLE 56-8		Swallowing Study Screening Protocol[a]

Start

Scout film: AP and Lateral

Position	Film	Maneuver
Stand R Lateral	**video**	Say "candy"
	video	One swallow thick barium (include palate on upper portion of view)
	video	One swallow thick barium (include upper larynx on lower portion of view)
	2/1	Quiet breathing (one exposure)
	2/1	Say long "eeeeeeeeeee" (one exposure)
Standing AP	**video**	Say short "ee"
	video	One swallow thick barium
	2/1	Quiet breathing (one exposure)
	2/1	Puff out cheeks as if blowing a balloon
Standing LPO	**video**	Esophagus: follow one swallow thick barium from thoracic inlet to GEJ
	2/1	Air esophagram with gas pills and thick barium (two exposures)
Prone RAO	**video**	Esophagus: follow one swallow thin barium from thoracic inlet to GEJ
	2/1	Drinking esophagram with thin barium [over bolster] (two exposures)
Supine AP		Check for GE reflux; try eliciting with cough, lateral position, Valsalva, and/or straight leg raise; document level if present
Stand LPO	**1/1**	Stomach (include fundus)

[a]Spot film (9" × 9") formats:

1/1   2/1   4/1

Contraindications.   Complete large bowel obstruction. Patient's inability to cooperate with the examination.

Patient Prep.   NPO for 6 hours.

Caution.   Barium is generally the contrast agent of choice. Use water-soluble iodinated contrast if perforation is suspected. Use nonionic water-soluble contrast if aspiration is also likely, because it is less likely than Gastrografin to cause chemical pneumonitis if aspirated.

Hints

- Collimate before each video sequence or spot film!
- For single swallows, have patient take mouthful, fluoro for position, then tell patient to swallow.

What to Look for:

- Posterior pharyngeal stripping wave (cricopharyngeal prominence).
- Soft palate elevation (nasopharyngeal regurgitation).
- Larynx elevation.
- Epiglottic tilt/cricoid motility (elevation).
- Aspiration/cough/clearing (laryngeal penetration).
- Pooling in hypopharynx after swallow (retention).
- Oromotor function (premature leakage, escape).

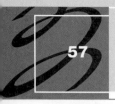

57 INTUSSUSCEPTION REDUCTION
Alexander M. Kowal

Indications. Enema reduction is the first line of treatment for intussusception in children. Enema reduction, when compared to surgery, is less invasive, decreases morbidity, costs, and length of hospitalization. Enema reduction is less successful when there is a pathologic lead point causing the intussusception, and therefore laparotomy is mandatory in adults. Children who fail enema reduction are reduced surgically.

Enema reduction is contraindicated in patients with dehydration, shock, sepsis, and suspected bowel perforation or necrosis. Therefore, patients with pneumoperitoneum or peritoneal signs on physical examination are reduced surgically. There is a decreased rate of successful reduction after 24 hours of symptoms and surgical reduction is often the choice after 48 hours, particularly if there is bright red blood per rectum. Infants younger than 3 months and children older than 5 years have an increased perforation rate. Small bowel obstruction decreases the success rate but is not a contraindication. The mean perforation rate during reduction is 0.8%. Partial reduction has been shown to reduce incision size at laparotomy.

Delayed attempts at reduction are considered safe and effective in stable patients who have been partially reduced on initial attempts. A 50% success rate has been observed. The optimal time delay between attempts has not yet been defined and varies from 15 minutes to 12 hours. Partial reduction of an initial attempt allows venous congestion and wall edema to subside, allowing for an easier subsequent reduction.

The recurrence rate for intussusception after air enema reduction is 5–15% and after barium reduction is 8–15%, compared to a 5% recurrence rate after surgical reduction. Fifty percent of recurrences present within 48 hours. Repeat enema is safe and effective with recurrent intussusceptions.

Air Versus Contrast. In the past, the decision to use air versus contrast was largely dependent on the preference of the institution and radiologist. Currently, air reduction has gained favor as a safer, more effective, and less expensive approach. Air reduction has a success rate of 76–90% versus a 55–90% success rate for contrast reduction, possibly due to higher intraluminal pressure with air. Air reduction is also a shorter procedure requiring less fluoroscopy time than contrast reduction. Although air enema is associated with a significantly higher risk of bowel perforation, probably due to higher luminal pressures during the procedure, the perforations are often smaller and cleaner with less fecal spillage and peritoneal contamination. Air reduction may be disadvantageous in patients with marked small bowel gas distention. Perforations secondary to contrast enema have increased morbidity and mortality. Water-soluble contrast is thought to have decreased morbidity in comparison to barium in case of perforation. Barium is avoided due to the risk of chemical peritonitis, infections, and adhesion formation.

 PREREQUISITES FOR ENEMA REDUCTIONS

- All patients should have a surgical consult before attempting enema reduction to ensure that preparations are made for surgery if enema reduction is unsuccessful.
- Informed consent should be obtained before procedure.
- Patient should have a good, working intravenous (IV) in place.
- Patient should be well hydrated and clinically stable.

CONTRAST REDUCTION

Equipment

- Pediatric enema (nonballoon) catheter, tubing, enema bag filled with either diluted, isotonic water-soluble contrast, or USP barium.
- Roll of surgical tape.
- Octagon board for immobilizing smaller patients.
- Optional: sedation medications such as 0.2 mg/kg morphine sulfate intramuscular (IM) or 2 mg/kg sodium pentobarbital (Nembutal) IV.

Procedure

1. Sedation can be given before procedure for agitated patients. This requires personnel trained in pediatric sedation and monitoring for the patient during the procedure.
2. Immobilize patient on octagon board.
3. Insert pediatric enema catheter into rectum and tape the buttocks together securely around the catheter.
4. Connect the catheter to a bag containing contrast.
5. Follow the "rule of 3's" described in the following steps. Of note, there is no direct evidence supporting the rule of 3's.
6. Suspend the enema bag 3 ft above the tabletop. If contrast fills the cecum and flows freely into the terminal ileum, intussusception is effectively ruled out.
7. If an intussusception is encountered, allow the bag to hang for 3 minutes at 3 ft above the tabletop in order to reduce the intussusception by hydrostatic pressure. (See Chap. 32, "Intussusception," for radiologic findings.)
8. If the intussusception is not reduced at the end of 3 minutes, lower the bag to siphon out the contrast and allow the patient to evacuate. Reinsert the catheter and repeat.
9. If the intussusception cannot be reduced after three attempts of 3 minutes duration, the patient is taken to the operating room (OR) for surgical reduction.
10. If the intussusception is successfully reduced as shown by visualization of a contrast-filled cecum with free flow of contrast into the terminal ileum, carefully examine the terminal ileum and cecum to look for a possible pathologic lead point.
11. Palpation should not be performed at any time duration enema.

 PNEUMATIC (AIR) REDUCTION

Equipment

- Pediatric enema (nonballoon) catheter, rubber surgical glove, and Shiels air insufflation device with manometer.
- Roll of surgical tape.
- Angiocath, 18 or 20 G.

Procedure

1. Sedation is not given before pneumatic reductions.
2. The patient is placed prone, which allows for manual compression of the buttocks.
3. Cut a hole in the center of the rubber glove, and pass the enema catheter through the hole and into the patient's rectum.
4. Fold the glove around the catheter in the natal crease and tape the buttocks firmly together. It is very important to make an airtight seal around the catheter.
5. Insufflate air rapidly into the colon while observing under fluoroscopy and monitoring the pressure reading on the Shiels device.
6. If no intussusception is present, air will reflux into the terminal ileum at approximately 30 mm Hg and intussusception is effectively ruled out. Spontaneous reduction may occur in up to 17% of cases.

7. If intussusception is encountered, insufflate air up to a maximum pressure of 120 mm Hg for a period of 3 minutes to attempt to reduce the intussusception.

8. If the intussusception is not reduced at the end of 3 minutes, decompress the colon through the valve on the Shiels device. Repeat the process.

9. If the intussusception is not reduced after three attempts of 3 minutes' duration at a maximum pressure of 120 mm Hg, the patient is taken to the OR for surgical reduction.

10. If free reflux of air into the terminal ileum and disappearance of the cecal soft tissue mass is seen, pneumatic reduction is considered successful. The pressure required is usually less than 100 mm Hg. Carefully look for a possible lead point in the ileum. An edematous ileocecal valve or feces may imitate a persistent intussusception.

11. During pneumatic reductions, frequently check for pneumoperitoneum under fluoroscopy. The procedure should be terminated and the patient taken to the OR at the first sign of pneumoperitoneum. Perforation can result from pressures as low as 60–80 mm Hg. A rare but potentially fatal complication of pneumatic reduction is tension pneumoperitoneum with increased intra-abdominal pressure compromising circulation. In the case of tension pneumoperitoneum, an 18 or 20 G Angiocath is inserted into the peritoneal cavity along the linea alba to achieve decompression.

12. Palpation should be avoided during pneumatic reduction.

 ULTRASOUND-GUIDED REDUCTION

Air reduction under ultrasound guidance has proved to be successful but is not widely practiced. Ultrasound-guided saline enema has had success rates of 77–96%. There is the advantage of avoidance of radiation with the elimination of time as a limiting factor.

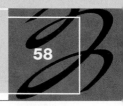
$\mathcal{T}$he role of percutaneous nephrostomy has expanded from that of a largely emergent procedure for the relief of acute supravesicular urinary tract obstruction to now include many elective indications in the initial percutaneous management of subacute or chronic upper urinary tract disease.

Indications. In most cases, percutaneous access to the urinary tract is clearly indicated to relieve acute or subacute obstruction occurring at the level of the ureteropelvic junction (UPJ) to the ureterovesicular junction (UVJ) when accompanied by pain, azotemia, and/or urosepsis. If these findings and symptoms are absent, one must proceed more cautiously to avoid draining the collecting system of a kidney that is permanently nonfunctional due to chronic obstruction. Such concerns can often be addressed by comparing the current computed tomography (CT) or ultrasonography with previous scans and evaluating renal cortical thickness as an approximate indicator of functioning renal parenchyma. Nuclear medicine studies of differential function can be misleading because an obstructed system can show markedly reduced function that can rebound immediately after the obstruction is relieved. When bilateral obstructions are encountered, old studies are also invaluable in deciding which side to drain first by showing progression of disease and parenchymal viability of each kidney. General indications for percutaneous nephrostomy are as follows:

- Relief of obstruction causing pain, azotemia, and/or urosepsis due to stone, neoplasm, blood clot, fungal ball, pyonephrosis, stricture, retroperitoneal fibrosis, or other lesion compressing the ureter. Iatrogenic causes of obstruction include inadvertant operative ligation of the ureter, complications of pyeloplasty, or postradiation fibrosis.
- Temporary urinary diversion following operative ureteral laceration, urinoma formation, or ureteric fistulas.
- Percutaneous access for pyeloplasty, operative or radiologic stone or foreign body removal, lithotripsy, nephroscopy, biopsy, and so on.
- Diagnostic puncture for antegrade pyelography and renal Whittaker test.

Contraindications. A significant bleeding diathesis is the only absolute contraindication to percutaneous nephrostomy. Overwhelming urosepsis is only a relative contraindication as percutaneous drainage may be lifesaving. Chronic obstruction with evidence of severe renal parenchymal loss is not an indication for percutaneous nephrostomy unless accompanied by pain, sepsis, or increasing azotemia.

Risks and Consent. The major risk of percutaneous nephrostomy is hemorrhage, with less than 1% incidence of life-threatening bleeding and 0.2% risk of death. It is normal to have gross hematuria for 1–2 days after the procedure, but excessive or persistent bleeding may require treatment with tube tract upsizing (to tamponade the bleeding), vascular embolization, or even surgery. Septic complications range from clinically evident bacteremia and fever in 1–9% to septic shock in approximately 0.1%. Other complications include colonic perforation (0.2%), pneumothorax, urinoma, urine peritonitis, pain, catheter malfunction, and contrast allergy.

PATIENT PREPARATION

- **Workup.** A directed workup should be obtained, including a history, physical, and pertinent laboratory data. As hemorrhage represents the most significant risk to the patient, the platelet count should be more than 50,000 and both the prothrombin time (PT) and partial thromboplastin time (PTT) should be no more than 1.3 times control. If not within acceptable limits, these values should be corrected with platelet and/or fresh frozen plasma (FFP) transfusion in every possible circumstance. A hemoglobin or hematocrit is important to establish a baseline. Blood urea nitrogen (BUN) and creatinine are important to document preprocedure renal impairment. Full urinalysis with urine cultures and, if necessary, blood cultures should be obtained before antibiotic therapy.
- **Antibiotics.** On the basis of experience at our institution, antibiotics should always be given before percutaneous nephrostomy. Give cefotetan 1 g IV approximately 1 hour before the procedure.
- **Sedation.** Depending on institutional policies, conscious sedation can be initiated either before or on the patient's arrival in the case room. Continuous monitoring of oxygen saturation, cardiac rhythm, and blood pressure must be performed during conscious sedation. Midazolam 1 mg and fentanyl 50 μg IV aliquots may be administered p.r.n before and during the procedure.
- **Imaging studies.** Prior imaging studies that could yield anatomic information on the position of the kidney relative to the ipsilateral 12th rib, pleura, liver, spleen, and colon as well as information on variant anatomy such as malrotation, duplication, or ectopia should be reviewed and posted in the case room.

Planning the Approach.   Ultimately, the final path of the percutaneous nephrostomy tube must meet a number of important anatomic criteria to be safe, effective, and comfortable to the patient. Additionally, if the nephrostomy tube is being placed to provide initial access for endoscopy, endopyelotomy, or other surgical intervention, it may be necessary to engage specific calices. For such cases, consult with the referring surgeon before proceeding. For routine nephrostomy, the following criteria, from deep to superficial, should be noted:

- **Kidney.** The renal cortex should be entered posterolaterally to engage a posterior middle-to-lower pole calyx. The normal kidney is rotated posteriorly 30 degrees relative to the coronal plane such that the renal pelvis is directed anteromedially. The lower pole also lies slightly more posterolateral than the upper pole. Most of the arterial supply of the kidney is divided into the anterior segmental divisions with the posterior kidney being largely supplied by a single divisional artery that passes behind the upper pole infundibulae. This leaves a relatively avascular plane or "watershed" along the posterolateral kidney (Brodel's line), which is least perfused inferiorly. This is the safest site through which to intubate the kidney, and it logically follows that posterior calyces will allow the most direct path to the renal pelvis from this approach. The desired posteroinferior calyces will be projected slightly more medially than anterior calyces in the anterior-posterior (AP) projection.
- **Soft tissues.** To meet the previous anatomic requirements, the skin entrance site is usually 30 degrees from the spine in the axial plane. If too far lateral, there is a risk of entering liver, spleen, or colon. Medially, the skin entrance site should remain lateral to the paraspinal musculature. A proper entrance site, in addition to being more comfortable by allowing the patient to lie supine, will also help prevent tube kinking. Superiorly, the path of the nephrostomy tube should pass below the 12th rib to avoid the pleural reflection. A path immediately subcostal could cause bleeding from the intercostal artery and should be avoided.

Positioning.   Place the patient in prone position with hands below chin or above head. Prep the involved side from T9 to below the iliac crest and from the mid-axillary line to the contralateral paraspinal musculature. If available, perform a renal ultrasonography to determine the renal position relative to the 12th rib, spine, liver, and spleen. While holding the transducer over the desired skin entrance site based on the above criteria, note the relative angulation and depth to the posteroinferior calyces. Make a skin mark at this site.

Visualization Options.   There are two main options for visualizing the collecting system before definitive puncture of a posteroinferior calyx.

"Single-stick" Option.   The first option is the "single-stick" technique whereby intravenous contrast is given to opacify the collecting system before definitive puncture. This technique should be reserved for those patients in whom the kidney in question is not completely obstructed and is capable of excretion and in whom the creatinine is less than 1.7 mg/dL. Occasionally, the patient will already have intrapelvic contrast from a recent intravenous urography (IVU) or CT. Ultrasonography can also be used exclusively on a single pass to engage the posteroinferior calyces, a preferred method in the pregnant patient.

"Double-Stick" Option.   The second and often only option is the "double-stick" technique whereby a first needle is passed under fluoroscopic or ultrasonographic guidance to engage the renal pelvis. A small amount of contrast is then injected to opacify the collecting system. A second definitive pass is made under fluoroscopic guidance allowing permanent access through a posteroinferior calyceal approach. If the degree of dilatation is sufficient and the patient's body habitus is suitable, some prefer ultrasonography for the first pass, especially if the patient is pregnant or diabetic.

Engagement of the renal pelvis can be done either under fluoroscopic or ultrasonographic control, as outlined in the preceding text.

■ **Fluoroscopic control.** Position the C-arm opposite the kidney in the axial plane. Identify the renal outline under fluoroscopy and position the tip of a metallic clamp over the junction of the medial and middle thirds of the kidney transversely and over its midportion craniocaudally. Mark this site on the skin. If this site lies above the 12th rib, position the clamp below the rib and angle the image intensifier (II) caudad until the clamp superimposes over the kidney mid-portion. Infiltrate the site with 1% lidocaine, make a small skin incision with a no. 11 blade, and advance a 22- or 23-gauge needle slowly, centimeter by centimeter, toward the target while confirming alignment with the x-ray beam by intermittent fluoroscopy. When a depth is reached roughly approximating that noted on the initial ultrasound, remove the needle stylet between each advancement and closely examine the hub for the presence of urine. Often a palpable "pop" or "give" (sudden loss of resistance) will be noted as the needle enters the renal pelvis. If the needle is significantly beyond the expected depth of the renal pelvis with no urine noted, slowly withdraw the needle while aspirating through a short extension tubing, as the needle may have passed through a collapsed renal pelvis. This process may have to be repeated several times before a "flash" of urine is obtained. Collect a urine specimen for Gram stain and culture.

■ **Ultrasonographic control.** Position the transducer on the skin to allow maximal visualization of the pelvis and calyces while repeating the anatomic criteria defined in the preceding text. Position a 21- or 22-gauge needle alongside the transducer (or better still, within a needle guide) and advance to the target along the image plane until urine is seen at the needle hub.

Opacification.   Once in the renal pelvis, there are several options for opacification. A small quantity of dilute contrast is often all that is required to visualize the pelvocalyceal system. Remove some urine before opacification to avoid contrast dilution and calyceal rupture and to lower the risk of bacteremia. In the prone patient, maximal visualization of the nondependent posterior calyces can be obtained with injection of carbon dioxide. An appropriate gas-filled calyx will appear as a low-density halo when seen end-on. Over the course of the case, more contrast and/or carbon dioxide will likely be needed as leakage occurs around the needle and down the ureter.

Skin Entry Site.   Sweep the C-arm around from the side opposite the kidney to a position approximately 30–45 degrees relative to the head on the same side of the kidney and angle the II approximately 45 degrees caudally. Place a metallic clamp tip on the patient at a desirable skin entry site (i.e., below 12th rib, lateral to paraspinal muscles, etc.). "Fine tune" the II position to superpose the clamp tip with a contrast- or gas-filled posteroinferior calyx. This may require minor adjustments in the clamp position as well. The site should roughly correlate with the earlier ultrasonographic site. If not, reevaluate the position. Once a skin entry site is chosen, generously infiltrate with 1% lidocaine and make a small skin incision with the No. 11 blade.

Needle Insertion.   A number of needle-wire-dilator-sheath combinations are commercially available, many of which work on the same basic principle. The Jeffrey Wire Guide Exchange Set (Cook, Inc., Bloomington, IN) will be used herein as an example. This kit consists of a 15-cm 21-gauge trocar needle, an 0.018-in. platinum-tipped Cope mandril wire, a 100-cm J-tipped 0.038-in. wire, and a three-piece assembly containing an inner metallic 20-gauge stiffening cannula, a 6.3-F dilator with a 3–4 cm long taper ending in a tip fitted to the 0.018 wire, and an 8.0-F outer sheath.

Seat the 21-gauge needle in the skin incision, align it with the x-ray beam, and advance it in small increments toward the selected lower pole calyx with intermittent fluoroscopy to confirm alignment. When 75% of the distance to the calyx is reached (based on the earlier ultrasonographic measurement), rotate the II cranially toward the contralateral side 60–90 degrees without moving the C-arm. This allows the operator to visualize the needle in profile instead of end-on as it approaches and engages the desired calyx. Again, a palpable "pop" will often be felt, and the calyx will suddenly "give" on fluoroscopy when the needle enters. Remove the stylet. Urine should be visible or able to be aspirated from the hub.

To perform a "single-stick" nephrostomy exclusively using real-time ultrasound, the same skin landmarks are chosen before advancing an 18- to 21-gauge needle along the image plane into a well-visualized posteroinferior calyx.

Securing Access.   Advance the 0.018 wire through the needle, calyx, infundibulum, and into the renal pelvis. This may require use of a torque device to negotiate the infundibulum. If possible, direct the 0.018 wire past the UPJ and into the ureter for more stable access. If not possible, coil the wire in the renal pelvis. Remove the needle while maintaining wire position and carefully advance the stiffener-dilator-sheath assembly over the wire under fluoroscopy, taking great care to avoid kinking the wire. Once the assembly reaches the calyx, disengage the metallic stiffening cannula and hold its position relative to the calyx while advancing the dilator-sheath components farther over the wire. Avoid applying undue pressure on the opposite wall of the renal pelvis during this advancement. Once the sheath and dilator are well inside the renal pelvis, remove the wire, dilator, and stiffening cannula, leaving the sheath. Advance the 0.038 wire and coil it in the renal pelvis. Remove the sheath.

Intubation.   Choose an 8- to 10-F "pigtail" type catheter with multiple side-holes confined to the loop. Advance the catheter over the 0.038 wire and coil it in the renal pelvis. A catheter with a self-retaining locking mechanism (e.g., a string) is preferable, as respiratory excursion can otherwise dislodge the catheter. Suture the catheter to the skin for 4–8 weeks until the tract is mature.

Patient Follow-up.   Place the percutaneous nephrostomy catheter to external gravity drainage. The patient's vital signs should be closely monitored for 4–6 hours after the procedure, and nephrostomy tube output should be charted. It is normal for the urine to be blood-tinged, often related to renal pelvis clot. This hematuria clears in 1–2 days in the vast majority of patients. A follow-up hematocrit may be helpful in evaluating patients with persistent hematuria. In a patient with impaired renal function, a follow-up BUN or creatinine may also be helpful. Routine post-procedure orders are as follows:

- Nephrostomy tube to gravity drainage. Record tube output q8h.
- Vital signs every 30 minutes × 4, q1h × 4, then routine (q8h).
- Bedrest or limited activity for 6–12 hours.
- Hematocrit and BUN/creatinine in the morning (optional).

SPINAL PUNCTURE AND MYELOGRAPHY

59

Note: Myelography is described herein. As a separate procedure, spinal puncture (lumbar or cervical) is carried out identically as described for myelography, except that contrast is not administered.

MATERIALS

- Spinal needle, 22 or 25 gauge, 9 cm length.
- Lidocaine, 1% (preferentially buffered with bicarbonate).
- Syringe, 20 mL, with extension tubing.
- Iohexol (Omnipaque) 180 or 240 or 300.

Indications. Magnetic resonance imaging (MRI) is the primary imaging modality of the spinal canal and its contents. Myelography should be performed in patients who are unable to undergo MRI, such as those with cardiac pacemakers, certain aneurysm clips, or those who have enough steel hardware to create unacceptable artifact over the areas to be imaged. Additionally, myelography should be undertaken in patients who are unable to tolerate MRI due to their size or to claustrophobia. Certain surgeons may prefer myelography to MRI preoperatively, as it gives better information regarding bony structures.

Consent. The main risks of the procedure include pain (possibly radicular), contrast reaction, headache, infection, or, rarely, hematoma. Seizures may occur as a very rare complication. The risk of seizure may be higher for cervical myelogram. The seizure threshold may be lowered by certain medications, including major tranquilizers, antidepressants, and central nervous system (CNS) stimulants; such medications should be discontinued 48 hours before the procedure. Diabetic patients taking metformin (Glucophage) should stop taking metformin. A blood creatinine level should be obtained 48 hours after the procedure and if this is comparable to baseline value, the patient can resume metformin. This is the general recommendation for intravenous (IV) injections. Considering the amount of contrast used for myelography and the time that it takes for contrast to enter the blood stream, this approach is probably over cautious but it is still recommended as most myelography examinations are elective.

Patient Position. Efforts should be made to position the patient's head to prevent contrast from reaching the basal cisterns, especially during rolling and other maneuvers potentially necessary for the procedure. If the patient remains prone, the neck should be extended.
Lumbar—prone. The patient may be slightly oblique to optimize access to the interlaminar space.
Cervical—prone. May also be done with patient in lateral decubitus position if lateral fluoroscopy is not available. A lumbar approach may be used if cervical access is limited. In that case, the contrast is moved to the cervical region using a tiltable myelography table or by elevating the pelvis, with the hip and knee joints.

Landmarks

Lumbar. The goal is to place the needle through the interlaminar space to access the subarachnoid space. In order to avoid the cord, access through the L2-3 interspace or below is recommended.

Cervical. The posterior, superior one third of the spinal canal between C1 and C2 is the needle insertion site.

Preparation. The patient should be well hydrated before and after the procedure (orally, if possible). Care must be taken to procure a coagulation profile (e.g., prothrombin time [PT], partial thromboplastin time [PTT], platelets) in patients with a suspected coagulopathy. Renal function (e.g., blood urea nitrogen [BUN], creatinine) should be ascertained. A steroid preparation is needed for patients who have a history of allergy to iodinated contrast material. Patients should not have eaten within approximately 4 hours of the procedure. Prep and drape the skin around the appropriate site.

Lumbar. Under fluoroscopic guidance, find the appropriate interlaminar space and make a skin indentation to mark it. After raising a skin wheal of lidocaine at that site (25-gauge needle), administer approximately 5 mL lidocaine (1%) through a 25-gauge needle into the subcutaneous and muscular tissues of the back.

Cervical. Under fluoroscopic guidance, locate the posterior, superior one third of the spinal canal between C1 and C2 and make a skin indentation to mark it. After raising a skin wheal of lidocaine at that site (25-gauge needle), administer approximately 5 mL lidocaine (1%) through a 25-gauge needle into the subcutaneous and muscular tissues of the neck. It may be helpful to leave in the anesthetizing needle as a landmark, which is then removed upon insertion of the spinal needle.

Insert Spinal Needle

Lumbar. Lay the needle on the patient's back with the tip directed toward the head and superimposed upon the interlaminar space. Check the position of the needle tip fluoroscopically. With position confirmed, raise the needle 90 degrees so that it is perpendicular to the table and image intensifier. Pierce the skin, inserting the needle approximately 1 cm, and check needle position. The needle bevel marker (indicating bevel up) should face the operator to minimize disruption of the collagen fibers of the dure. Advance the needle, removing the stylet as necessary to check for return of cerebrospinal fluid (CSF). A "pop" will often be felt upon access to the subarachnoid space. If CSF is not accessed after three or four attempts, try another level.

Cervical. Use a direct lateral approach. If necessary, the patient may be placed in the lateral decubitus position. Insert the spinal needle until CSF return or a "pop" is felt upon access to the subarachnoid space. Patient cooperation is critical.

Remember that the needle will travel slightly away from the direction of the bevel marker as the needle is advanced. For either lumbar or cervical punctures the needle depth should be visualized when appropriate. After accessing the subarachnoid space, collect CSF for analysis, if requested by the referring physician.

Contrast Selection and Dose. The most critical point in performing myelography is to be certain that a nonionic agent, specifically approved for intrathecal administration, is used. Fatalities have resulted from inadvertent use of ionic agents. Contrast misadministration may not be readily apparent, with symptoms and signs (dizziness, nausea, diaphoresis, lower extremity paresthesias, seizures, and death) appearing anywhere from 30 minutes to 6 hours after administration. During myelography, contrast flow may be very slow due to decreased blood pressure if contrast misadministration occurs. The contrast bottle must be visualized by the radiologist before withdrawal of contrast into the syringe for injection into the subarachnoid space. Iohexol (Omnipaque) comes in densities of 140, 180, 210, 240, 300, and 350 mg iodine/mL. The 140 and 350 mg iodine/mL are NOT approved for intrathecal administration. Iopamidol (Isovue) may also be used in densities approved for intrathecal administration. Iohexol 180 is generally a good choice for routine lumbar studies whereas 300 may be necessary to perform panmyelography from a lumbar approach.

The maximum permissible contrast load to the subarachnoid space is approximately 3 g iodine (12 mL iohexol 180, 2.2 g, is a routine standard dose).

Contrast Administration. After access to the subarachnoid space has been achieved, attach a short extension tubing to the hub of the needle, taking care not to disturb the needle position. Next, gently pulse a minimal amount of contrast under fluoroscopy to assure subarachnoid administration. The contrast should flow freely away from the needle tip. If there is uncertainty, that is, possible subdural administration, try looking lateral and reposition the needle if necessary. For a routine lumbar myelogram, place the patient in a slight reverse Trendelenberg position so that contrast may be seen to flow into the terminus of the thecal sac. After all the contrast is administered, detach the extension tubing and remove the needle after reinserting the stylet.

Films. Begin radiograph myelography immediately after contrast administration.

Lumbar. Obtain standing (if possible) AP and lateral as well as approximately 45-degree bilateral obliques of the lower lumbar region. Then, take prone AP, lateral, and bilateral oblique images of the upper lumbar region. Lastly, obtain an AP image of the conus medullaris, for a total of nine images. CT: 3 × 3 mm slices from L3 to S1 0.5 to 4 hours after contrast administration.

Cervical—AP, lateral, and bilateral approximately 45-degree obliques (four images, total). CT: 1.5 × 1.5 mm slices from C3 to T1 immediately after contrast administration.

Of course, imaging is tailored to the clinical question and correlated to previous imaging studies. One of the greatest uses of myelography is that it may give dynamic information. For example, if the patient has pain only when standing or flexed in a certain position, perform imaging in that position.

If a block to contrast flow occurs: many obstructions which appear total are not. CT often shows flow of contrast around the cord (cervical) or throughout the thecal sac (lumbar) when such was not visualized on the radiographs. Delayed images may be helpful, sometimes up to 24 hours. If a total block is strongly suspected, first try positional maneuvers, for example, contrast may be unable to negotiate a pronounced kyphosis when attempting a cervical (or pan) myelogram from a lumbar approach in the prone patient. If a block is confirmed after various positional maneuvers, an additional bolus of contrast may be administered through a second puncture on the opposite side of the block, taking care not to exceed a total of 3 g iodine.

After the Procedure. Myelography is an outpatient procedure. The patient may be discharged 4 hours after the procedure. The most frequent adverse reaction is headache (~20% in one series), which is believed to be due to CSF leak and not contrast toxicity. Finer needles (25 or 26 G) appear to confer protection against postmyelography headache. If the patient complains of headache beyond 24 hours after the procedure, continued CSF leakage near the needle insertion site may be present, and a reparative measure such as a blood patch may be necessary.

Further Readings

Harrison PB. The contribution of needle size and other factors to headache following myelography. *Neuroradiology* 1993;35:487–489.

Shapiro R. *Myelography*, 4th ed. Chicago: Mosby–Year Book, 1984.

Tamura T. A simple technique for cervical myelography. *Spine* 1991;16:1267–1268.

Wang H, Binet EF, Gabrielsen TO, et al. Lumbar myelography with iohexol in outpatients: prospective multicenter evaluation of safety. *Radiology* 1989;173:239–242.

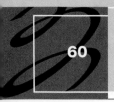

60 RETROGRADE URETHROGRAM

 MATERIALS

- Small Foley catheter.
- Small (5 mL) syringe for inflating Foley catheter balloon.
- Water-soluble iodinated contrast, ionic or nonionic, such as Renografin or Omnipaque.
- Syringe (with catheter tip) for injecting contrast.

Indications.   Retrograde urethrography is commonly performed by urologists using a penile clamp. In the emergent setting, usually during evaluation for traumatic urethral tear, the radiologist may be asked to perform the procedure without the clamping device.

Scout Film.   Coned anteroposterior (AP) view of the urethra and bladder base.

Insert catheter into the urethra, using sterile technique, until the balloon is in the fossa navicularis (just inside the urethral meatus). Inflate the balloon with 1–2 mL water, or until patient expresses discomfort, to form a seal around the catheter.

Inject contrast to fill the urethra while obtaining films in three positions: (1) left anterior oblique (LAO) with right leg flexed at hip, (2) AP supine, and (3) right anterior oblique (RAO) with left leg flexed. This is best done using fluoroscopic guidance and spot films, but the urethral injections can also be done (preferably by a nonradiologist wearing a lead apron) while overhead films are being taken.

Hints.   The entire contrast-filled urethra should be visualized on the films without evidence of extravasation into the soft tissues. Proper filling of the urethra requires more than gentle pressure when pushing contrast with the syringe.

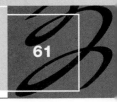
 PROCEDURE

See Figure 61-1 for normal urethral anatomy.

1. Empty the bladder.
2. Catheterize bladder, record residual volume (normal <100 mL).
3. Fill bladder with contrast by gravity, fluoro intermittently, look for vesicoureteral reflux.
4. Spot film 1/1 bladder, partially filled.
5. Spot film 1/1 anteroposterior (AP) full bladder.
   Spot film 1/1 obliques of both lower ureters (include ureterovesical junctions [UVJs]).
   (Spot film 1/1 AP both kidneys if reflux and/or hydronephrosis is present.)
   (Spot film 1/1 lateral bladder if study to rule out fistulae.)
6. Fluoro urethra for position (oblique position for males).
   Cone down!
   Have patient void around catheter.
   (Remove catheter, if there is time.)
7. Spot film 1/1 voiding urethra.
   (Include entire urethra, especially in males.)
8. Fluoro both kidneys (look for postvoid vesicoureteral reflux).
9. (Postvoid KUB.)

Spot film (9" × 9") formats:

1/1	2/1	4/1

 UROLOGIST'S TRICKS FOR CATHETERIZING THE BLADDER IN MALES

■ **Catheter.** Use a stiff catheter (white silastic or clear plastic) rather than red rubber. Use as large a diameter catheter as can comfortably fit in the meatus.

■ **Lidocaine.** If necessary, inject 10 mL lidocaine gel into the meatus and urethra using syringe tip or syringe plus large intravenous (IV) catheter (≥18 G). Have patient or parents hold meatus closed for 5 minutes.

■ **Relaxation.** The patient must be relaxed. A crying child is very difficult to catheterize even with these tricks.

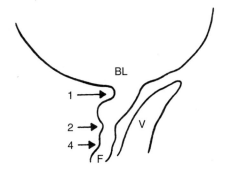

Female–lateral

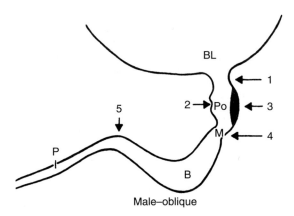

Male–oblique

Figure 61-1. Normal female and male urethra.
BL, bladder
1 Bladder neck or urethrovesical junction
2 Intermuscular incisura
3 Verumontanum (male)
4 Membranous urethra at the level of the urogenital diaphragm
5 Suspensory ligament of the penis (male)
Po Posterior (prostatic) urethra (male)
M Membranous urethra (male)
B Bulbous urethra (male)
P Penile urethra (male)
F Fossa navicularis (female)
V Vagina (female)
(Kirks DR, ed. *Practical pediatric imaging: diagnostic radiology of infants and children*, 2nd ed. Boston: Little, Brown and Company, 1991:921, Fig. 8-8.)

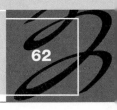

SALINE INFUSION SONOHYSTEROGRAPHY

Laura Amodei

$\mathcal{S}$aline infusion sonohysterography (SIS) is known by several other names, including sonohysterosalpingography and hysterosonography. SIS involves the acquisition of multiple endovaginal ultrasonographic (EVS) images of the uterus and endometrial cavity during the infusion of sterile saline.

ROLE OF SALINE INFUSION SONOHYSTEROGRAPHY AND COMMON INDICATIONS

SIS is most commonly used in one of two ways. The first is for the evaluation of endometrial abnormalities. In this case, patients are often peri- or postmenopausal and may have postmenopausal or other abnormal uterine bleeding. These patients should always have an EVS before SIS. Other patients will have undergone pelvic ultrasonography for another indication and will have been found to have an abnormal endometrium. Endometrial abnormalities on EVS include thickening (normal endometrium: premenopausal $\leq$15 mm; postmenopausal asymptomatic, on HRT $\leq$8 mm; and postmenopausal with symptoms $\leq$5 mm), endometrial distortion, suspected mass/focal abnormality, and poor visualization. The role of SIS in the evaluation of endometrial abnormalities is presented in Figure 62-1. The second application of SIS is in the evaluation of suspected congenital anomalies or variants (e.g., bicornuate uterus) or acquired abnormalities (e.g., uterine synechiae). These patients are younger and are usually being evaluated for infertility or repeated spontaneous abortions.

ALTERNATIVE TECHNIQUES

Evaluation of Endometrial Abnormalities

- EVS is very sensitive for endometrial thickening, but is often nonspecific. Occasionally, on EVS, findings are sufficiently specific to warrant proceeding directly to hysteroscopy without SIS (Fig. 62-1).
- **Hysteroscopy** is performed by gynecologists; it allows direct visualization of the uterine cavity and targeted biopsy or resection of abnormalities, but is invasive and requires anesthesia.
- **Blind endometrial biopsy and dilatation and curettage (D&C)** are also performed by gynecologists; they provides tissue for pathologic diagnosis, but can be prone to sampling error and false negatives, particularly in the case of focal abnormalities.
- **Pelvic magnetic resonance imaging (MRI)** is occasionally used to evaluate causes of abnormal uterine bleeding or pelvic pain.

Evaluation of Congenital Variants/Anomalies or Acquired Abnormalities

- **Hysterosalpingography** is an older technique in which contrast material is introduced into the uterine cavity and x-ray images are obtained for evaluation of the morphology or the uterine cavity and fallopian tubes. It is particularly useful in the evaluation of fallopian tube patency.
- **Pelvic MRI** can be used to evaluate suspected congenital anomalies or variants.

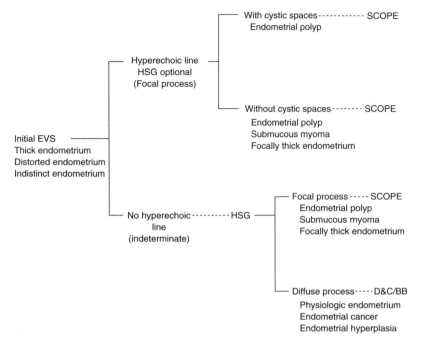

Figure 62-1. Diagram illustrates a method of triage for patients with suspected endometrial pathology. In this flowchart, hysterosonography (HSG) is used only selectively and as a complement to the initial endovaginal ultrasonography. SCOPE, hysteroscopy; EVS, endovaginal ultrasonography; D&C, dilatation and curettage; BB, blind endometrial biopsy. (Reprinted with permission from Dudiak KM. Hysterosonography: a key to what is inside the uterus. *Ultrasound Q* 2001;17(2):73–86.)

 ## CONTRAINDICATIONS OF SALINE INFUSION SONOHYSTEROGRAPHY

- **Pregnancy or possible pregnancy.** SIS. should be performed in the follicular portion of cycle after menstruation has ended, but before ovulation, and should generally not be performed after the 10th day of the menstrual cycle.
- **Pelvic inflammatory disease (PID).** Patients should be assessed for unexplained pelvic or cervical motion tenderness, which could be a sign of PID during the manual examination described in the subsequent text.
- The theoretic risk of spread of endometrial cancer through the fallopian tubes into the abdomen during SIS has not been supported by the literature.

 ## PHYSICIAN'S QUALIFICATIONS

In addition to their general guidelines for ultrasonography, the American College of Radiology (ACR) recommends that physicians performing SIS have at least 3 months of formal training and ongoing experience in the performance in interpretation of gynecologic examinations, as well as familiarity with cervical cannulation techniques.

 ## SUPPLIES

- Speculum.
- 5 F (occasionally 7 F) balloon catheter.

- Cervical dilators.
- Long ring forceps.
- Povidone/iodine (Betadine) swabs.
- Sterile saline.
- Two 10-mL syringes.
- Endovaginal probe cover.
- Sterile ultrasonographic gel.

 TECHNIQUE

Timing

The patients should be 7–10 days into their cycle.

Preparation

If the patient usually takes prophylactic antibiotics before an invasive procedure (e.g., patient with artificial heart valves), these should be administered before SIS. If there is any concern for pregnancy, a pregnancy test should be performed or the examination should be rescheduled in the first half of the menstrual cycle as discussed in preceding text. Assess for latex allergy. Obtain written informed consent.

Place patient in the lithotomy position. Standard EVS should be performed before all SIS procedures, including measurement of dual-layer endometrial thickness. Manual examination should be performed to assess for pelvic or cervical motion tenderness (as signs of possible contraindication due to PID) and to assess the location and orientation of the cervix.

Speculum Insertion. Place patient in lithotomy position with the buttocks at the end of the table. Lubricate speculum. Using the index and middle finger of dominant hand, separate labia from below to visualize introitus. Insert speculum obliquely at a 15-degree angle while maintaining a posterior direction toward the rectum. Always apply pressure downward during insertion. (Pressing upward pushes the urethra against the symphysis pubis, causing pain or discomfort to the patient.) Rotate the speculum to a horizontal position and grasp handle with nondominant hand. Continue to insert the speculum until flush against perineum. Open and position speculum by depressing the thumb rest slowly, approximately 2–3 cm or until the cervix is visible between the blades. If cervix is not visualized, pull the speculum back approximately 2–3 cm, then release thumb pressure. Maintain pressure on thumb rest to prevent bills from closing on cervix, and once you are sure that the cervix is not between the blades you can close completely and reposition closed speculum. If necessary, repeat manual examination to clarify location and orientation of cervix before replacing speculum.

Catheter Insertion. Clean cervix with Betadine swabs held in ring forceps. Insert catheter through cervical canal into endometrial cavity. If catheter will not pass, cervical dilators can be gently used. Once catheter is well into endometrial canal, inflate catheter balloon.

Exchanging Speculum and Probe. Take care not to dislodge the catheter; special care must be taken with multiparous patients who are more prone to catheter dislodgement. To remove speculum, place thumb of dominant hand on thumb rest, grasp handles in hand and release the secured position by loosening the bolt. Rotate clockwise, applying posterior pressure on the pelvic floor. Remove the blades at an oblique angle. Carefully insert EVS probe (in probe cover with sterile ultrasonographic gel). Withdraw the catheter so that the balloon is just above in the internal cervical os.

Saline Infusion. Using the 10-mL syringes under sonographic visualization, infuse just enough sterile saline to distend the endometrial cavity, usually 5–15 mL. In certain patients, the saline will continuously leak through the cervical canal, requiring constant or near constant infusion.

Imaging.   The entire endometrial cavity should be assessed with EVS in at least two planes. If the uterus is too large, supplemental transabdominal ultrasonography may also be necessary. The most important determination is whether a visualized abnormality is focal (hysteroscopy would be best if further evaluation/treatment is needed) or diffuse (blind endometrial biopsy or dilatation and curettage should be adequate). If an abnormality is focal, its relationship to the endometrial wall (e.g., broad base or narrow stalk) should be assessed. Remember that endometrial lesions can be multiple or multifocal. Doppler imaging should be performed to determine whether there is a single feeding vessel or diffuse vascularity. Near the end of the examination, the catheter balloon should be deflated so that the lower endometrial cavity can be completely evaluated, then the catheter and probe can be removed.

 ## POTENTIAL COMPLICATIONS

SIS is usually very well tolerated. Patients may experience cramping. Very rare potential complications include infection, bleeding, and uterine perforation.

 ## SALINE INFUSION SONOHYSTEROGRAPHIC IMAGE INTERPRETATION

Determine whether an endometrial abnormality is focal or diffuse to guide further evaluation and/or treatment (Fig. 62-1).

Possible Findings

DDx Focal Lesions.   Polyp(s) (Fig. 62-2), submucosal fibroid(s), focal endometrial thickening, and endometrial wrinkle (in redundant benign proliferative endometrium).

■ **Polyps.** Usually attached to cavity wall by a narrow stalk with a single feeding vessel. Usually hyperechoic relative to the endometrium, but can be heterogeneous or hypoechoic. Often have appearance of cystic spaces due to dilated glands.

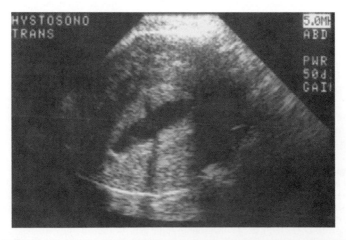

Figure 62-2. Elderly patient with atrophic endometrium and two discrete polyps on this sagittal image from a saline infusion sonohysterography (SIS). One polyp is slightly smaller and hyperechoic relative to the larger polyp on this single sagittal image. Both polyps have a narrow attachment to the adjacent endometrium that is otherwise thin and atrophic. These polyps would be at risk of evading a blind biopsy device. (Reprinted with permission from Dudiak KM. Hysterosonography: a key to what is inside the uterus. *Ultrasound Q* 2001;17(2):73–86.)

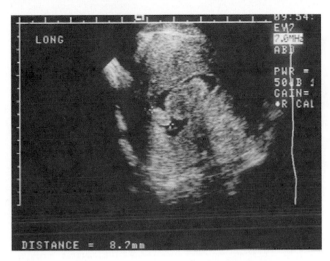

Figure 62-3. Elderly patient with postmenopausal bleeding and endometrial hyperplasia. Transverse scan performed during hysterosonography (HSG) shows a globally thickened endometrial lining. This appearance can be seen with physiologically triggered processes or may be caused by underlying pathology, such as endometrial carcinoma or hyperplasia. In this case, the endometrial myometrial interface is intact. In a patient with endometrial cancer, this information would indicate minimal or no myometrial invasion of tumor. (Reprinted with permission from Dudiak KM. Hysterosonography: a key to what is inside the uterus. *Ultrasound Q* 2001;17(2):73–86.)

■ **Submucosal fibroids.** Usually broad base of attachment. Heterogeneous echogenicity. Can usually identify a think echogenic rim of endometrial tissue around the fibroid. Blood flow is usually more random (i.e., not single feeding vessel).

■ **Diffuse lesions.** Endometrial carcinoma, proliferative endometrium, and endometrial hyperplasia (Fig. 62-3). SIS often cannot differentiate between these causes of diffuse endometrial thickening, but can triage these patients to blind endometrial biopsy or D&C.

■ **Endometrial carcinoma.** Usually demonstrates heterogeneous central blood flow.

■ **Congenital anomalies or variants.** In patients being evaluated for infertility or repeated spontaneous abortions, SIS may demonstrate congenital anomalies or variants (e.g., bicornuate, didelphic, or septate uterus) or acquired abnormalities (e.g., uterine synechiae).

■ **Adenomyosis.** Occasionally, what was suspected to be an endometrial polyp with cystic spaces on EVS will be shown to represent intramural adenomyosis on SIS.

■ **Arteriovenous malformation.** Detection of uterine arteriovenous malformation (AVM) with SIS has also been reported.

Further Readings

American College of Radiology. *ACR Practice guidelines for the performance of saline infusion sonohysterosalpingoraphy (SIS)*. Reston: American College of Radiology, 2002.

Corticelli A, Podesta M, Pedretti L, et al. Uterine arteriovenous malformation: a case report diagnosed by sonohysterography. *Clin Exp Obstet Gynecol* 2005;32(2):132–134.

Dudiak KM. Hysterosonography: a key to what is inside the uterus. *Ultrasound Q* 2001;17(2):73–86.

de Kroon CD, de Bock GH, Dieben SW, et al. Saline contrast hysterosonography in abnormal uterine bleeding: a systematic review and meta-analysis. *BJOG* 2003;110(10):938–947.

Valenzano MM, Mistrangelo E, Lijoi D, et al. Transvaginal sonohysterographic evaluation of uterine malformations. *Eur J Obstet Gynecol Reprod Biol* 2005;124:246–249. [Epub ahead of print]

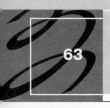

63 BONES

 ACCESSORY OSSICLES

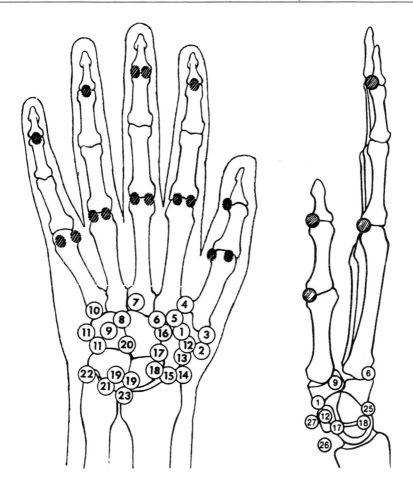

Figure 63-1. Accessory ossicles of the hand. The *shaded circles* indicate locations of sesamoid bones.

1. Epitrapezium
2. Calcification (bursa, flexor carpi radialis)
3. Paratrapezium (petrapezium)
4. Trapezium secundarium
5. Trapezoides secundarium
6. Os styloideum
7. Ossiculum Gruberi
8. Capitatum secundarium
9. Os hamuli proprium
10. Os vesalianum
11. Os ulnare externum (calcified bursa or tendon)
12. Os radiale externum
13. Fissure of traumatic origin
14. Persisting ossification center of the radial styloid process
15. Intercalary bone between the navicular and the radius (paranavicular)
16. Os carpi centrale
17. Hypolunatum
18. Epilunatum
19. Accessory bone between the lunate and the triangular bone
20. Epipyramis
21. So-called "os triangulare"
22. Persisting center of the ulnar styloid
23. Small ossicle at the level of the radioulnar joint
24. None
25. Avulsion from the triangular bone; no accessory ossicle
26. Tendon or bursal calcification
27. Calcification of the pisiform

(Keats TE. *Atlas of normal Roentgen variants that may Simulate disease, 5th ed.* St. Louis: Mosby–Year Book, 1992:420–430. Fig. 6-139, p. 430).

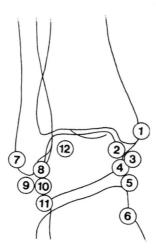

Figure 63-2. Accessory ossicles of the ankle.

1. Accompanying shadow on the internal malleolus (patella malleoli)
2. Intercalary bone (or sesamoid) between the internal malleolus and the talus
3. Os subtibiale
4. Talus accessorius
5. Os sustentaculi
6. Os tibiale externum
7. Os retinaculi
8. Intercalary bone (or sesamoid) between the external malleolus and the talus
9. Os subfibulare
10. Talus secundarius
11. Os trochleare calcanei
12. Os trigonum

(Keats TE. *Atlas of normal Roentgen variants that may simulate disease*, 5th ed. St. Louis: Mosby–Year Book; 1992:614. Fig. 7-321, p. 614).

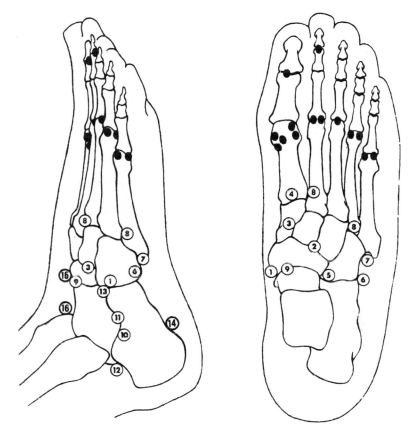

Figure 63-3. Accessory ossicles of the foot. The *shaded circles* indicate locations of sesamoid bones.

1. Os tibiale externum
2. Processus uncinatus
3. Os intercuneiforme
4. Pars peronea metatarsalia
5. Cuboides secundarium
6. Os peroneum
7. Os vesalianum
8. Os intermetatarseum

9. Os supratalare
10. Talus accessorius
11. Os sustentaculum
12. Os trigonum
13. Calcaneus secundarius
14. Os subcalcis
15. Os supranaviculare
16. Os talotibiale

(Keats TE. *Atlas of normal Roentgen variants that may simulate disease*, 5th ed. St. Louis: Mosby–Year Book, 1992:615. Fig. 7-322, p. 615).

BONES OF THE ELBOW, WRIST, AND FOOT

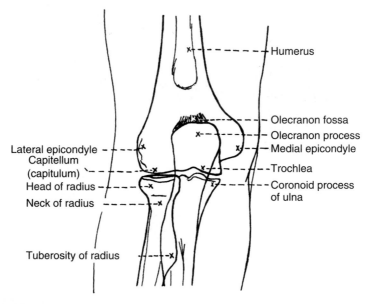

Figure 63-4. Bones of the elbow. (Meschan I. *An atlas of normal radiographic anatomy*, 2nd ed. Philadelphia: WB Saunders, 1959:101. Fig. 4-22, p. 101.)

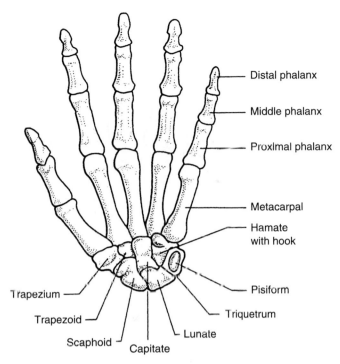

Distal phalanx

Middle phalanx

Proximal phalanx

Metacarpal

Hamate
with hook

Pisiform

Triquetrum

Lunate

Trapezium

Trapezoid

Scaphoid

Capitate

Figure 63-5. Bones of the wrist and hand. (Modified from Ryan SP, McNicholas MMJ. *Anatomy for diagnostic imaging*. London: W B Saunders, 1994:242. Fig. 7-8, p. 242.)

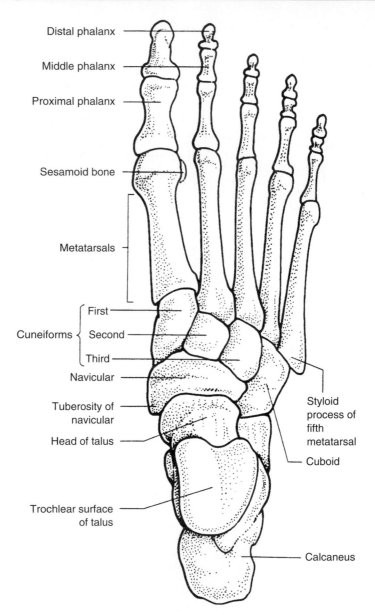

Figure 63-6. Bones of the foot. (Modified from Ryan SP, McNicholas MMJ. *Anatomy for diagnostic imaging*. London: W B Saunders, 1994:258. Fig. 8-3, p. 258.)

Order of Appearance of Ossification Centers of the Elbow

The *order* of appearance is more important than the absolute age of appearance, which varies widely. Remember "**CRITOE**":

	Approximately average age (years)
Capitellum	1
Radial head	3–6
Internal (medial) epicondyle	4
Trochlea	8
Olecranon	9
External (lateral) epicondyle	10

EPIPHYSEAL OSSIFICATION CENTERS

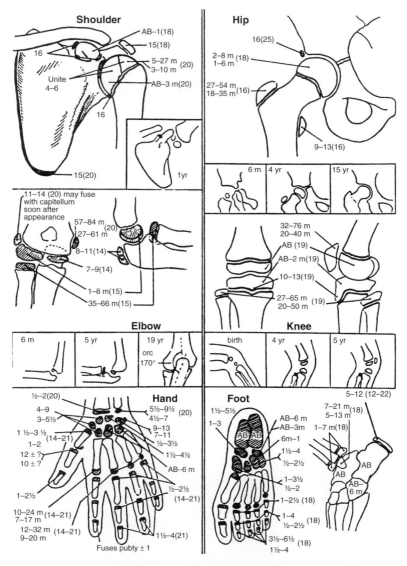

Figure 63-7. Epiphyseal ossifications centers. For each ossification center, a range is given for the time of appearance. Numbers in parentheses indicate approximate time of fusion. Some ossification centers are labelled with two ranges, one set for males (*upper*) and one set for females (*lower*). All numbers are in years except for those labelled "m" for months. "AB" indicates ossifications centers visible at birth. (Girdany BR, Golden R. Centers of ossification of the skeleton. *Am J Roentgenol* 1952;68:922–924. Charts I and II, pp. 922–923.)

Vertebrae

ossify from three primary centers and nine secondary centers–any of these secondary centers, except for annular epiphyses, may fail to fuse.

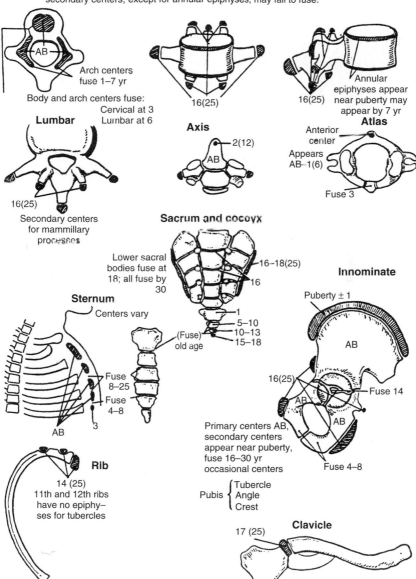

Arch centers fuse 1–7 yr

Body and arch centers fuse:
Cervical at 3
Lumbar at 6

Lumbar

16(25)

Axis

16(25)

Annular epiphyses appear near puberty may appear by 7 yr

Atlas

Anterior center

Appears AB–1(6)

Fuse 3

2(12)

AB

16(25)

Secondary centers for mammillary processes

Sacrum and cocoyx

Lower sacral bodies fuse at 18; all fuse by 30

16–18(25)

16

1
5–10
10–13
15–18

(Fuse) old age

Innominate

Puberty ± 1

AB

16(25)

Fuse 14

AB

AB

Fuse 4–8

Primary centers AB, secondary centers appear near puberty, fuse 16–30 yr occasional centers

Sternum

Centers vary

Fuse 8–25

Fuse 4–8

AB

3

Rib

14 (25)
11th and 12th ribs have no epiphyses for tubercles

Pubis { Tubercle
Angle
Crest

Clavicle

17 (25)

Figure 63-7. *(continued)*

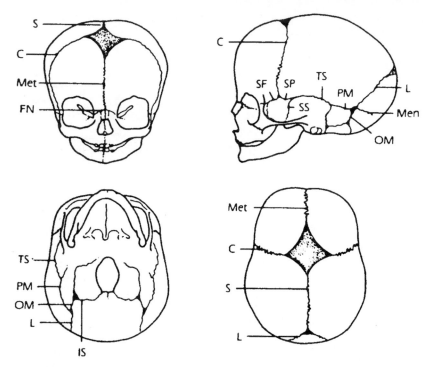

Figure 63-8. Normal neonatal sutures and synchondroses. S, sagittal suture; C, coronal suture; Met, metopic suture; FN, frontonasal suture; SF, sphenofrontal suture; SP, sphenoparietal suture; SS, sphenosquamosal suture; TS, temporosquamosal suture; PM, parietomastoid suture; L, lambdoid suture; Men, mendosal suture; OM, occipitomastoid suture; IS, innominate synchondrosis. (Kirks DR, ed. *Practical pediatric imaging: diagnostic radiology of infants and children*, 2nd ed. Boston: Little, Brown and Company, 1991:65. Fig. 2-6, p. 65.)

EPIPHYSEAL PLATE FRACTURES (SALTER — HARRIS CLASSIFICATION)

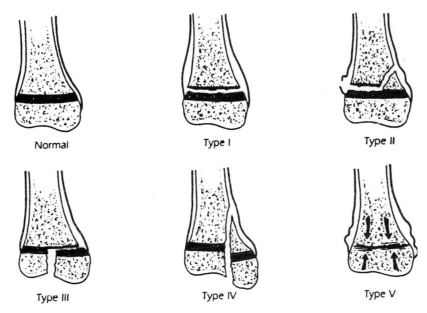

Normal	Type I	Type II
Type III	Type IV	Type V

Figure 63-9. Epiphyseal plate fractures. Salter-Harris classification system. (Kirks DR, ed. *Practical pediatric imaging: diagnostic radiology of infants and children*, 2nd ed. Boston: Little, Brown and Company, 1991:348. Fig. 4-60C, p. 348.)

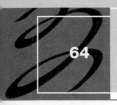

CONTRAST
Kenneth C. Wang

 PREMEDICATION PROTOCOL FOR HISTORY OF INTRAVENOUS CONTRAST REACTION

Please note: Premedication is indicated in patients who have had a history of mild/moderate contrast reactions (urticaria/pruritus/erythema). Patients who have had prior severe contrast reaction (bronchospasm/hypotension/anaphylaxis) do not receive contrast at our institution, as prophylaxis has not been shown to be effective.

- Prednisone 40 mg PO per protocol, for premedication before IV contrast examination; two-dose protocol: one dose 12–18 hours and one dose 2 hours before examination; three-dose protocol: 24, 12, and 2 hours before examination.
- Optional: Benadryl 50 mg PO 1 hour before examination (no proven benefit).
- Use nonionic contrast.

 CUSTOMARY CONTRAST DOSES FOR COMPUTED TOMOGRAPHY

Body or Head Computed Tomography

1 mL/lb or 2 mL/kg up to 100 mL IV.

Myelography

3 g iodine intrathecal, such as:
        10 mL Omnipaque 300 (cervical puncture) or
        12 mL Omnipaque 240 (thoracic puncture) or
        16 mL Omnipaque 180 (lumbar puncture).

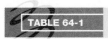

TABLE 64-1	Intravenous Contrast Dosages, Formulations, and Premedications	

Tradename	Iodine Content (mg/mL)	Comments
Angiovist 282, 292, 370	282, 292, 370	
Conray 30, 43, 325, 400	141, 202, 325, 400	
Conray (plain), Cysto, Angio	282, 81, 480	
Diatrizoate meglumine 76%	358	
Gastroview	367	
Hexabrix	320	Low osmolality, but ionic
Hypaque meglumine 30%, 60%	141, 282	
Hypaque sodium 25%, 50%	150, 300	
Hypaque 76	370	
Hypaque-M 75%, 90%	385, 462	
Imagopaque 150, 200, 250, 300, 350	150, 200, 250, 300, 350	Nonionic
Isovue 128, 200, 300, 370	128, 200, 300, 370	Nonionic
MD 60, 76	292, 370	
Omnipaque 180, 240, 300, 350	180, 240, 300, 350	Nonionic
Optiray 160, 240, 300, 320, 350	160, 240, 300, 320, 350	Nonionic
Osmovist	240	Nonionic
Oxilan 300, 350	300, 350	Nonionic
Renografin 60, 76	292, 370	
Reno-M DIP, 60	141, 282	
Renovue DIP, 65	111, 300	
Renovist II	309	
Renovist	370	
Ultravist 150, 240, 300, 370	150, 240, 300, 370	Nonionic
Urovist meglumine (Cysto-141)	141	
Urovist sodium 300	300	
Vascoray	400	
Visipaque 270, 320	270, 320	Nonionic, isosmolar

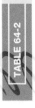

TABLE 64-2 Commonly Used Intravenous Contrast Agents: Formulations and Properties

Brand name	Compound	mOsm/kg H$_2$O	Viscosity at room temperature	Viscosity at 37°C	Iodine (mg/mL)	Sodium (mEq/L)
Hypaque-76[a]	Sodium-meglumine diatrizoate	2,160	13.3	9.0	370	160
Renografin-76[b]	Sodium-meglumine diatrizoate	1,940	10.0	8.4	370	190
Hexabrix	Sodium-meglumine ioxaglate	600	15.7	7.5	320	150
Isovue	Iopamidol	796	20.7	9.4	370	2
Omnipaque	Iohexol	844	20.4	10.4	350	5
Optiray	Ioversol	702	9.9	5.8	320	2
Visipaque[c]	Iodixanol	290	26.0	11.8	320	19

[a]Formulated with the additives of calcium disodium EDTA.
[b]Originally formulated with the additives of sodium citrate, sodium EDTA.
[c]Formulated with the addition of a "balanced" sodium and calcium salts to bring to isotonicity.
All nonionic contrasts have additives of tromethamine and calcium disodium EDTA.
Courtesy of Jeff Brinker MD, FACC, FSCAI, Johns Hopkins University, Department of Medicine, Division of Cardiology and Department of Radiology.

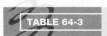

TABLE 64-3	Predicting the Risk of an Acute Decline in Kidney Function after Percutaneous Coronary Intervention[a]

Risk factor	Score
Systolic pressure <80 mm Hg for >1 h and patient requires inotropic support or an intra-aortic balloon pump within 24 h of the procedure	5
Use of intra-aortic balloon pump	5
Heart failure (New York Heart Association class III or IV), history of pulmonary edema, or both	5
Age older than 75 yr	4
Hematocrit <39% for men or <36% for women	3
Diabetes	3
Volume of contrast medium	1 for each 100 mL
Serum creatinine level >1.5 mg/dL (133 μmol/L)	4
or	
Estimated GFR[b] <60 mL/min/1.73 m^2 body-surface area	2, 40 to <60 mL/min/1.73 m^2
	4, 20–39 mL/min/1.73 m^2
	6, <20 mL/min/1.73 m^2

Total risk score[c]	Risk of an increase in serum creatinine levels of >0.5 mg/dL (44 μ mol/L) or >25% (%)	Risk of dialysis (%)
≤5	7.5	0.04
6–10	14.0	0.12
11–15	26.1	1.09
≥16	57.3	12.6

[a]Adapted from Mehran et al.
[b]Estimated glomerular filtration rate (GFR) = 186 × (serum creatinine in mg/dL)$^{-1.154}$ × age$^{-0.203}$ × 0.742 if female ×1.21 if black.
[c]The total risk score is determined by adding the scores for each factor.
(Adapted from Barrett BJ, Parfrey PS. Preventing Nephropathy Induced by Contrast Medium. *N Engl J Med* 354;4:379–386.)

NEPHROGENIC SYSTEMIC FIBROSIS/NEPHROGENIC FIBROSING DERMOPATHY (NSF/NFD)

NSF/NFD was first described in the medical literature in 2000. The first case of NSF/NFD was seen in 1997. The disease is seen after the administration of Gadolinium in patients that have noticeably advanced renal failure. The disease causes fibrosis of the skin and connective tissues throughout the body. Patients develop skin thickening that may prevent bending and extending joints, resulting in decreased mobility of joints. In addition, patients may experience fibrosis that has spread to other parts of the body such as the diaphragm, muscles in the thigh and lower abdomen, and the interior areas of lung vessels. The clinical course of NSF/NFD is progressive and may be fatal. The primary risk factor is reduced renal function.

Creatinine/eGFR is to be obtained for patients at risk for reduced renal function, including:

- Age *65 years
- Diabetes
- History of renal disease/renal transplantation
- History of liver transplantation, hepato-renal syndrome
- Other medical conditions as determined by attending radiologist

In acute renal failure, eGFR may be inaccurate and gadolinium use should be avoided.

Indications for Nonionic Contrast

- Previous significant allergic reaction to IV contrast
- History of anaphylaxis or non-trivial allergy to anything.
- Chronic urticaria or angioedema.
- Diagnosis of sickle cell, multiple myeloma, or renal disease.
- History of asthma.
- Anhistoric patient.

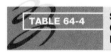 **TABLE 64-4** **Suggested Guidelines for Use of Gadolinium in Chronic Renal Failure Patients**

Patient on dialysis, or estimated GFR <30 mL/min/1.73 m^2

1. Radiologist to determine if gadolinium use is essential for diagnosis. Confirm that alternative tests are not available.
2. Patient consent for gadolinium is obtained.
3. Maximum recommended dose is 0.1 mmol/kg gadolinium.
4. Contrast agent other than gadodiamide is preferred and may have a lower risk of NSF/ NSD.
5. If patient is on hemodialysis: dialysis to be scheduled same day. Dialysis to be repeated 24 hours later. For outpatients who are on dialysis, there must be verification that the patient will receive dialysis as soon as possible after the MRI. 2 dialysis sessions separated by 1 day are recommended.
6. If patient is on peritoneal dialysis, use of gadolinium contrast is strongly discouraged unless highly necessary for diagnosis. Nephrology should be consulted to determine if hemodialysis can be performed.

GFR, glomerular filtration rate; NSF, nephrogenic systemic fibrosis; NSD, nephrogenic fibrosing dermopathy.
Adapted from Johns Hopkins. MRI Policy in relationship to nephrogenic systemic fibrosis/nephrogenic fibrosing dermopathy.
http://www.rad.jhmi.edu/mri/MRI_dialysis_gadolinium.htm. 2007.

- Severe cardiac dysfunction or general debilitation.
- Age >70 yrs, <1 yr.

 INTRAVENOUS CONTRAST IN THE PREGNANT PATIENT

There are few studies of the placental transmission of intravenous iodinated contrast agents. An ionic contrast agent was shown to cross the human placenta to the fetus in one frequently cited study. Regarding nonionic agents, the limited evidence is mixed. Investigators using an animal model in one study found that maternal injection of a nonionic agent led to no detectable contrast in fetal plasma or amniotic fluid. However, anecdotal evidence of fetal uptake of a nonionic agent has been reported in a case of maternal contrast CT for pulmonary embolism evaluation.

The safety of fetal exposure to contrast materials is also not well-described in the literature. However one study of the effects of a nonionic agent in rabbit and rat models found no significant abnormalities in either the fetus or post-partum offspring on a range of physical and developmental criteria.

Based on this limited evidence, which neither confirms nor refutes a relationship between iodinated contrast agents in pregnancy and risk of harm to a fetus, contrast studies in pregnant patients should be approached on a case-by-case basis. In conjunction with the referring physician, the following factors should be considered. (1) necessity of contrast (and ionizing radiation) in obtaining the desired information, (2) relevance of results to management decisions during the pregnancy, (3) urgency of obtaining the desired information prior to the end of pregnancy, and (4) informed consent of patient regarding risks, benefits and alternatives.

Gadolinium-based MR contrast agents have been shown to cross the placenta to the fetus in a monkey model, though risks to the fetus of exposure to these agents or to the MR imaging environment have not been well characterized. Current recommendations are to avoid routine administration of MR contrast agents in pregnant patients, and to consider the use of contrast on a case-by-case basis in a manner similar to that described above. In particular, modalities which do not employ ionizing radiation should be considered as potential alternatives to the contrast MR study. That is, given the known risks of exposure to ionizing radiation and the unknown risks of the MR imaging environment and MR contrast, alternatives such as ultrasound should be considered when appropriate.

Further Readings

ACR Committee on Contrast Media. *ACR Manual on Contrast Media*, 5th ed. Reston, Virginia: American College of Radiology; 2004.

Kanal E, Borgstede JP, Barkovich AJ, et al. American College of Radiology white paper on MR safety. *AJR Am J Roentgenol.* 2002;178:1335–1347.

Moon AJ, Katzberg RW, Sherman MP. Transplacental passage of iohexol. *J Pediatr.* 2000;136:548–549.

Morisetti A, Tirone P, Luzzani F, et al. Toxicological safety assessment of iomeprol, a new X-ray contrast agent. *Eur J Radiol.* 1994;18:S21–S31.

Thomsen HS, Muller RN, Mattrey RF eds. *Trends in Contrast Media.* Berlin Germany: Springer-Verlag New York; 1999.

*T*wo **dermatome charts** are in common use, and they have significant differences. In the diagram according to Keegan (Fig. 65-1), the dermatomes are shown to extend in continuous strips along the entire length of the limbs, following a regular, logical pattern. In the diagram according to Foerster (Fig. 65-2), some of the dermatomes are isolated to the distal portion of the limbs.

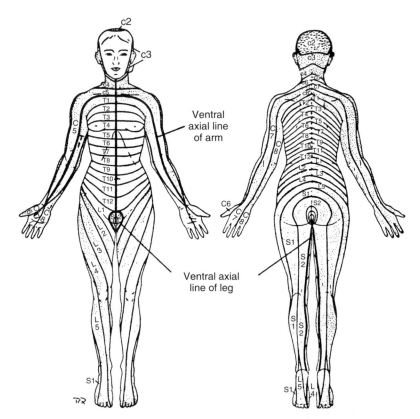

Figure 65-1. Dermatomes according to Keegan. This and Fig. 65-2 are the two dermatome charts in common use, and there are significant differences. In this diagram, the dermatomes are shown to extend in continuous strips along the entire length of the limbs. The extension of C5 and T1 across the upper chest is erroneous because C3 and C4 innervate this area. (Hollinshead WH. Textbook of anatomy, 3rd ed. Hagerstown: Harper & Row, 1974:54. Fig. 4-8, p. 54.)

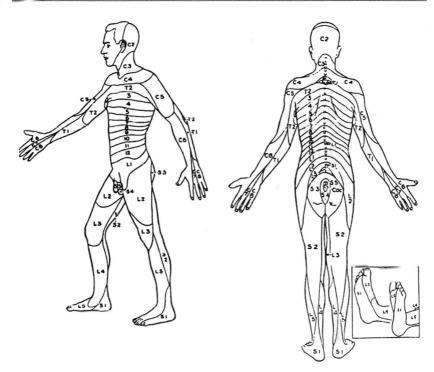

Figure 65-2. Dermatomes according to Foerster. This and Fig. 65-1 are the two dermatome charts in common use, and there are significant differences. In this diagram, some of the dermatomes are isolated to the distal portion of the limbs. (Hollinshead WH. Textbook of anatomy, 3rd ed. Hagerstown: Harper & Row, 1974:55. Figs. 4-9 and 4-10, p. 55.)

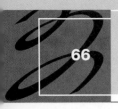
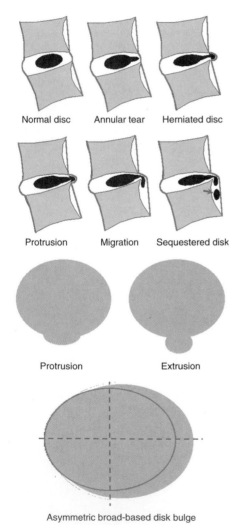

Normal disc   Annular tear   Herniated disc

Protrusion   Migration   Sequestered disk

Protrusion   Extrusion

Asymmetric broad-based disk bulge

Adapted from Fardon DF, Milette PC. Nomenclature and classification of lumbar disc pathology. 2001.http://www.asnr.org/.

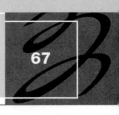
 DEFINITIONS AND UNITS

- **Exposure** is a measure expressing the intensity, strength, or amount of radiation in an x-ray beam, based on the ability of radiation to ionize air. It is a measure of the total charge of electrons liberated per unit mass of air by the x-ray photons. Conventional units are the roentgen (R); SI units are coulombs per kilogram (C/kg).
  Key concept: exposure follows the inverse square law, and decreases with the square of the distance from the source.
- **Absorbed dose,** (D) is a measure of radiation energy deposited per unit mass of a medium such as human tissue. It is expressed in gray (Gy). One gray is equivalent to an energy deposition of 1 joule per kilogram (J/kg) of medium. The conventional unit is the rad, and 100 rad = 1 Gy.
  Key concept: human tissue damage from radiation depends not only on the *absorbed dose* (D) of the radiation, but also the type of radiation affecting the tissue. For example, an α-particle is much more damaging than an x ray. This is taken into consideration by *equivalent dose*.
- **Equivalent dose** (H) is the absorbed dose (D) multiplied by a weighting factor for each type of radiation W_R and allows comparison of biological damage caused by different types of radiation. It is given by the equation $H = D \times W_R$. X-rays, γ rays, and β particles have a W_R of 1, whereas α particles have a W_R of 20, as they are more damaging. It is expressed in rem or Sieverts (Sv), and 1 rem = 0.01 Sv.
  Key concept: just as each different type of radiation causes a different biological effect on tissue, each tissue has a different sensitivity to the radiation it is exposed to. In other words, the same radiation to the gonads is more damaging than to the hands. This brings in the concept of *effective dose*.
- **Effective dose** (E) is the equivalent dose H times a weighting factor W_T for each organ that is being exposed to the radiation. $E = H \times W_T$. The W_T for the gonads is 0.25, whereas the W_T for bone is only 0.03.
  Key concept: as radiologists choosing an appropriate study for a patient, we require a measurement that allows us to compare the radiation exposure to the entire patient to evaluate the potential risks and benefits of the study. The *effective dose equivalent* is the measurement that allows us to do so.
- **Effective dose equivalent** (H_E) is a weighted sum of the individual organ doses of the entire body taking into account the type of radiation and also the sensitivity of each organ to that radiation. The *effective dose equivalent* is expressed in rem or Sv.
  Key concept: a table of effective dose equivalents such as the one provided in this chapter (Table 67-1), allows a comparison of common procedures used in radiology. With this table, the radiologist can give clinicians and patients a relative comparison of the radiation exposure resulting from a radiograph of the chest compared with that from a computed tomography (CT) of the chest.

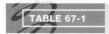

TABLE 67-1 Effective Dose Values for Common Radiographic Procedures[a]

Modality	Effective dose equivalent in mrem
Natural background yearly	360
Chest PA	2
Chest lateral	4
Chest PA and lateral	6
Abdomen	53
Pelvis AP	70
Skull lateral	10
Skull PA or AP	10
Thoracic spine AP	40
Thoracic spine lateral	70
Lumbar spine AP	30
Lumbar spine lateral	70
Barium swallow 24 images, 106-s fluoroscopy	150
Barium enema 10 images, 137-s fluoroscopy	100
CT head	200
CT chest	800
CT abdomen	1000
CT pelvis	1000
Coronary angiogram	460–1580
Lung perfusion/ventilation scan	150
CT angiogram for PE	800
Hepatobiliary scan	370

Individual patient dose varies according to multiple factors and should be reviewed with your institutions health physicist to determine the specific dose an individual will receive
PA, posteroanterior; AP, anteroposterior; CT, computed tomography; PE, physical examination.
[a]Table from personal correspondence with Mahadevappa Mahesh, M.S., Ph.D. at The Russel H. Morgan Department of Radiology and Radiological Science, The Johns Hopkins University and The Health Physics Society.
(Kelly classic Certified Medical Health Physicist for the Health Physics Society. *Effective doses for single x-ray films, table 2 effective doses for complete x-ray procedures, and effective doses for routine nuclear medicine studies.* Compiled by Kelly Classic Certified Medical Health Physicist for the Health Physics Society, posted online March 30, 2001.)

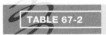

TABLE 67-2 Estimated Fetal Exposure for Common Radiographic Procedures[a]

Modality	Effective dose equivalent in mrem
Environmental background (9 mo)	100
Chest two views	0.07
Abdominal x-ray	245
Pelvis	40
Upper or lower extremity	1
CT head (ten slices each 10 mm thick)	<50
CT chest (ten slices each 10 mm thick)	<100
CT abdomen (ten slices each 10 mm thick)	2600
HIDA scan	150
V/Q scan (perfusion)	175
V/Q scan (ventilation with xenon)	40

Individual fetal dose varies according to multiple factors and should be reviewed with your institutions health physicist to determine the specific dose a fetus will receive
CT, computed tomography; HIDA, hepatobiliary scan; V/Q, ventilation/perfusion.
[a]Table from data published by Toppenberg KS, Hill AD, Miller DP. *Safety of radiographic imaging during pregnancy American family physician.* Vol. 59, no. 7, 1999.

Further Readings

Brateman L. The AAPM/RSNA physics tutorial for residents: radiation safety considerations for diagnostic radiology personnel. *RadioGraphics* 1999;19:1037–1055.

Huda Walter, Slone Richard. *Review of radiologic physics second edition.* Philadelphia: Lippincott Williams & Wilkins, 2003.

Kelly classic Certified Medical Health Physicist for the Health Physics Society. *Effective doses for single x-ray films, table 2 effective doses for complete x-ray procedures, and effective doses for routine nuclear medicine studies.* Compiled by Kelly Classic Certified Medical Health Physicist for the Health Physics Society, posted online March 30, 2001.

Parry RA, Glaze SA, Archer BR. The AAPM/RSNA physics tutorial for residents: typical patient radiation doses in diagnostic radiology. *RadioGraphics* 1999;19:1289–1302.

Toppenberg KS, Hill AD, Miller DP. *Safety of radiographic imaging during pregnancy American family physician.* Vol. 59, no. 7, 1999.

RADIONUCLIDES AND RADIOPHARMACEUTICALS

TABLE 68-1 Commonly Used Radionuclides and Radiopharmaceuticals

Nuclide	Half-life	Energy (keV)	Tracer	Applications	Dose (mCi)	Time to imaging
99mTechnetium (99mTc)	6 h	140	Pertechnetate	**Thyroid** — diagnostic imaging	5	20 min
				GI — Meckel scan[a]	5	0
				Testes — torsion	10	0
			HMPAO	**Brain** — perfusion SPECT	20	20 min
			Pyrophosphate	**Cardiac** — infarct	15	2 h
			RBC	**Cardiac** — gated ventriculography (MUGA)	20	0
				GI — bleeding scan	20	0
				Liver — SPECT for hemangioma	20	0
			Sestamibi	**Cardiac** — perfusion[b]	25	30–60 min
				Parathyroid — adenoma	20	0 + 2 h
			Teboroxime	**Cardiac** — perfusion	25–30	0
			Sulfur colloid	**GI** — gastric/esophageal emptying for liquids	1	0
				GI — gastric/esophageal emptying for solids	0.5	0
				Liver — SPECT for mass	5	5 min
			IDA derivative	**Liver** — cholecystitis, biliary atresia[c]	5	0
			MAA	**Lung** — perfusion	3	0
			DTPA	**Brain** — perfusion	30	0 + 2 h
				Kidney — perfusion, filtration	10 or 20	0
			DMSA	**Kidney** — parenchyma	5	3 h
			Glucoheptonate	**Kidney** — like DMSA + DTPA	10	0
			MAG3	**Kidney** — blood flow, clearance (like hippuran)	10	0
			MDP	**Bone** — infection, metastasis[d]	20	[0] + 3 h

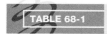

TABLE 68-1   *(Continued)*

Nuclide	Half-life	Energy (keV)	Tracer	Applications	Dose (mCi)	Time to imaging
			WBC	**Infection** — labelled with HMPAO[e]	3–10	1+ [24] h
^{123}Iodine (^{123}I)	13 h	159	Sodium	**Thyroid** — diagnostic imaging	0.4	6 h
^{111}Indium (^{111}In)	67 h	172, 247	DTPA	**CSF** — cisternogram, shunt patency	0.5	4 + 24 h
				CSF — shunt patency	0.5	0 + 2 h
			WBC	**Infection**[e,f]	0.5	24 h
^{201}Thallium (^{201}Tl)	73 h	71, 135, 167	Chloride	**Cardiac** — stress + rest perfusion[g]	3 + 1	0 + 3 h
^{67}Gallium (^{67}Ga)	78 h	93, 184, 296, 388	Citrate	**Infection**[f]	5	24 h
				Tumor	5	48 h
^{133}Xenon (^{133}Xe)	5.3 d	81	Gas	**Lung** — ventilation	10–30	0
^{131}Iodine (^{131}I)	8 d	284, 364, 637	Sodium	**Thyroid** — diagnostic (postthyroidectomy), therapeutic (192 keV β emission)	5	48 h
			MIBG	**Tumor** — pheo, neuroblastoma, carcinoid, medullary thyroid, paraganglioma, and chemodect	1.5	48 h
			Hippuran	**Kidney** — blood flow, clearance (like MAG3)	0.25	0
^{18}Fluorine (^{18}F)	2 h	511	FDG	**PET tracer**	15	45–60

Half-lives are given as the physical half-life in hours (h) or days (d). "Image Time" is the time from radiotracer injection to the start of image acquisition, given in minutes (min) or hours (h).

HMPAO, hexamethylpropyleneamine oxime; SPECT, single photon emission computed tomography; RBC, red blood cell; MUGA, multiple gated acquisition; GI, gastrointestinal; IDA, iminodiacetic acid; MAA, macroaggregated albumin; DTPA, diethylenetriamine-pentaacetic acid; DMSA, 2,3-dimercaptosuccinic acid; MAG3, mercaptoacetyltriglycine; MDP, methylene diphosphonate; WBC, white blood cell; MIBG, metaiodobenzylguanidine; FDG, fluorodeoxyglucose; PET, positron emission tomography.

[a]**Preparation for Meckel scan.** To enhance uptake of pertechnetate by the ectopic gastric mucosa, administer pentagastrin 6μg/kg SQ 15 minutes before study. To block release of pertechnetate by the ectopic gastric mucosa, administer cimetidine 300 mg PO q6h beginning 12–24 hours before study.

[b]**Sestamibi versus thallium.** Cardiac imaging with sestamibi is preferred over thallium in three situations: (1) obese patient, (2) history of previous nondiagnostic thallium study, and (3) acute or emergent setting. When sestamibi is used in the acute or emergent setting, imaging does not have to take place immediately following injection because sestamibi does not redistribute. This allows time for the patient to be stabilized. Thallium is preferred over sestamibi when myocardial viability is the main question (status post myocardial infarction or known severe coronary artery disease).

[c]**Jaundice and hepatobiliary scans.** For each mg/dL that the bilirubin is above normal, 1 mCi is added to the normal radiotracer dose up to a maximum of 10 mCi.

[d]**Three-phase bone scan indications.** In addition to 2-hour delayed imaging, images are also obtained immediately postinjection to obtain blood flow and blood pool images. These early images are indicated when evaluating for infection, stress fracture, avascular necrosis, or primary bone tumor.

[e]**WBC count and leukocyte scans.** For an adequate study, the patient's WBC count must be greater than 3,000 WBC/mm^3.

[f]**Indium versus gallium** for inflammation imaging. Indium-labelled WBCs are less sensitive for vertebral osteomyelitis or for chronic infections of any kind (possibly due to altered WBC function). Gallium may be preferable in these cases. Gallium activity is normally present in bowel on delayed imaging, making gallium less desirable in the evaluation of abdominal inflammation, but the use of SPECT may at least partially compensate for this problem.

[g]**Thallium reinjection** (for reperfusion imaging after thallium stress imaging) is indicated when myocardial viability is being evaluated, such as in patients who are status post myocardial infarction or have known severe coronary artery disease.

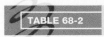

| TABLE 68-2 | Abbreviations and Common Trade Names for Radiopharmaceuticals |

Name	Full name
Cardiolite	Sestamibi (see MIBI)
Cardiotec	Teboroxime
Ceretec	HMPAO (hexamethylpropyleneamine oxime)
Choletec	TMB-IDA (*m*-bromotrimethyl IDA)
DISIDA	Diisopropyl IDA
DMSA	2,3-Dimercaptosuccinic acid
DTPA	Diethylenetriamine-pentaacetic acid
HIDA	2,6-Dimethyl IDA
HMPAO	Hexamethylpropyleneamine oxime
IDA	Iminodiacetic acid
MAA	Macroaggregated albumin
MAG3	Mercaptoacetyltriglycine
MDP	Methylene diphosphonate
Mebrofenin	TMB-IDA (*m*-bromotrimethyl IDA)
MIBG	Metaiodobenzylguanidine
MIBI	Methoxyisobutylisonitrile (sestamibi)
PIPIDA	Paraisopropyl IDA
Sestamibi	See MIBI
TMB-IDA	*m*-Bromotrimethyl IDA

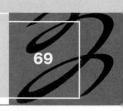

ATELECTASIS, ROENTGENOGRAPHIC PATTERNS

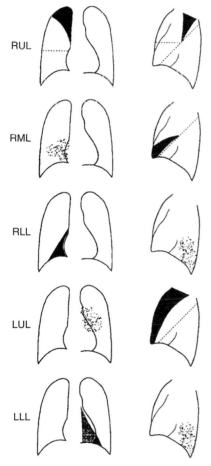

RUL

RML

RLL

LUL

LLL

Figure 69-1. Patterns of lobar atelectasis.
Roentgenographic Signs of Atelectasis

Direct
- **Displacement of interlobar fissures** — the only direct sign of atelectasis.

Indirect
- **Focal increase in density.**
- **Hemidiaphragm elevation** — more prominent in lower lobe atelectasis than in upper lobe atelectasis.
- **Tracheal shift** — occurs only with upper lobe atelectasis.
- **Cardiac shift** — occurs variably with lower lobe atelectasis.
- **Hilar displacement** — more prominent in upper lobe atelectasis than in lower lobe atelectasis.
- **Absence of air bronchogram** — only if resorptive type atelectasis.
- **Nonvisualization of interlobar artery** — differentiates lower lobe atelectasis from pleural effusion.

FLEISCHNER SOCIETY GUIDELINES FOR PULMONARY NODULES

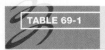 **TABLE 69-1** | **Recommendations for Follow-up and Management of Nodules Smaller Than 8 mm Detected Incidentally at Nonscreening Computed Tomography (CT)**

Nodule size (mm)[a]	Low-risk patient[b]	High-risk patient[c]
<4	No follow-up needed[d]	Follow-up CT at 12 mo; if unchanged, no further follow-up[e]
>4–6	Follow-up CT at 12 mo; if unchanged, no further follow-up[e]	Initial follow-up CT at 6–12 mo, then at 18–24 mo if no change[e]
>6–8	Initial follow-up CT at 6–12 mo, then at 18–24 mo if no change	Initial follow-up CT at 3–6 mo, then at 9–12 and 24 mo if no change
>8	Follow-up CT at approximately 3, 9, and 24 mo, dynamic contrast-enhanced CT, PET, and/or biopsy	Same as for low-risk patient

PET, positron emission tomography.
Newly detected indeterminate nodule in persons 35 years of age or older.
[a]Average of length and width.
[b]Minimal or absent history of smoking and of other known risk factors.
[c]History of smoking or of other known risk factors.
[d]The risk of malignancy in this category (<1%) is substantially less than that in a baseline CT scan of an asymptomatic smoker.
[e]Nonsolid (ground-glass) or partly solid nodules may require longer follow-up to exclude indolent adenocarcinoma.
Adapted from MacMahon H, Austin JHM, Gamsu G, et al.. Guidelines for management of small pulmonary nodules detected on CT scans: a statement from the Fleischner society. *Radiology* 2005;237:395–400.

**MODIFIED PROSPECTIVE INVESTIGATION OF
PULMONARY EMBOLISM DIAGNOSIS (PIOPED) CRITERIA**

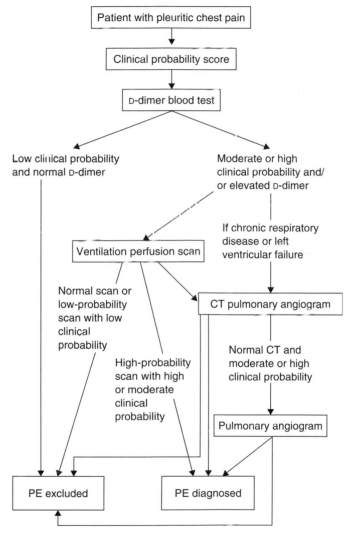

Figure 69-2. Prospective investigation of pulmonary embolism diagnosis chart. CT, computed tomography; PE, pulmonary embolism.
Adapted from Hogg K, Dawson D, Mackway-Jones K. Investigating pulmonary embolism in the emergency department with lower limb plethysmography: the Manchester Investigation of Pulmonary Embolism Diagnosis (MIOPED) study. *Emerg Med* J 2006;23;94–98.

Further Reading
Fraser RG, Paré JAP, Paré PD, et al. *Diagnosis of diseases of the chest*, 3rd ed. Philadelphia: WB Saunders, 1988:494–534.

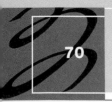

70 ULTRASOUND

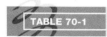

CAROTID DUPLEX ULTRASONOGRAPHY

TABLE 70-1 Gray Scale and Doppler Ultrasound (US) Criteria for Diagnosis of Internal Cartoid Artery (ICA) Stenosis

| Degree of stenosis (%) | Primary parameters | | Additional parameters | |
	ICA PSV (cm/s)	Plaque estimate (%)	ICA/CCA PSV ratio	ICA EDV (cm/s)
Normal	<125	None	<2.0	<40
<50	<125	<50	<2.0	<40
50–69	125–230	≥50	2.0–4.0	40–100
≥70 but less than near occlusion	>230	≥50	>4.0	>100
Near occlusion	High, low, or undetectable	Visible	Variable	Variable
Total occlusion	Undetectable	Visible, no detectable lumen	Not applicable	Not applicable

PSV, peak systolic velocity; CCA, common cartoid artery; EDV, end diastolic ratio.
(From Grant EG, Benson CB, Moneta GL, et al. Radiology 2003;229:340–346.)

ABDOMINAL DUPLEX ULTRASONOGRAPHY

Renal Transplant

Parenchymal resistive indices (RIs) (arcuate and intralobar arteries):

- Less than or equal to 0.7 normal.
- 0.7–0.8 indeterminate.
- Greater than 0.8 abnormal.

    Reversal of diastolic flow in the venous system often indicates **renal vein thrombosis**. Renal artery anastomosis:

- Equal to or greater than 3:1 ratio of PSV between anastomosis: iliac artery equal to stenosis or kinked vessel.
- PSV greater than 180–210 cm/second is suggestive of stenosis.
- RI is less important.

(Adapted from Friedewald SM, Molmenti EP, Friedewald JJ, et al. *J Clin Ultrasound* 2005;33:127–139.)

Liver Transplant

Hepatic artery resistive index less than 0.5 suggests central hepatic artery thrombosis or stenosis.

Transjugular Intrahepatic Portosystemic Shunt

Shunt velocity

- 50–200 cm/second is normal.
- Greater than 200 cm/second is abnormal.

Left portal flow should be **toward the shunt.**
Main portal vein velocity should be **more than 40 cm/second.**
(Adapted from Middleton WD, Teefey SA, Darcy MD, et al. *Ultrasound Q* 2003; 19:56–70.)

Appendicitis

- Appendiceal thickness more than 6 mm is abnormal.

 OBSTETRIC ULTRASONOGRAPHY

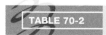

TABLE 70-2	First Trimester Obstetric Ultrasonography

βhCG:

- Need more than 1,000–1,500 to see gestational sac.
- Should double every 48 hours.

Nonviable gestation:

Parameter	Transabdominal US	Transvaginal US
Gestational sac	—	Present at 5 wk
Yolk sac	Present with an MSD of >20 mm	Present with an MSD of >8 mm
Embryo	Present with an MSD of >25 mm	Present with an MSD of >16 mm
Embryonic cardiac activity	CRL of >5 mm	CRL of >5 mm

β-hCG, β-human chorionic gonadotropin; US, ultrasound; MSD, mean sac diameter; CRL, crown rump length.
Advise using more conservative numbers than mentioned in the preceding text, for example:
- MSD greater than 20 mm for fetal pole.
- CRL greater than 9 mm for fetal heart movement (FHM).
(From Dogra V, Paspulati RM, Bhatt S, et al. First trimester bleeding evaluation. *Ultrasound Q* 2005;21:69–85.)

PEDIATRIC ULTRASONOGRAPHY VALUES

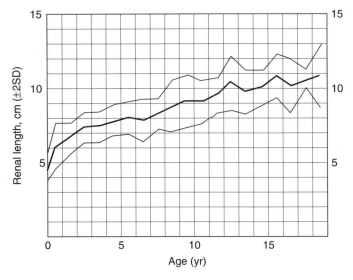

Figure 70-1. Renal length in children. (From Rosenbaum DM, Korngold E, Teele RL. Sonographic assessment of renal length in normal children. *Am J Roentgenol* 1984;142:467–469.)

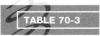

TABLE 70-3	Summary of Grouped Observations — Mean Renal Length			
Average age[a]	**Interval[a]**	**Mean renal length (cm)**	**SD**	**N**
0 mo	0–1 wk	4.48	0.31	10
2 mo	1 wk–4 mo	5.28	0.66	54
6 mo	4–8 mo	6.15	0.67	20
10 mo	8 mo–1 yr	6.23	0.63	8
11/2	1–2	6.65	0.54	28
21/2	2–3	7.36	0.54	12
31/2	3–4	7.36	0.64	30
41/2	4–5	7.87	0.50	26
51/2	5–6	8.09	0.54	30
61/2	6–7	7.83	0.72	14
71/2	7–8	8.33	0.51	18
81/2	8–9	8.90	0.88	18
91/2	9–10	9.20	0.90	14
101/2	10–11	9.17	0.82	28
111/2	11–12	9.60	0.64	22
121/2	12–13	10.42	0.87	18
131/2	13–14	9.79	0.75	14
141/2	14–15	10.05	0.62	14
151/2	15–16	10.93	0.76	6
161/2	16–17	10.04	0.86	10
171/2	17–18	10.53	0.29	4
181/2	18–19	10.81	1.13	8

SD, standard deviation.
[a]Years unless specified otherwise.
(From Rosenbaum DM, Korngold E, Teele RL. Sonographic assessment of renal length in normal children. *Am J Roentgenol* 1984;142:467–469.)

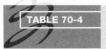

TABLE 70-4	Hypertrophic Pyloric Stenosis	
	Measurements (mm)	**Score**
Pyloric diameter	<10	0
	10.1–15	1
	15.1–17	2
	>17.1	3
Muscular thickness	<2.5	0
	2.51–3.5	1
	3.51–4.5	2
	>4.5	3
Pyloric length	<13	0
	13.1–19	1
	19.1–22	2
	>22	3

Scores of normal group, 2 or less; scores of PS group, 3 or more.
PS, pyloric stenosis.
(From Ito S, Tamura K, Nagae I, et al. Ultrasonographic diagnosis criteria using scoring for hypertrophic pyloric stenosis. *J Ped Surg* 2000 35:1714–1718.)

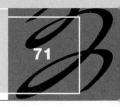
 CEREBRAL VASCULAR TERRITORIES

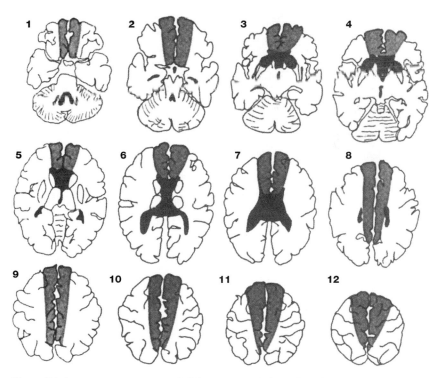

Figure 71-1. Anterior cerebral artery (ACA) territory, axial plane. The ACA territory is divided into three regions: *light shading* = hemispheric, *medium shading* = medial lenticulostriate, and *dark shading* = callosal. (Berman SA, Hayman LA, Hinck VC. Cerebral vascular territories: anatomic-functional correlation with axial and coronal images. In: Latchaw RE, ed. *MR and CT imaging of the head, neck, and spine*, 2nd ed. St. Louis: Mosby–Year Book, 1991:48–53. Figs. 3-1 and 3-2, pp. 48–49.)

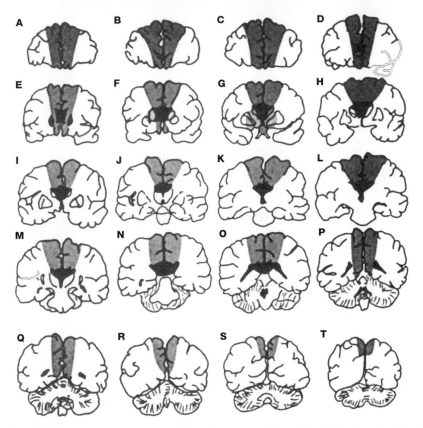

Figure 71-2. Anterior cerebral artery (ACA) territory, coronal plane. The ACA territory is divided into three regions: *light shading* = hemispheric, *medium shading* = medial lenticulostriate, and *dark shading* = callosal. (Berman SA, Hayman LA, Hinck VC. Cerebral vascular territories: anatomic-functional correlation with axial and coronal images. In: Latchaw RE, ed. *MR and CT imaging of the head, neck, and spine*, 2nd ed. St. Louis: Mosby–Year Book, 1991:48–53. Figs. 3-1 and 3-2, pp. 48–49.)

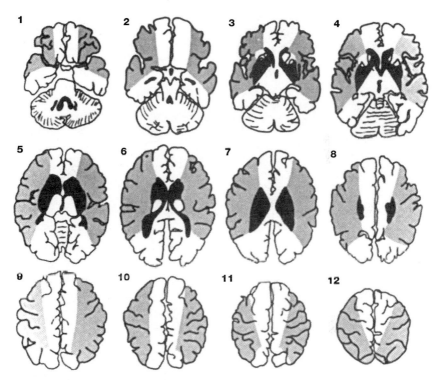

Figure 71-3. Middle cerebral artery (MCA) territory, axial plane. The MCA territory is divided into two regions: *light shading* = hemispheric and *dark shading* = lateral lenticulostriate. (Berman SA, Hayman LA, Hinck VC. Cerebral vascular territories: anatomic-functional correlation with axial and coronal images. In: Latchaw RE, ed. *MR and CT imaging of the head, neck, and spine*, 2nd ed. St. Louis: Mosby–Year Book, 1991:48–53. Figs. 3-4 and 3-5, pp. 50–51.)

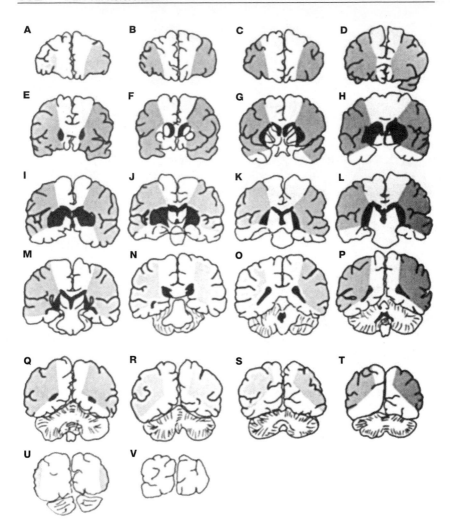

Figure 71-4. Middle cerebral artery (MCA) territory, coronal plane. The MCA territory is divided into two regions: *light shading* = hemispheric and *dark shading* = lateral lenticulostriate. (Berman SA, Hayman LA, Hinck VC. Cerebral vascular territories: anatomic-functional correlation with axial and coronal images. In: Latchaw RE, ed. *MR and CT imaging of the head, neck, and spine*, 2nd ed. St. Louis: Mosby–Year Book, 1991:48–53. Figs. 3-4 and 3-5, pp. 50–51.)

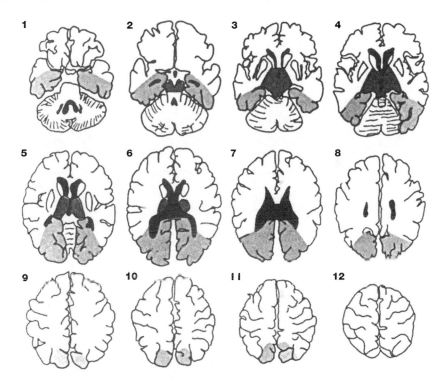

Figure 71-5. Posterior cerebral artery (PCA) territory, axial plane. The PCA territory is divided into three regions: *light shading* = hemispheric, *medium shading* = thalamic and midbrain perforators, and *dark shading* = callosal. (Berman SA, Hayman LA, Hinck VC. Cerebral vascular territories: anatomic-functional correlation with axial and coronal images. In: Latchaw RE, ed. *MR and CT imaging of the head, neck, and spine*, 2nd ed. St. Louis : Mosby–Year Book, 1991:48–53. Figs. 3-7 and 3-8, pp. 52–53.)

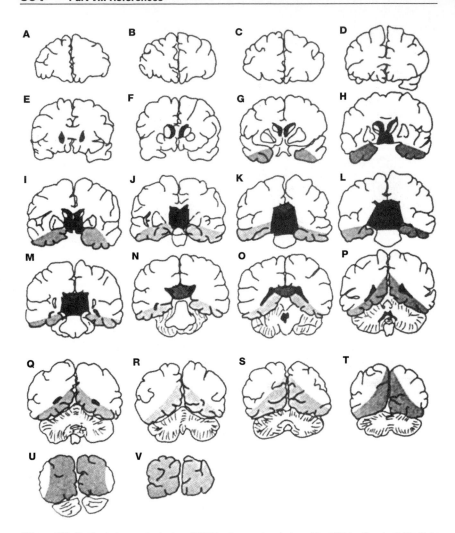

Figure 71-6. Posterior cerebral artery (PCA) territory, coronal plane. The PCA territory is divided into three regions: *light shading* = hemispheric, *medium shading* = thalamic and midbrain perforators, and *dark shading* = callosal. (Berman SA, Hayman LA, Hinck VC. Cerebral vascular territories: anatomic-functional correlation with axial and coronal images. In: Latchaw RE, ed. *MR and CT imaging of the head, neck, and spine*, 2nd ed. St. Louis: Mosby–Year Book, 1991:48–53. Figs. 3-7 and 3-8, pp. 52–53.)

CORONARY ARTERY ANATOMY

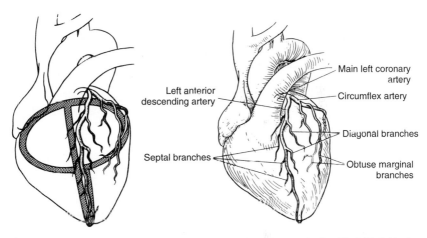

Figure 71-7. Left coronary artery (LCA) in the left anterior oblique projection. The LCA divides into the circumflex artery, which makes up the left side of the circle, and the left anterior descending artery, which makes up the anterior portion of the loop. Obtuse marginal branches extend from the circumflex artery; diagonal and septal branches extend from the left anterior descending artery. (Reproduced with permission from Kubicka RA, Smith C. How to interpret coronary arteriograms. *Radiographics* 1986;6:661–701.)

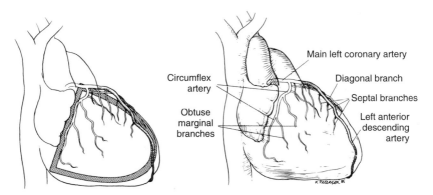

Figure 71-8. Left coronary artery in the right anterior oblique projection. The loop is more open in this projection, whereas the circle is superimposed. The left anterior descending artery makes up the anterior portion of the loop. The circumflex artery and its obtuse marginal branches make up the left side of the circle. (Reproduced with permission from Kubicka RA, Smith C. How to interpret coronary arteriograms. *Radiographics* 1986;6:661–701.)

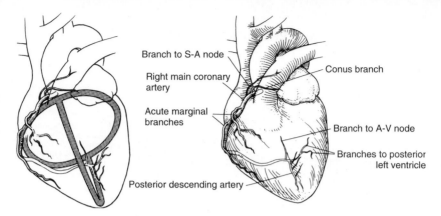

Figure 71-9. Right coronary artery (RCA) in the left anterior oblique projection. The right portion of the circle represents the RCA, and the posterior portion of the loop represents the posterior descending artery. S-A, sinoatrial; A-V, atrioventricular. (Reproduced with permission from Kubicka RA, Smith C. How to interpret coronary arteriograms. *Radiographics* 1986;6:661–701.)

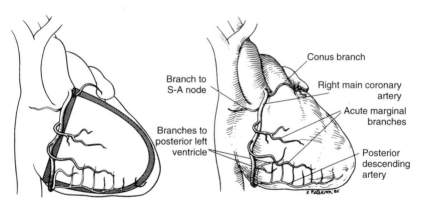

Figure 71-10. Right coronary artery (RCA) in the right anterior oblique projection. The RCA forms the atrioventricular circle. The loop is more opened in this projection with the posterior descending artery making up its inferior margin. S-A, sinoatrial. (Reproduced with permission from Kubicka RA, Smith C. How to interpret coronary arteriograms. *Radiographics* 1986;6:661–701.)

ABDOMINAL VASCULAR ANATOMY

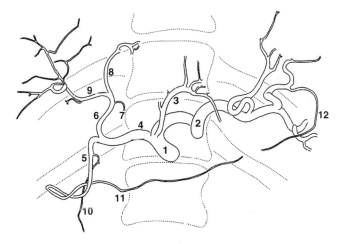

Figure 71-11. Celiac artery and branches. (Drawn from Meschan I. *An atlas of normal radiographic anatomy*, 2nd ed. Philadelphia: WB Saunders, 1959. Fig. 12-11c, p. 561.)

1 Celiac artery
2 Splenic artery
3 Left gastric artery
4 Common hepatic artery
5 Gastroduodenal artery
6 Hepatic artery (proper)
7 Right gastric artery
8 Left hepatic artery
9 Right hepatic artery
10 Superior pancreaticoduodenal artery
11 Right gastroepiploic artery
12 Left gastroepiploic artery

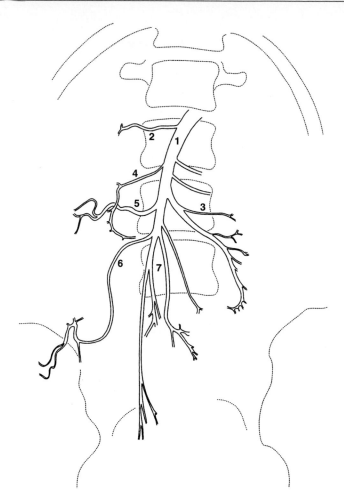

Figure 71-12. Superior mesenteric artery and branches. (Drawn from Meschan I. *An atlas of normal radiographic anatomy*, 2nd ed. Philadelphia: WB Saunders, 1959. Fig. 12-11d, p. 561.)

1 Superior mesenteric artery
2 Inferior pancreaticoduodenal artery
3 Jejunal branches
4 Middle colic artery
5 Right colic artery
6 Ileocolic artery
7 Ileal branches

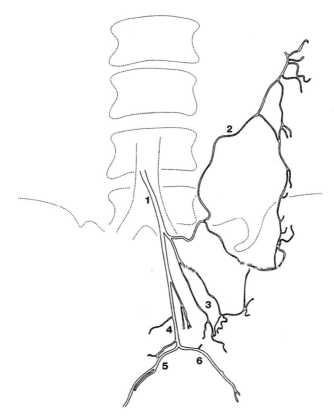

Figure 71-13. Inferior mesenteric artery and branches. (Drawn from Meschan I. *An atlas of normal radiographic anatomy*, 2nd ed. Philadelphia: WB Saunders, 1959. Fig. 12-11e, p. 561.)
1 Inferior mesenteric artery
2 Left colic artery
3 Sigmoid arteries
4 Superior rectal artery
5 Superior rectal artery, right branch
6 Superior rectal artery, left branch

PERIPHERAL VASCULAR ANATOMY

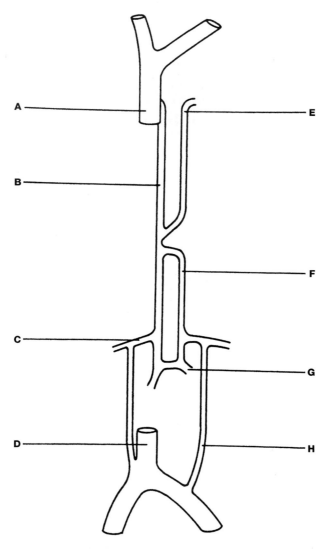

Figure 71-14. Azygos system. (Westacott S, Hall JRW. *Key anatomy for radiology*. Oxford: Heinemann Professional Publishing, 1988. Fig. 1-21, p. 37.)

A Superior vena cava
B Azygos vein
C Subcostal vein
D Inferior vena cava
E Accessory hemiazygos vein
F Hemiazygos vein
G Lumbar azygos vein
H Ascending lumbar vein

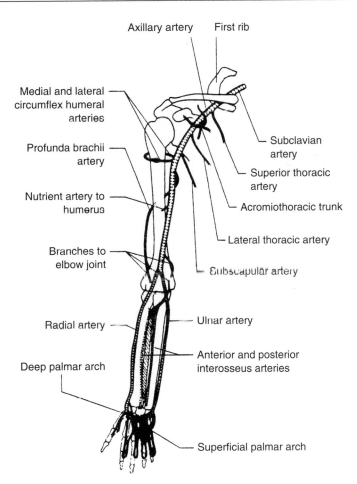

Axillary artery   First rib

Medial and lateral circumflex humeral arteries

Profunda brachii artery

Nutrient artery to humerus

Branches to elbow joint

Radial artery

Deep palmar arch

Subclavian artery

Superior thoracic artery

Acromiothoracic trunk

Lateral thoracic artery

Subscapular artery

Ulnar artery

Anterior and posterior interosseus arteries

Superficial palmar arch

Figure 71-15. Arteries of the upper extremity. (Ryan SP, McNicholas MMJ. *Anatomy for diagnostic imaging*. London: WB Saunders, 1994. Fig. 7-16, p. 251).

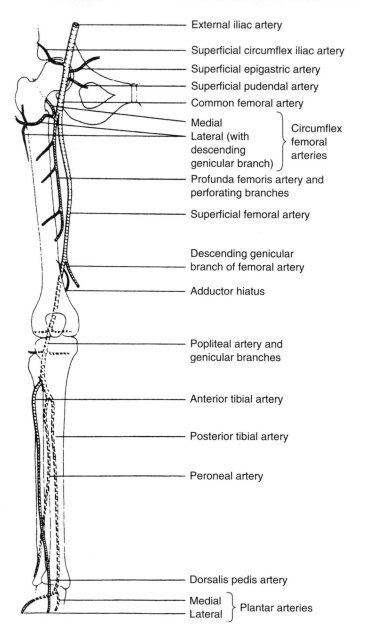

External iliac artery

Superficial circumflex iliac artery

Superficial epigastric artery

Superficial pudendal artery

Common femoral artery

Medial
Lateral (with
descending
genicular branch)

Circumflex
femoral
arteries

Profunda femoris artery and
perforating branches

Superficial femoral artery

Descending genicular
branch of femoral artery

Adductor hiatus

Popliteal artery and
genicular branches

Anterior tibial artery

Posterior tibial artery

Peroneal artery

Dorsalis pedis artery

Medial
Lateral

Plantar arteries

Figure 71-16. Arteries of the lower extremity. (Ryan SP, McNicholas MMJ. *Anatomy for diagnostic imaging*. London: WB Saunders, 1994. Fig. 8-19, p. 271).

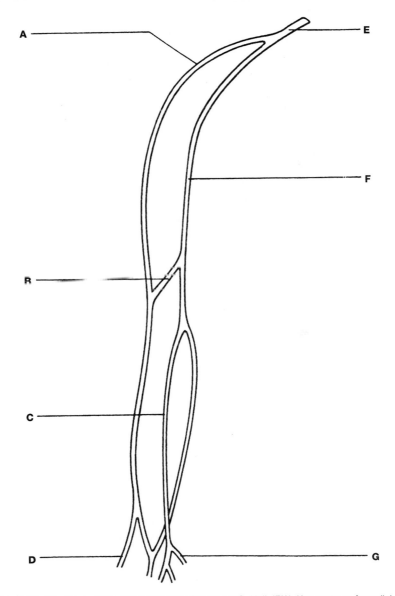

Figure 71-17. Veins of the upper extremity. (Westacott S, Hall JRW. *Key anatomy for radiology.* Oxford: Heinemann Professional Publishing, 1988. Fig. 7-17, p. 190.)
A Cephalic vein
B Median cubital vein
C Median vein of the forearm
D Dorsal network
E Axillary vein
F Basilic vein
G Palmar plexus

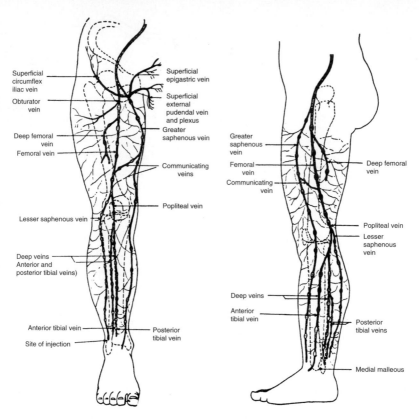

Figure 71-18. Veins of the lower extremity. (Meschan I. *An atlas of normal radiographic anatomy*, 2nd ed. Philadelphia: WB Saunders, 1959. Fig. 12-14, p. 571).

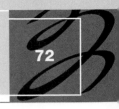
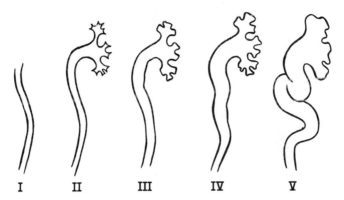

I   II   III   IV   V

Figure 72-1. Classification of reflux. Distal ureteral reflux is termed *grade I*. Reflux into the upper collecting system with no dilation of the upper tract is *grade II*. *Grade III* reflux is similar to grade II, but with mild blunting of the calices. *Grade IV* reflux demonstrates marked hydroureter and caliceal dilatation. *Grade V* reflux is seen when the ureter is massively dilated and tortuous and the upper tract is markedly dilated. (International classification modified after: International Reflux Study Committee. Medical versus surgical treatment of primary vesicoureteral reflux: report of the International Reflux Study Committee. *Pediatrics* 1981;67:392–400.)

Abdominal abscess, 131–135
Abdominal aortic aneurysm and dissection, 136–141
Abdominal duplex ultrasonography, 354–355
Abdominal pseudocyst, 76
Abdominal trauma, 142–146
Abdominal vascular anatomy, 367–369
Abscess
  abdominal, 131–135
  appendicitis and, 152
  Brodie's, 270, 271
  dental abscess, 53
  epidural intracranial, 40
  epidural spinal, 86, 90
  liver, 160
  orbital/periorbital infection and, 48
  percutaneous drainage of, 135
  pericolic, 160
  renal transplantation and, 201, 203
  retropharyngeal, 51–52
  spinal epidural, 40–41
  tonsillar/peritonsillar, 51
  tubo-ovarian, 255–260
  urinary tract, 226, 227
Absorbed dose, 345
Acute tubular necrosis (ATN), 200–201
Adenomyosis, 323
Adynamic ileus, 168–169, 175
Aerophagia, 171
Air/pneumatic reduction of
    intussusception, 306–308
Alar herniation, 85
Aneurysm
  abdominal aortic, 136–141
  false, 138, 140, 184
    peripheral vascular injury, 279
    renal transplantation, 201–203
  ruptured, 137–138
  saccular, 66
  subarachnoid, 66–70
  thoracic aortic, 110–116
  traumatic transection or tear, 138
Angiography
  abdominal aortic aneurysm, 140–141
  computed tomography, 122–128

intracranial venous thrombosis, 74
myocardial ischemia/infarction, 128–129
renal failure, 198–199
thoracic aortic aneurysm and dissection, 115–116
thoracic aortic injury, 119–120
Ankle, accessory ossicles of, 326
Anterior pararenal space, 208
Aorta
  abdominal, aneurysm and dissection of, 136–141
  graft infection, 138
  postoperative, 138
  thoracic
    aneurysm and dissection, 110–116
    injury of, 117–120
Aortoenteric fistula, 138–139
Aortography, thoracic aortic injury, 119–120
Appendicitis, 147–152, 355
Arrowhead sign, 160
Arterial dissection, 60–61
Arterial injury, neck, 33–35
Arteriography, 285–287
  femoral artery puncture, 286
  gastrointestinal hemorrhage and, 165–166
  hemostasis, 286
  imaging protocols, 287
  indications for emergent, 285
  patient management in, 285
  pelvic fracture and, 246–247
  peripheral vascular injury, 279–280
  postprocedure patient management, 287
  preprocedure consult for, 285
Arteriovenous fistula, 201–202
Arteriovenous malformations (AVMs), 166, 323
Arthritis, septic, 281–284
Arthrography
  hip, 288–290
  magnetic resonance, 292
  shoulder, 291–294
Ascites, ovarian torsion and, 240, 243
Aspergillosis, 42

Aspiration, foreign body, 97–101
  clinical information, 97–98
  computed tomography, 100
  fluoroscopy, 99–100
  intrathoracic, 96
  magnetic resonance imaging, 100
  nuclear medicine imaging, 100
  radiograph imaging, 98
  upper airway, 94
Asthma, 95
Atelactasis, 351
Axonal shearing injury, 5

Baker's cyst, 264
Barium studies
  colostomy enema, 300–301
  lower GI, 297–299
  small bowel series, 301–303
  swallowing study screening series,
    303–305
  T-tube cholangiogram series, 303
  upper GI, 295–297
  Whipple, 297
Beak sign, 222
Bell clapper deformity, 249, 250
Biliary complications, 184–185
Bilomas, 185
Biopsy, image-guided renal, 199
Bladder catheterization, 317–318
Bladder injury, 231–235, 247
Bone scans, 274
Bones, 324–335
  accessory ossicles, 324–327
  elbow, wrist, foot, 328–331
  epiphyseal ossification centers,
    332–334
  epiphyseal plate fractures, 335
Bowel. *See also* Gastrointestinal tract
  diverticulitis, 159–161
  gas patterns and, 170–171
  injury to, 145
  intussusception, 176–180
  malrotation and midgut volvulus,
    215–219
  obstructions, 159, 167–175
Brain
  axonal shearing injury, 5
  computed tomography and magnetic
    resonance imaging, 1
  deep gray matter injury, 5
  extracerebral/extra-axial hemorrhage,
    1–4
  intracranial trauma in children, 6
  intraparenchymal/intra-axial
    hemorrhage, 4
  parenchymal abscess, 38
  traumatic injury, 1–6
  vascular anatomy, 359–364

Brain herniation, 80–85
  alar, 85
  extracranial, 85
  subfalcine, 80–81
  tonsillar, 84–85
  transtentorial, 81–84
Brodie's abscess, 270, 271
Bronchoscopy, 100–101
Burst fracture, thoracolumbar spinal, 29

Calcium pyrophosphate dihydrate
  deposition (CPPD) syndrome, 281
Calcium scoring, 123
Candidiasis, intracranial, 44
Carotid artery stenosis, 354
Caterpillar stomach, 222
Catheterization
  bladder, 317–318
  saline infusion sonohysterography and,
    321
Cavernous sinus thrombosis, 48
Cecal volvulus, 171
Cellulitis, 264
Cellulosis, orbital and periorbital, 46, 47
Cerebral intracranial venous thrombosis,
  71–75
Cervical puncture, 313–315
Cervical spine trauma, 17–25
  computed tomography, 23
  epidemiology of, 17
  mechanism of, 17
  mechanism of injury in, 17–20
  radiograph imaging, 17, 21–23
  stability of, 17
Chance fracture, of thoracolumbar spine,
  30
Chiari I malformation, 85
Children
  barium studies in, 295, 297
  epiglottitis, 93–94
  foreign body aspiration, 97–101
  hydrocephalus in, 76
  hypertrophic pyloric stenosis in,
    220–222
  intestinal obstructions, 167, 168
  intracranial trauma in, 6
  intussusception, 176–180
  reduction of, 306–308
  necrotizing enterocolitis, 212–214
  ultrasonography values, 356
Cholangiography, T-tube, 183, 297,
  303
Cholangiopancreatography, 158
Cholecystitis, 153–158
Choledocholithiasis, 153
Coccidioidomycosis, 40
Colostomy enema, 300–301
Compartment syndromes, 264

Compression
  cervical spine injury and, 17, 19
  spinal cord, 86–90
Computed tomography. *See also*
    Arteriography
  abdominal abscess, 132
  abdominal aortic aneurysm, 136–140
  abdominal trauma, 142–146
  angiography, 122–128, 276–278
  appendicitis, 148–150
  aspirated foreign bodies, 100
  bladder/ureteral injury, 233–235
  cervical spine trauma, 23
  cholecystitis, 154–157
  contrast dosages for, 336–337
  deep venous thrombosis, 266–267
  diverticulitis, 160
  four-dimensional cardiac, 127–128
  headache, 91, 92
  hydrocephalus, 77
  intestinal obstruction, 173–175
  intracranial venous thrombosis, 72–73
  intussusception, 178–179
  myocardial ischemia/infarction,
      122–128
  nephrolithiasis, 189, 191–192
  noncontrast, 189
  orbital fracture, 13–15
  orbital/periorbital infection, 47–48
  osteomyelitis, 275
  ovarian torsion, 241–242
  pelvic fracture, 246–247
  peripheral vascular injury, 276–278
  pulmonary embolism, 103–104
  renal failure, 196–197
  renal transplantation, 203–205
  retroperitoneal hemorrhage, 209–210
  skull fracture, 8–9
  stroke, 57–59
  subarachnoid hemorrhage, 67
  thoracic aortic aneurysm and dissection,
      111–114, 116
  thoracic aortic injury, 119
  thoracolumbar spinal trauma, 27, 28
  traumatic brain injury, 1–4
  tubo-ovarian abscess, 257–258
  urinary tract infection, 226–229
Conception, retained products of, 261–263
Contrast agents, 336–341
  doses for computed tomography,
      336–337
  formulations and properties of, 337–338
  kidney function and, 339
  myelography, 314–315
  nephrogenic systemic
      fibrosis/nephrogenic fibrosing
      dermopathy and, 340–341
  in pregnant patients, 341

premedication protocols for, 336
renal transplantation and, 204–205
Contrast enema. *See* Enema, contrast
Cord sign, 92
Coronary artery disease, 121–130
Coronary artery vascular anatomy,
    365–366
Crescent sign, 177
Croup, 93
Cryptococcosis, 44
Cystography, retrograde, 232
Cystourethrogram, voiding, 317–318

DDx focal lesions, 322–323
DeBakey system of dissection, 110
Deep venous thrombosis (DVT), 102, 108,
    264–269
Dental abscess, 53
Digital subtraction angiography (DSA), 33,
    68–69
Dimercaptosuccinic acid scintigraphy, 229
Diplopia, with orbital fracture, 13
Discitis, 87, 89
Disk disease nomenclature, 344
Dislocation
  cervical spinal, 20
  thoracolumbar spinal, 30
Dissection
  abdominal aortic, 136–141
  arterial, 277, 278
  thoracic aortic, 110–116
Diverticulitis, 159–161
Dosimetry, 345–347
Double bubble sign, 171
Double-stick nephrostomy, 311
Double track sign, 221

Ectopic pregnancy, 236–239
Effective dose, 345, 346
Effective dose equivalent, 345
Elbow
  bones of, 328
  ossification centers of, 331
Electrocardiography (ECG), myocardial
    ischemia/infarction and, 121–122
Embolism, pulmonary, 102–109, 264
Embolotherapy, 166
Embryology, malrotation and, 215–216
Emphysematous cholecystitis, 153
Encephalopathy, intracranial venous
    thrombosis and, 71
Endometrium
  carcinoma, 323
  retained products of conception and,
      261–263
  saline infusion sonohysterography and,
      319–323

Endoscopic retrograde
  cholangiopancreatography (ERCP),
  158
Enema, contrast
  appendicitis, 151–152
  colostomy, 300–301
  double-contrast barium, 297–300
  intestinal obstruction, 172–173
  intussusception, 179
Enema reduction of intussusception,
  306–308
Enterocolitis, necrotizing, 212–214
Entrapment, with orbital fracture, 13–16
Epididymitis, 253
Epidural abscess, spinal, 40–41, 89–90
  orbital/periorbital infection and, 48
  treatment of, 90
Epidural hematoma, 1–2
Epiglottitis, 93–94
Epiphyseal plate fractures, 335
Equivalent dose, 345
Excretory urography, 232–233
Exposure, 345
Extracranial herniation, 85
Extraluminal gas, 171–172
Extraperitoneal rupture, 231
Extremities
  deep venous thrombosis of, 264–269
  vascular anatomy of, 370–374

Facial injury, 10–12
Fentanyl, 285
Fibroids, submucosal, 323
Fistula
  aortoenteric, 138–139
  peripheral artery injury and, 279
FLAIR
  headache and, 92
  subarachnoid hemorrhage and, 67, 68
Flumazenil, 285
^{18}Fluorine, 349
Fluoroscopy
  of aspirated foreign bodies, 99–100
  hypertrophic pyloric stenosis, 221–222
  nephrostomy, 311
Foot
  accessory ossicles of, 327
  bones of, 330
Foreign bodies
  aspiration of, 97–101
  intrathoracic, 96
  upper airway, 94
Fractures
  burst, thoracolumbar spinal, 29
  chance, thoracolumbar spinal, 30
  epiphyseal plate, 335
  facial, 10–12
  mandibular, 11–12
    midfacial, 10–11
    nasal, 12
    nasoethmoidal-orbital, 11
    orbital, 13–16
    pelvic, 244–248
      retroperitoneal hemorrhage and, 209,
        210
    rib, spleen injury and, 143
    skull, 7–9
    thoracolumbar spinal, 29–30
    wedge compression, thoracolumbar
      spinal, 29
Fungus balls, 226

Gadolinium, 340–341
Gallbladder perforation, 153
^{67}Gallium, 349
^{67}Gallium citrate, 135
Gallium scans, 274
Gallstone ileus, 168–169
Gallstones, 153–158
Gangrenous cholecystitis, 153
Gastrointestinal hemorrhage, 162–166
Gastrointestinal tract
  colostomy enema, 300–301
  lower, barium studies, 297–300
  upper, barium studies, 295–297
Graft infection, aortic, 138
Grey-Turner sign, 208
Gunshot wound, thoracolumbar spinal, 30

Hand
  accessory ossicles of, 325
  bones of, 329
Harris ring, 23
Head and neck infection, 51–55
  dental abscess, 53
  Ludwig's angina, 54
  parotitis and submandibular sialadenitis,
    54–55
  retropharyngeal abscess, 51–52
  tonsillar/peritonsillar abscess, 51
Headache, 91–92
  acute, 91
  chronic/recurrent, 91
  hydrocephalus and, 77
  subarachnoid hemorrhage and, 66
Hematoma
  epidural, 1–2
  intrahepatic, 144
  intramural, 115
  intrasplenic, 143
  mesenteric, 145
  pelvic fracture and, 247
  perivesical, 232
  renal transplantation and, 201, 203
  retroperitoneal, 140
  scalp, 4

subcapsular, 143
subdural, 2–3
Hemobilia, 186
Hemoperitoneum, 142
Hemorrhage
  extracerebral/extra-axial, 1–4
  gastrointestinal, 162–166
  headache and, 92
  intraparenchymal/intra-axial, 4
  intraventricular, 4
  nephrostomy and, 309
  peripheral vascular injury and, 276
  retroperitoneal, 140, 208–211
  subarachnoid, 4, 66–70
Hemorrhagic stroke, 61–64
Hepatic abscess, 131
Hepatic artery thrombosis, 183
Herniation
  alar, 85
  brain, 80–85
  extracranial, 85
  internal hernias, 169
  sphenoid, 85
  subfalcine, 80–81
  tonsillar, 84–85
  transtentorial, 81–84
Herpes simplex, intracranial, 38–39
Herpes zoster, intracranial, 42
Hip arthrogram, 288–290
HIV/AIDS
  cholecystitis and, 153
  intracranial infection and, 41–42
Hydrocephalus, 76–79
  computed tomography, 77
  magnetic resonance imaging, 78
  nuclear medicine imaging, 78–79
  radiographic imaging, 77
  shunt complications, 76–77
  signs and symptoms of, 77
Hydronephrosis, 187, 189, 203, 225
Hydroureter, 189
Hyperextension, cervical spine injury and, 17, 19
Hyperflexion, cervical spine injury and, 17, 18
Hypermotility disorders, 167
Hypertension, renovascular, 198
Hypertrophic pyloric stenosis, 220–222, 358
Hysterosalpingography, 319–323
Hysterosonography, 319–323

Ileus, 173–175
  gallstone, 168–169
Image-guided renal biopsy, 199
Indinavir, 187
[122]Indium, 349
[111]Indium-labeled leukocytes, 135

Infarcts
  acute/subacute, 59
  bowel, 166
  brain, 4–5
  chronic, 59
  early, 56, 57
  intracranial venous, 74
  lacunar, 56
  myocardial, 121–130
  renal transplantation and, 201–202
  splenic, 143
  testicular torsion and, 249
  watershed, 56
Infection
  aortic graft, 138
  head and neck, 51–55
  intracranial, 36–45
  liver transplantation, 186
  orbital/periorbital, 46–50
  osteomyelitis, 270–275
  skull fracture and, 7
  urinary tract, 223–230
Inflammatory bowel disease, 163, 167, 281
Infundibular dilatation, 69
Intestinal obstruction, 167–175
Intracranial infection, 36–45
  aspergillosis, 42
  brain parenchymal abscess, 38
  candidiasis, 44
  coccidioidomycosis, 40
  cryptococcosis, 44
  herpes simplex, 38–39
  herpes zoster, 42
  HIV and, 41–42
  meningitis, 36–38
  mucormycosis, 44
  norcardiosis, 44
  toxoplasmosis, 42–44
  tuberculosis, 39–40
Intracranial venous thrombosis, 71–75
  angiography, 74
  clinical information on, 71
  computed tomography, 72–73
  etiology and epidemiology of, 71–75
  magnetic resonance imaging, 73–74
Intramural hematoma, 115
Intraperitoneal abscess, 131
Intraperitoneal rupture, 231
Intrathoracic foreign body, 96
Intravenous pyelography, 232–233, 248
Intravenous urogram, 190–191
Intraventricular hemorrhage, 4
Intraventricular shunts, 76–77
Intussusception, 167, 176–180
  air/pneumatic reduction, 306–308
  contrast reduction, 306, 307
  reduction of, 306–308

[123]Iodine, 349
[131]Iodine, 349
Ischemia
    liver transplantation, 183
    myocardial, 121–130
    peripheral vascular injury and, 276
Ischemic stroke, 56–60

Kidneys
    function of after percutaneous coronary
        intervention, 339
    injury to, 145–146
    nephrolithiasis, 187–193
    nephrostomy and, 310
    renal failure, 194–199
    transplantation, 200–207

Lacunar infarcts, 56
Laparoscopic cholecystectomy, 158
Laryngotracheal injury, 35
Lateral flexion, cervical spine injury and,
    17
Le-Fort fracture variations, 10–11
Leptomeningeal cyst, 7
Leukocytosis, 281
Liver abscess, 160
Liver, anatomy of, 181–182
Liver, injury to, 143–144
Liver transplantation, 181–186, 355
Lower extremity deep venous thrombosis,
    264–269
Ludwig's angina, 54
Lumbar puncture, 313–315
Lumenography, 129
Lungs. *See also* Pulmonary embolism
    atelactasis, 351
    pulmonary nodules, 352
Lymphocele, 201, 203

Macroaggregated albumin (MAA), 104
Magnetic resonance imaging, 197–198
    abdominal abscess, 134
    abdominal aortic aneurysm, 140
    appendicitis, 151
    arthrography, 292
    aspirated foreign bodies, 100
    brain, 1
    cervical spine trauma, 23–24
    cholecystitis, 158
    deep venous thrombosis, 267–268
    diffusion-weighted, 198
    headache, 91, 92
    hydrocephalus, 78
    intracranial venous thrombosis, 73–74
    intussusception, 179
    liver transplantation, 183
    myocardial ischemia/infarction, 128
    of neck soft tissue injury, 33

nephrolithiasis, 192
orbital/periorbital infection, 48–50
osteomyelitis, 272–273
ovarian torsion, 242–243
peripheral vascular injury, 279–280
renal failure, 198
retained products of ultrasonography,
    263
septic arthritis, 282, 284
spinal cord compression, 87–90
stroke, 59–60
subarachnoid hemorrhage, 67–68
thoracic aortic aneurysm and dissection,
    114–115
thoracic aortic injury, 119
thoracolumbar spinal trauma, 27, 29
tubo-ovarian abscess, 258–260
Malrotation, bowel, 215–219
Malrotation, 215–219
Mandibular fracture, 11–12
Meckel's diverticulum, 163, 164, 176
Meningeal injury, 7
Meningitis, 36–38, 48
Meniscus sign, 177
Metastases, spinal, 86–90
Metformin, 204–205
Midazolam, 285
Midfacial fracture, 10–11
Migraine, 57
[99m]Tc diethylenetriamine penta-acetate
    (DTPA), 206
[99m]Technetium, 206, 229, 348–349
Mucormycosis, 44
Murphy's sign, 154
Myelography, 313–315
Myocardial ischemia/infarction, 121–130
    angiography, 128–129
    clinical information, 121
    computed tomography imaging,
        122–128
    magnetic resonance imaging, 128
    nuclear medicine imaging, 129
Myositis, 264

Naloxone, 285
Nasal fracture, 12
Nasoethmoidal-orbital fracture, 11
Neck. *See also* Cervical spine trauma
    anatomy of, 32
    soft tissue injuries, 32–35
Necrotizing cholecystitis, 153
Necrotizing enterocolitis, 212–214
Neisseria gonorrhoeae, 281
Nephrocalcinosis, 196
Nephrogenic systemic fibrosis/nephrogenic
    fibrosing dermopathy (NSF/NFD),
    198, 340–341
Nephrolithiasis, 187–193, 224

Nephrostomy, 309–312
Newborns, necrotizing enterocolitis in,
   212–214
Norcardiosis, 44
Nuclear medicine imaging
   abdominal abscess, 135
   aspirated foreign bodies, 100
   cholecystitis, 157–158
   gastrointestinal hemorrhage, 164–165
   hydrocephalus, 78–79
   myocardial ischemia/infarction, 129
   osteomyelitis, 274–275
   pulmonary embolism, 104–107
   renal failure, 197–198
   renal transplantation, 205–207
   testicular torsion, 252–253

Obstructions
   biliary, 185–186
   bowel, 159
   closed-loop, 167–168
   intestinal, 167–175
   nephrolithiasis, 187–193
   nonmechanical, 175
   renal failure and, 198
   renal transplantation and, 201, 206
   urinary tract, 226
      nephrostomy, 309–312
Occlusion, arterial, 277, 278
Opacification, nephrostomy, 311
Orbital fracture, 13–16
Orbital/periorbital infection, 46–50
   anatomy and, 46
   clinical information, 46
   computed tomography, 47–48
   magnetic resonance imaging, 48–50
   pathophysiology and, 46
Orchiopexy, 253–254
Orchitis, 253
Orthotopic liver transplantation, 181–186
Ossification centers, 331–334
Osteomyelitis, 87, 89, 270–275
Ovaries
   torsion, 240–243
   tubo-ovarian abscess, 255–260

Pancreas, injury to, 144
Pancreatic abscess, 131
Papillary necrosis, 226
Paralytic ileus, 175
Parenchymal injury, 7
Parotitis, 54–55
Pelvic fractures, 244–248
   retroperitoneal hemorrhage and, 209,
      210
Pelvic inflammatory disease (PID),
   255–260, 320

Penetrating trauma, peripheral vascular
   injury and, 276–280
Percutaneous abscess drainage, 135
Percutaneous coronary intervention,
   kidney function after, 339
Perihepatic fluid collection, 185–186
Peripheral vascular injury, 276–280
Perirenal space (PRS), 208
Pharyngoesophageal injury, 35
Phlegmon
   appendicitis and, 152
   bladder injury and, 231
PIOPED. See Prospective Investigation of
   Pulmonary Embolism Diagnosis
   (PIOPED)
Pneumatosis, 171–172
Pneumobilia, 172
Pneumonitis, viral, 95
Pneumoperitoneum, 145, 159, 172
Polyps, uterine, 322–323
Portal vein complications, 184
Posterior pararenal space, 208
Pregnancy
   contrast agents in, 341
   ectopic, 236–239
   fetal exposure for radiographic
      procedures, 346
   retained products of conception,
      261–263
   saline infusion sonohysterography and,
      320
   ultrasonography, 355
Prospective Investigation of Pulmonary
   Embolism Diagnosis (PIOPED),
   104–108
Pseudoaneurysm, 138, 140, 184
Pseudofracture, renal, 146
Pseudosubluxation, of cervical spine, 23
Pulmonary embolism, 102–109
   clinical information, 102
   computed tomography, 103–104
   deep venous thrombosis and, 108,
      264
   nuclear medicine imaging, 104–107
   PIOPED criteria for, 104–108, 353
   radiograph imaging, 102–103
Pulmonary nodules, 352
Pyelography, intravenous, 232–233,
   248
Pyelonephritis, 224–229, 226
   xanthogranulomatous, 228
Pyloric stenosis, hypertrophic, 220–222
Pylorospasm, 222

Radiation, nephrolithiasis and, 192
Radiograph imaging
   abdominal abscess, 132
   appendicitis, 150–151

Radiograph imaging (*contd.*)
  arthrogram
    hip, 288–290
    shoulder, 291–294
  aspirated foreign body, 98
  bladder and urethral injury, 232
  cervical spine trauma, 17, 21–23
  diverticulitis, 159
  dosimetry, 345–347
  hydrocephalus, 77
  intestinal obstruction, 169–172
  intussusception, 176–177
  malrotation/midgut volvulus, 216
  myelography, 315
  necrotizing enterocolitis, 212–213
  nephrolithiasis, 187, 189, 192
  osteomyelitis, 270–272
  pelvic fracture, 244–246
  pulmonary embolism, 102–103
  radionuclides/radiopharmaceuticals,
    348–350
  renal failure, 194–195
  retroperitoneal hemorrhage, 209
  septic arthritis, 282, 283
  skull injury, 7–8
  spinal cord compression, 87
  stridor/wheezing, 93, 94, 96
  thoracic aortic aneurysm and dissection,
    111
  thoracic aortic injury, 117–119
  thoracolumbar spinal, 27
  thoracolumbar spinal trauma, 27
Radionuclides/radiopharmaceuticals,
  348–350
Reflux grading, vesicoureteral, 375
Reiter's syndrome, 281
Rejection
  liver transplantation, 183
  renal transplantation, 202
Renal colic, 187
Renal cortical abscess, 131
Renal failure, 194–199
  gadolinium and, 340–341
Renal medullary abscess, 131
Renal stones. *See* Nephrolithiasis
Renal transplantation, 200–207
  pediatric ultrasonography values, 356
  ultrasonography, 354–355
Renal vein thrombosis, 354
Renovascular hypertension, 198
Retained products of conception (RPOC),
  261–263
Retrograde cystography, 232
Retrograde urethrogram, 316
Retroperitoneum
  abscess, 131
  anatomy of, 208
  hemorrhage, 140, 208–211

Retropneumoperitoneum, 145
Rigler's triad, 169
Rim sign, renal artery occlusion and, 146
Rotation, cervical spine injury and, 17, 18

Saline infusion sonohysterography,
  319–323
Scalp hematoma, 4
Scintigraphy, dimercaptosuccinic acid,
  229
Seizures
  intracranial venous thrombosis and, 71
  subarachnoid hemorrhage and, 66
Sentinel clots, 145
Sentinel loop sign, 171
Septic arthritis, 281–284, 288
Septic cavernosa sinus thrombosis, 71
Seroma, 201
Shoulder arthrogram, 292–294
Shunts
  complications of, 76–77
  failure of, 76–77, 78
  hydrocephalus and, 76–79
  intraventricular, 76
  overshunting, 77, 78
Single-stick nephrostomy, 311
Skull fracture, 7–9
Small bowel series, 173, 301–303
Soft tissue injury
  neck, 32–35
  pelvic fracture and, 247
Sonohysterography, saline infusion,
  319–323
Sphenoid herniation, 85
Spinal cord compression, 86–90
  clinical presentation of, 86–87
  clinical significance of, 86
  magnetic resonance imaging, 87–90
  radiograph imaging, 87
Spinal puncture, 313–315
Spinal trauma
  cervical, 17–25
  thoracolumbar, 26–31
Spine, disk disease nomenclature, 344
Spleen, injury to, 142–143
Splenic abscess, 131
Splenic laceration, 143
Stanford system of dissection, 110
Stenosis
  hepatic artery, 183–184
  hypertrophic pyloric, 220–222
  internal carotid artery, 354
  quantification of, 125–126
  renal transplantation and, 201–202
Stress ECG, 121–122
Stridor and wheezing, 93–96
  croup, 93
  epiglottitis, 93–94

expiratory, 94–95
foreign body aspiration, 97–101
String sign, 222
Stroke, 56–65
  arterial dissection, 60–61
  hemorrhagic, 61–64
  ischemic, 56–60
Subarachnoid hemorrhage, 4, 66–70
  clinical information on, 66–67
  computed tomography, 67
  digital subtraction angiography imaging,
    68–69
  etiology and epidemiology of, 66
  magnetic resonance imaging, 67–68
Subcapsular hematoma, 143
Subdural empyema, spinal, 40, 48
Subfalcine herniation, 80–81
Submandibular sialadenitis, 54–55
Superior ophthalmic vein, 48
Swallowing study screening series,
  303–305

Testicular torsion, 249–254
201Thallium, 349
Thoracic aortic aneurysm and dissection,
  110–116
  angiography, 115–116
  clinical information, 110–111
  computed tomography, 111–114,
    116
  magnetic resonance imaging, 114–115
  radiograph imaging, 111
  transesophageal echocardiography, 114
Thoracic aortic injury, 117–120
Thoracolumbar spinal trauma, 26–31
  classification of, 26
  common fracture types, 29–30
  complications of, 26
  computed tomography, 27, 28
  epidemiology of, 26
  location of, 26
  magnetic resonance imaging, 27, 29
  mechanism of, 26
  radiographic imaging, 27
Thorax, 351–353
Thrombophlebitis, 264
Thrombosis
  cavernous sinus, 48
  deep venous, 102, 108, 264–269
  hepatic artery, 183
  intracranial venous, 71–75
  ovarian vein, 263
  renal transplantation and, 201–202,
    354
  renal vein, 196
TIA. See Stroke
Tonsillar herniation, 84–85
Tonsillar/peritonsillar abscess, 51

Torsion
  ovarian, 240–243
  testicular, 249–254
Toxic megacolon, 171
Toxoplasmosis, 42–44
Transesophageal echocardiography
  thoracic aortic aneurysm and dissection,
    114
Transient ischemic attack (TIA). See Stroke
Transjugular intrahepatic portosystemic
  shunt, 355
Transplants
  liver, 181–186
  renal, 200–207
Transtentorial herniation, 81–84
Trauma, abdominal, 142–146
  retroperitoneal hemorrhage and, 208
Traumatic transection or tear, abdominal
  aortic, 138
T tube cholangiography, 183, 297, 303
Tubal pregnancy, 236–239
Tuberculosis
  disc edema and, 89
  intracranial, 39–40
Tubo-ovarian abscess, 255–260

Ultrasonography, 354–358
  abdominal abscess, 132–134
  abdominal duplex, 354–355
  appendicitis, 150
  carotid duplex, 354
  cholecystitis, 154
  color Doppler, 250–252
  deep venous thrombosis, 264–266
  ectopic pregnancy, 236–238
  hypertrophic pyloric stenosis, 220–222,
    358
  intussusception, 176
  intussusception reduction, 308
  malrotation/midgut volvulus, 218–219
  mean renal lengths, 357
  of neck soft tissue injury, 33
  nephrolithiasis, 189–190
  nephrostomy, 311
  obstetric, 355
  ovarian torsion, 240–241
  pediatric, 356
  peripheral vascular injury, 278–279
  renal failure, 195–196
  renal transplantation, 202–203
  retained products of ultrasonography,
    261–263
  saline infusion sonohysterography,
    319–323
  septic arthritis, 282
  testicular torsion and, 250–252
  tubo-ovarian abscess, 255–257
  urinary tract infection, 225–226

Upper airway foreign body, 94
Upper extremity
    deep venous thrombosis, 264
Upper gastroesophageal series
    malrotation/midgut volvulus,
        216–217
Ureteral injury, 231–235
Ureteral reflux grading, 375
Urethritis, 224
Urethrography
    pelvic fracture and, 247
    retrograde, 316
    voiding cystourethrogram, 317–318
Urinary tract
    infection, 223–230
    nephrostomy, 309–312
    obstruction, 187–193
    retrograde urethrogram, 316
    structural abnormalities of, 225, 229
    ureteral injury, 231–235
    voiding cystourethrogram, 317–318
Urinoma, 201, 203
Urography
    excretory, 232–233
    intravenous, 190–191
    pelvic fracture and, 247–248
Urolithiasis, 187, 188, 196. *See also*
    Nephrolithiasis

Vaginitis, 224
Vascular anatomy, 359–374
    abdominal, 367–369
    brain, 359–364

coronary artery, 365–366
    extremity, 370–374
Vascular injury, 7
Vascular loop, 68
Vasopressin, 166
Vasculitis, 202
Vesicoureteral reflux grading, 375
Vesicoureteral reflux (VUR), 224–229
Viral pneumonitis, 95
Virchow's triad, 264
Visceral abscess, 131
Voiding cystourethrogram, 317–318
Volvulus, 168
    cecal, 171
    malrotation and midgut, 215–219
    sigmoid, 171
V/Q (ventilation and perfusion) imaging,
    102–108

Watershed infarcts, 56
Wedge compression fracture,
        thoracolumbar spinal, 29
Wheezing, 93–96
Whipple study, 297
White blood cell (WBC) scans, 274–275
Wrist, bones of, 329

Xanthogranulomatous pyelonephritis, 228
[133]Xenon, 349

Yin-Yang flow pattern, 279

ZMC fracture, 11